Study Manual for the

Test of Essential Academic Skills (TEAS®)

Reading, Mathematics, Science, and English and Language Usage

Version V

Editor

Amanda Wolkowitz, PhD
Psychometrician
Assessment Technologies Institute®, LLC

Associate Editors

Amanda Lehman, BA
Test Developer

Brant Stacy, BS
Product Developer

ATI would like to thank the following individuals for their contributions:

Susan Adams, MA
Mathematics Teacher
Cranford, NJ

Erika Archer, BS
Test Developer, ATI

Michele Bach, MS
Professor of Mathematics
Kansas City Kansas Community College
Kansas City, KS

Brenda Ball, MEd, BSN, RN
Nursing Education Specialist, ATI

Joseph Bell, BA
Technical Writer
Madison, WI

Wendy Cain, MS
Instructor of Science
Ivy Tech Community College
Columbus, IN

Mechel Camp, PhD
Instructor of English
Jackson State Community College
Jackson, TN

Jennifer Champion, MEd
Client Service and Sales Representative, ATI

Michelle Dunham, PhD
Research Specialist, ATI

Chuck Duske, BA
Vice President of Sales: Southeast Region, ATI

Ryan Elsenpeter, PhDc
Department of Cell Biology and Biophysics and
    Molecular Biology
University of Missouri–Kansas City
Kansas City, MO

Thor Garber, PhD
Assistant Professor of Physics and Astronomy
Pensacola Junior College
Adjunct Instructor of Physics
University of West Florida
Pensacola, FL

Justin Grasso, BA
Lead Graphic Designer, ATI

Louise Groth, MBA
Instructor of Science
South College
Knoxville, TN

Sheri Harshaw, BS
English Teacher
Williamsburg, KS

Mary Jones, Layout
Springfield, MO

Tony Juve, PhD
Psychometrician, ATI

Kim Miller, MS
Associate Professor of Mathematics
Labette Community College
Parsons, KS

Brooke Nash, MSEd
Doctoral student in Psychology and Research
    in Education
University of Kansas
Lawrence, KS

Nicole Reynolds, BA
Assistant to Psychometric Services, ATI

Karin Roberts, PhD, RN, CNE
Nursing Education Coordinator, ATI

Matt Scaruto, MA
Research Associate, ATI

Rebecca Schantz, MS
Instructor of Mathematics
East Central College
Union, MO

Quin Showalter, MS
Science Teacher
De Soto School District
De Soto, KS

Heather Stenmark, BS
Attorney
Allstate Insurance
Chicago, IL

Linda Stenmark, MS
(Retired) Science Teacher
Franklin High School
Franklin, WI

Oather Strawderman, MS
Science Teacher
Lawrence Free State High School
Lawrence, KS

Kristen Waggener, BA
Test Developer, ATI

Jaime Walla, MS
Lenexa, KS

Karen Wood, BS
Administrative Assistant for Nursing Curriculum &
    Educational Services, ATI

Mendy Wright, MSN, RN, DNP
Nursing Education Specialist, ATI

table of contents

Thank you for purchasing the Test of Essential Academic Skills (TEAS®) Pretest Study Manual. This book contains instructional material for each of the four subject areas assessed, practice problems with explanatory answer keys, two comprehensive practice tests with explanatory answer keys, and a detailed glossary of terms used throughout the guide.

When creating the TEAS® Pretest Study Manual, the developers' primary objectives were to write a guide that was easy to follow and to design a guide that paralleled the proctored TEAS®.

About the Proctored TEAS®

The proctored TEAS® measures basic essential skills in the academic content area domains of reading, mathematics, science, and English and language usage. The test is intended for use primarily with adult nursing program applicant populations. Each question on the TEAS® (version V and later) is mapped to one of 115 objectives, all of which address topics presented in grades 7 to 12. The objectives assessed are those which nurse educators deemed most appropriate and relevant to measure entry-level skills and abilities of nursing program applicants.

The TEAS® is a 170-item, four-option, multiple-choice examination offered in both paper and pencil and computer-administered formats. To prepare in an organized and efficient manner, it is important to know what to expect from the proctored examination. Table I.1 lists the number of items and time limits allotted for each section of the TEAS® (version V and later) examination:

Table I.1 Content Areas, Number of Items, and Time Limit on the Proctored TEAS® (version V and later)

Content areas	Number of items	Time limit
Reading	48	58 minutes
Mathematics	34	51 minutes
Science	54	66 minutes
English and Language Usage	34	34 minutes
TOTAL	170	209 minutes

Although the TEAS® consists of 170 items, 20 of these items are unscored pretest items. Therefore, the number of scored items on the test is 150. Table I.2 details the number of scored items in each content area and subcontent area of the test:

Table I.2 Content and Subcontent Areas and the Number of Items on the Scored Portion of the Proctored TEAS® (version V and later)

Content and subcontent areas	Number of scored items	Percent of test items
Reading	**42**	**28%**
Paragraph and Passage Comprehension	19	12.7%
Informational Source Comprehension	23	15.3%
Mathematics	**30**	**20%**
Numbers and Operations	19	12.7%
Measurement	4	2.7%
Data Interpretation	3	2.0%
Algebraic Applications	4	2.7%
Science	**48**	**32%**
Scientific Reasoning	11	7.3%
Human Body Science	15	10.0%
Life Science	14	9.3%
Earth and Physical Science	8	5.3%
English and Language Usage	**30**	**20%**
Grammar and Word Meanings in Context	15	10.0%
Spelling and Punctuation	9	6.0%
Structure	6	4.0%
	150*	**100%**

*There are an additional 20 unscored pretest items.

About the TEAS® Study Manual

This study manual is similar to the TEAS® (version V and later) produced by Assessment Technologies Institute® (ATI) in that the 115 objectives explained in this manual are the same 115 objectives from which the test items were written. This study guide is organized by the objectives. The topics to review list on the score reports of the TEAS® (version V and later) map directly to the subheadings of this study guide.

The explanation provided for each objective contains at least two practice problems. The majority of these questions are open-ended. Solutions to these practice problems, as well as explanations for the solutions, are provided at the end of this book.

Within each section, words may be bolded. If a word is in bold, then that word is defined for the first time in the explanation. All bolded words are also defined in the glossary found at the end of this book.

Prior to the glossary are two comprehensive TEAS® practice tests. Each of these tests contains 150 items that are representative of the types of questions that appear on the proctored examination. Keep in mind that the proctored TEAS® (version V and later) contains an additional 20 unscored pretest items. Solutions and explanations for the solutions to the practice tests are given at the end of each test.

About the Online Practice TEAS®

To help prepare for taking the proctored TEAS®, two online practice versions of the TEAS® (version V and later) are also available. Each of these tests contains 150 scored items. Upon completing the online practice test, a score report will appear with your results and with a list of topics to review. Again, the list of topics to review corresponds to the subheadings found in this study guide for reading, mathematics, science, and English and language usage.
For more information, please visit www.atitesting.com.

Feedback

All feedback is welcome - suggestions for improvement, reports of mistakes (small or large), and testimonials of effectiveness. Please address feedback to: comments@atitesting.com.

SECTION 1: READING

The reading portion of the TEAS® contains questions related to paragraph and passage comprehension, as well as informational source comprehension. In paragraph and passage comprehension questions, it will be necessary to read a given text and answer questions related to that text. In informational source comprehension questions, a graphic or statement may be provided and questions will be related to the graphic or statement.

PARAGRAPH AND PASSAGE COMPREHENSION

Primary Sources

When reading about a topic, it is important to understand the type of source from which the information comes. **Primary sources** are firsthand records of events, theories, opinions, or actions. These records may come in the form of either published or unpublished documents, recordings, or artifacts, and they must be contemporary to the events, people, or information that is at issue.

Although the use of primary sources is important, there are some challenges that come with it. First of all, sometimes the only information available about an event was written hundreds of years after the event occurred. Anything written hundreds of years after an event occurred is not a primary source. Second, primary sources may not always be accurate, especially if the source contains a person's perception of an event. Lastly, primary sources are oftentimes ambiguous and fragmentary, making them difficult to analyze.

Primary sources don't come only from physical artifacts and writings. Oftentimes, a primary source can be found on the internet. Web site information may not always be accurate, so it is important to first examine the purpose of the Web site containing the information. While the purpose may not affect the accuracy of the information, the material can be altered in such a way as to persuade the reader to a particular viewpoint. Generally, Web sites with a nonbiased approach to presenting sources are more reliable. These types of Web sites include government sites, organization sites, and educational institution sites.

 Practice problems

Solutions to the practice problems are located in the back of this book.

1. Name three different types of primary sources.

2. Provide an example of a primary source in each of the following fields:
    A) Archaeology
    B) Art
    C) History
    D) Journalism
    E) Law
    F) Literature
    G) Music
    H) Political science
    I) Rhetoric
    J) Sociology

Facts, Opinions, Biases, and Stereotypes

An important part of reading comprehension is distinguishing between fact and opinion. **Facts** are information based on real, provable events, or situations. **Opinions** are beliefs based on personal judgments, rather than on indisputable facts. Sometimes the difference between fact and opinion is easy to spot; other times facts and opinions are mixed together in the same article, book, or paper; this type of writing demands careful reading.

Writers with particularly strong or closely held opinions may believe their opinions to be facts, and may present them as such in their writing. Again, in this case it is the reader's job to analyze the writing and make his or her own decision about whether the material is fact, opinion, or a mixture of both.

Biases and stereotypes can cloud a writer's judgment or ability to draw accurate conclusions. **Biases** are opinions or beliefs that affect a person's ability to make fair, unclouded judgments or decisions, whereas **stereotypes** are oversimplified opinions, that do not account for individual differences, about an entire group of people or things. Much discussion of bias and stereotype centers on controversial political or social issues. For example, a magazine might be perceived as having a liberal or conservative political bias, or a book might be seen as stereotyping members of a particular ethnic group. However, biases and stereotypes are not confined to hot-button issues. For example, a carpenter whose father always used a certain brand of tools might have a strong bias toward that brand, even though its products are essentially the same as those offered by another brand.

Critical reading, a reading style in which the reader carefully analyzes the text, judging its credibility and the author's intentions, rather than simply accepting the material as fact, is generally preferable to passive reading. A passive reader simply absorbs the text and assumes that it contains facts. A critical reader, on the other hand, analyzes the material as it is read, considering both the text itself and the author's possible biases. In this way the critical reader decides what is fact, what is opinion, and ultimately, how much trust to place in the written material.

(P) *Practice problems*

Solutions to the practice problems are located in the back of this book.

1. Read the following text:

    > Two vehicles, a minivan and a pickup truck, collided on Highway 16 at 6:45 p.m. last Saturday. The driver of the pickup truck was thrown from his vehicle and taken to Mercy Presbyterian Hospital, where doctors say he remains in critical but stable condition. The occupants of the minivan, a father, a mother, and three young children, escaped with only cuts and bruises. Police report that slippery road conditions contributed to the accident. Another contributing factor: the driver of the pickup truck was just 17 years old.

    Identify the elements of fact, opinion, bias, and stereotype in the passage above.

2. A blogger has just tried a new allergy medication called Allergone, and is reviewing it based on his personal experiences.

    Identify which statement(s) contains only facts, without a trace of the blogger's opinions.

    A) Last year, *Pharmaceutical Insider* magazine reported that Allergone faced a bumpy approval process. However, Allergone got approval in March and hit the shelves in early May.
    B) Allergone comes in three different dosages. The pill that is 10 milligrams is yellow and is the lowest available dose. The pill that is 20 milligrams is white and works best for most people. The pill that is 30 milligrams is pale pink and is too strong for most patients.
    C) Considering all the other excellent allergy medications on the market, Allergone will struggle to find an audience.
    D) Allergone is produced by a reputable, high-quality medication manufacturer in Iceland.

3. An opinion poll asked sports fans to guess which football team would win a college bowl game: Midland State University or Southeast Central University. Following are the responses of four people who picked Midland State.

    One of these four respondents revealed a bias. Which one was it?

    A) "Their quarterback won the Heisman Trophy, and their defensive line was rated 'superb' by the local paper."
    B) "The sportswriters picked the other team to win, but they're wrong so often. I tend to put my money on the guys they say will lose."
    C) "All the sportswriters say they're a 'lock' to win, so I'd imagine they're the heavy favorites."
    D) "Their running back just returned from an injury, so that's one more player they can put on the field."

Characteristics of Different Passage Types

Several common adjectives are used to explain an author's **purpose**, or main reason for writing a particular piece. Terms like narrative, expository, technical, and persuasive are labels that help the reader understand what to expect from a text.

Narrative text tells a story, or relates a chain of events. An **expository** passage introduces or explains a subject, gives groundwork information that is necessary for understanding later ideas, or analyzes information objectively. **Technical** writing passes along precise information, usually about a specific topic, and usually in a formal or semi-formal style. **Persuasive** writing tries to get the reader to agree with the author.

These terms may be applied to an entire text, or just to a part of that text (see Example 1.1). For example, an economist writing an article about his new economic theory might be writing a persuasive article – after all, he wishes his colleagues to agree with his theory. However, even though the article as a whole is persuasive, it may begin with an expository section that explains certain economic principles to less-experienced readers, and it may also contain a narrative section that tells the story of how he arrived at his theory. In this case, the scientist wrote a persuasive article that happened to contain expository and narrative elements.

(E) *Example 1.1:*   *Read the following passage. Then, answer the question.*

> - Open the program and select File > Preferences.
> - When the Preferences pane appears, select the Other Options tab.
> - Click on Save Progress, and then click Apply.
> - Return to the main window and verify that the Auto-Save icon is now green.

What type of writing is this: narrative, persuasive, technical, or expository?

This text is technical writing: its purpose is to pass along very specific information to the reader. In this case, the information explains how to change a preference setting in a computer program.

Notice that the text is in the form of a bulleted list, instead of a typical paragraph. Technical writing often (but not always) uses lists, text boxes, varying font sizes and colors, and many other kinds of text formatting. The goal of the text formatting is to make individual bits of information easier to read, and also to make them easier to find quickly.

Technical writing is a bit like expository writing, since both types of writing present the reader with facts. The main difference between the two lies in the purpose those facts serve. Facts in technical writing are written to teach the reader how to use a specific object or perform a specific action. Expository writing uses facts to inform or explain something to the reader in a more general sense.

(P) *Practice problems*

Solutions to the practice problems are located in the back of this book.

1.   Read the following passage. Then, answer the question.

> The ship ran aground on a great slab of ice. It had smashed its way almost to the Arctic Circle, but could press no further. It made a terrible grating sound as it slid up onto the ice: it was the sound of absolute finality. We knew we could not break free.
>
> We settled down to wait; we had no choice. We ran the ship's engines to produce heat, and whiled away the days with card games and old magazines. But days turned into weeks, and soon the reserves were low. We had neither the fuel nor the food to keep this up indefinitely.
>
> On the third week the captain made his decision: we loaded up the sled dogs and set out across the ice. We were apprehensive about leaving the ship, but we also knew that we could not stay. Every man – even those who professed no religion – prayed like a saint as we rode our sleds off into the gray distance.

What type of writing is this: narrative, persuasive, technical, or expository?

2. Read the following passage. Then, answer the question.

> The Russian icebreaker *Vladimir Karamenov* attempted a scientific expedition to the Arctic Circle in 1954. It was an ill-fated trip; after countless delays and obstacles, the ship was stuck in the ice and abandoned by the crew. Only about half the crew survived the experience.
>
> What lessons were learned from this expedition? How could such a tragedy be avoided? For one thing, the trip began far too late in the year. The trip would have been reasonably safe at the height of summer, but the ship got a late start, and autumn had taken hold by the time the ship neared its destination.
>
> More supplies could have been taken. A larger ship packed with more fuel and more food, and with fewer crew members to consume that food, could have waited out the winter and freed itself the next spring. The wait would have been tedious, but the cost in human life would have been minimized, or eliminated.
>
> Finally, a second ship could have accompanied the *Vladimir Karamenov*. Then, if the lead ship became stuck, the rear ship could have halted, attached chains to the stuck ship, and then towed it back into safer waters.

What type of writing is this: narrative, persuasive, technical, or expository?

3. Read the following passage. Then, answer the question.

> Since the late sixteenth century, the public has had a strange fascination with arctic expeditions. These expeditions are launched for many ostensible reasons: to chart new territory, to conduct scientific research, to search for oil, or simply to have an adventure.
>
> Consider the many hardships and tragedies of these expeditions: Franklin's memorable disaster, Shackleton's famous wreck, or the more recent tragedy of the *Vladimir Karamenov*. Ask yourself: is all this loss of life worthwhile? What real, tangible gains have been made from these expeditions? A few more marks and scribbles on our world maps? A few more frozen, useless islands that now possess explorers' names?
>
> The entire concept of the arctic expedition is folly. The subject, and indeed, this entire area of the world, should be abandoned until such time as fully automated research ships can be sent into the polar wastes. Only then, when no human life is at risk, should these dangerous efforts resume.
>
> In the meantime, we should not look back at the early arctic explorers as heroes or legends. We should not honor them with statues, plaques, or lengthy entries in our history books. Rather, we should shake our heads at their foolishness, and transfer our admiration to people who have made real discoveries in other, more practical fields of knowledge.

What type of writing is this: narrative, persuasive, technical, or expository?

Topic, Main Idea, Supporting Details, and Themes

Special terms are used to discuss written works. Understanding these terms can be an essential step toward understanding the works themselves. Here is a look at some of the most common terms.

Every written work has a **topic**. The topic is the *general* subject matter covered by the work. For example, consider a book called *Depression: the Rational Solution*. This book discusses the problem of depression, and offers a specific treatment for people dealing with depression. What is this book's topic? There are several possible answers. Good answers would be depression, mental health, or psychology. Or, consider the article about microchips in the practice problems. The topic for this article might be microchips or technology. Both answers are correct; one answer is just more general than the other.

Whereas the topic is the general subject of a written work, the **main idea** is the work's specific message. It is the reason the text was written. In the case of *Depression: the Rational Solution*, the main idea might be, "To erase depression, one must engage the rational part of the brain, and ignore the emotional part."

Supporting details flesh out, and explain, the main idea. Without these details, the reader has very little reason to believe the main idea. For example, *Depression: the Rational Solution* would not be very convincing if the only words in the book were, "Try to be more logical and less emotional, and you will then be less depressed. The End." This would not only be one of the world's shortest books, it would also be poor writing, because it would lack the supporting details to explain the book's controversial main idea.

Themes are subjects that a written work frequently touches upon. For example, *Depression: the Rational Solution* might touch upon themes of despair, hope, redemption, and self-improvement. Themes are simply ideas or concepts that the book comes back to again and again.

(P) *Practice problems*

Solutions to the practice problems are located in the back of this book.

Read the following passage. Then, answer the questions.

Microchip Production

There was a time – as recently as the 1990s – when dozens of factories produced microchips. Large American and European brands designed the microchips, and then produced the chips in their own, highly guarded factories. (They did not trust anyone else to have the necessary secrecy, know-how, or quality control to manufacture their products.) Meanwhile, these heavyweight brands competed with dozens of no-name Asian factories producing microchips of their own. Both the name-brand chips and the no-name chips found their way into thousands of products: computers, cordless phones, microwaves, and answering machines at first; then, more recently, into ever-growing numbers of cellular phones and digital cameras.

Recent years have shown a trend toward microchip consolidation, with manufacturing centered on a few giant, modern Asian factories, many in Taiwan. Many of the smaller factories – both no-name and name-brand – have shut down. In their place, the gleaming new mega-factories produce silicon chips for a vast array of brands. Major American and European brands have experienced the convenience of allowing these factories to manufacture their chips, rather than investing the cash, time, and labor to build factories of their own. These days, it is not uncommon for two bitter rivals, their products directly in competition with one another, to have their products manufactured side-by-side on the assembly lines of the same Taiwanese chipmaker.

At first there were concerns about confidentiality and quality. Could these independent factories be trusted with a major brand's newest products and secrets? Could they produce microchips that demanded a high degree of precision? The answer, learned from the experiences of the past decade, has been a resounding "Yes." The major brands have largely given up their factories, and have wholeheartedly embraced the new model of subcontracting chip production. The world's computers, cellular phones, and digital devices may still have American, European, or Japanese brand names, but the guts of those devices are almost always made in independent factories, often based in Taiwan.

What does the future hold? One new development is that Taiwan's largest factories have started producing their own products, in addition to continuing to manufacture products for established foreign brands. In the coming decades, the manufacturing clout of the mega-factories, combined with their growing engineering know-how, may turn the mega-factories' home-grown products into new household brands. The future looks bright indeed for the largest chip manufacturers.

Correctly identify each of the following elements as either a topic, a theme, a main idea, or a supporting detail.

1. Microchips are increasingly manufactured in a few giant Asian factories.

2. A few large factories versus many small factories

3. Technology and industry

4. The new Asian factories can be trusted to keep major brands' secrets.

Topic and Summary Sentences

Good writing often makes use of topic sentences. Without topic sentences, the reader can easily become confused: What is the writer trying to say? What is the point of a specific paragraph, or of the text as a whole? Topic sentences answer these questions.

Topic sentences express the main point of a paragraph, or of a larger text structure (such as an essay or a book chapter). Usually, a paragraph starts with a topic sentence. Then it goes on to back up that sentence with supporting ideas, or to explore the topic in greater detail. The same pattern holds true when a topic sentence applies to a larger text structure: the topic sentence appears early in the structure (say, in the first paragraph of an essay), and then the remainder of the text goes on to expand upon, and illustrate, the topic.

Summary sentences generally appear at (or near) the end of a paragraph, chapter, section, or document. Sometimes they sum up the point of the earlier text, driving the message home so that the reader does not forget it or miss it. Other times, they draw a conclusion that goes one step further than the topic sentence. In this type of summary sentence, instead of just reiterating the topic, the sentence draws a conclusion based on that topic.

Summary sentences are also useful for providing closure to a piece of text. Failure to include summary sentences can result in a document that seems chopped-off, abrupt, or unfinished. On the other hand, summary sentences can be overkill if they are used too often, so do not expect them to appear quite as frequently as topic sentences. Individual paragraphs often skip summary sentences, because using too many of them can make a document unnecessarily wordy and repetitive. However, expect summary sentences to appear at the end of a document, or at the end of any major piece of that document (such as a chapter).

Identifying topic and summary sentences is a useful skill. When looking for the topic sentence of any piece of text, look near the beginning of that text first. The topic sentence usually makes a statement that the remaining sentences will explain, discuss, or elaborate upon. When looking for a summary sentence, look near the end of the given text first. The summary sentence may reiterate the topic, and may draw a conclusion that was not fully explained in the topic sentence. This conclusion is based on the discussions and explanations found in the main body of the text.

(P) *Practice problems*

Solutions to the practice problems are located in the back of this book.

Read the passage titled, "Microchip Production" that appears in the previous section. Then, answer the questions.

1. What is the topic sentence of this passage?

2. What is the summary sentence of the last paragraph?

Logical Conclusions of a Reading Selection

One of the most important reading skills is the ability to draw **logical conclusions**. A logical conclusion is an idea that follows from the facts or ideas presented in the text. Note that a logical conclusion does not need to be factual or true; it may be completely illogical when viewed on its own. For example, a wild conspiracy theory is almost certain to be *illogical*. However, after reading this theory, the reader may be able to draw a logical conclusion from it. The conclusion merely has to be consistent with the ideas in the text; the reader is not obliged to agree.

When seeking logical conclusions, it may be helpful to ask questions, such as, "Assuming that everything I just read is true, what follows?" or, "Based on the ideas in the text, what is the author's point?" One of these questions usually produces the text's logical conclusion.

Some writing is very explicit about its purpose, and the logical conclusion is there for all to see. For example, consider a political flyer that accuses the local mayor of corruption and demands his impeachment. There is no need to guess at this flyer's logical conclusion. It's very clearly saying, "The mayor is corrupt and should be thrown out of office."

Other writing is much less explicit, forcing the reader to think in order to reach a conclusion. For example, a home remodeling journal might tell the story of a family who had problems with contractors as they tried to get their house remodeled. Careful reading of the article might reveal a logical conclusion: *always get personal references about a contractor; never just hire one from the phone book*. Or, the logical conclusion might be more general: *home remodeling can be a difficult and trying experience*. The actual conclusion depends entirely upon the facts or ideas presented in the article, and how those facts or ideas were presented.

(P) *Practice problems*

Solutions to the practice problems are located in the back of this book.

1. Read the following passage. Then, answer the question.

    > I heard that last year there were more than a hundred bike accidents in this city. They just opened a new set of bike lanes on the north side of town, but they're too small and too close to the main traffic lanes, so that won't help. Even worse, I saw a statistic about how bike accidents are much more likely to be fatal than car accidents. Wearing a helmet helps, but not enough. Cars protect you in a thick layer of steel and plastic; bikes just leave you hanging out there in the open.

    What is the logical conclusion of the above quote?

2. Read the following excerpt from a local newspaper. Then, answer the question.

    > As most readers are aware, our city has been struggling over the last several years to keep downtown businesses thriving. Locals often report that access issues prevent them from shopping downtown. Last week the city of Clarion reported in their local newspaper that the addition of two new parking lots in their downtown area increased the surrounding business revenue by 7% in the last year. It is also well known that Moville and Clarion are similar in terms of population and city characteristics. Moville is currently looking for ways to increase downtown revenue and is open to the public for suggestions.

    What is the logical conclusion of the above text?

Predictions, Inferences, and Conclusions

Some text is best read with as little judgment as possible. For example, a scientist reading a new theory is best served by keeping an open mind, and not making any predictions (or drawing any conclusions) – at least, not until she has read the entire theory and considered it on its own merits.

On the other hand, many times it *is* useful to "read between the lines," drawing **inferences** (an inference is a next step or logical conclusion that is not actually written in the text; rather, it is deduced by the reader, based on information that *is* in the text) and conclusions, and making predictions. There are many reasons to do this. For instance, if an article is written from a very distinct point of view, to get the maximum value from the article, the reader needs to make inferences from the text and draw conclusions about the author's viewpoint and possible biases. If the reader does not do this, he or she runs the risk of accepting opinionated writing as fact.

There are other reasons to draw inferences and make conclusions. For example, consider a set of poorly written instructions on how to rewire an electrical outlet. Even though these instructions might not say a thing about safety, a smart reader should infer that, because electricity is involved, certain precautions must be taken. The reader might draw the conclusion that the home's main electrical switch should be turned off before she starts working on the outlet. In this example, inferences and conclusions are not just handy – they could also save a life.

Here is another example: a reader picks up a novel and reads the first few pages. They are poorly written, and the reader finds that she is not at all interested in the plot. In this case the reader has two options: she can continue reading until the bitter end, or she can draw the conclusion that if the first few pages are bad, the rest of the book probably won't be any better. Drawing this conclusion allows the reader to put down the book, and avoid many hours of unpleasant, wasted activity.

Predictions, conclusions, and inferences are based on personal judgment and prior experience. Because of this, they can be risky, as personal biases may cloud the reader's conclusions. However, the benefits of making these kinds of judgments tend to outweigh the risks. In most cases it is useful for a reader to use his or her personal judgment to draw logical conclusions, make inferences, and make predictions, rather than to passively read a text and accept it at face value.

(P) *Practice problems*

Solutions to the practice problems are located in the back of this book.

1. Read the following text from a brochure. Then, answer the question.

   > Do you want to increase your IQ dramatically in just one short month?
   >
   > Become smarter by following my simple brain-energizing program. This program includes daily mental exercises, nutrition and fitness guides, and daily vitamin and nutrient supplements, all of which will help boost your IQ.
   >
   > With five easy payments of $19.99, we can guarantee that you will impress your friends and family with your new-found intelligence in just four weeks.

   What should the reader conclude about this brochure?

2. Read the following excerpt from a person's blog. Then, answer the question.

   > As of this morning, the president's approval rating decreased by 3%, which indicates that citizens are not pleased with the work he has done since he took office. The president has had 2½ years to work on his agenda with nothing to show for it. He has not met any of the goals he proposed while running for office. Furthermore, his actions have led to increased unemployment rates, increased poverty rates, a struggling economic system, and a failing educational system.

   What inferences or conclusions can the reader make about the excerpt above?

Position and Purpose

Determining an author's intentions may be the most important reading skill of all. Knowing (or guessing at) the author's position, and knowing (or guessing at) why the text was written, helps the reader decide whether the text is truthful or deceptive, worthwhile or pointless (see Example 1.2).

While some writers state their intentions and beliefs up front, others hide that information and force the reader to judge. Writers may hide their motives for a variety of reasons. A political columnist, for example, may conceal some of her strongly held beliefs to appear more fair and evenhanded. A writer in a scholarly publication may conceal opinions that may seem inappropriate in an academic context. A poor writer who *intends* to make a point may fail to express that point in a sufficiently clear fashion, unintentionally leaving the reader to figure it out on her own.

Sometimes it is impossible to decide on the author's position, as the text may not provide enough information. In these cases, the reader may have to refer to other sources (such as other works by the same author, or personal knowledge about the author) to make a judgment about what the author intended.

(E) Example 1.2: *Read the following note that was found in a factory worker's locker:*

> *Hey Bill –*
>
> *I've really been enjoying working on the third shift. It's very quiet and very relaxing. The pace is a lot slower than what you're used to on the second shift. I really think you'd like it. By the way, I have an appointment on Thursday. Can you trade your shift with mine that day? You'd get to work third shift and see what I'm talking about.*
>
> *Thanks,*
>
> *Jack*

What is the author's purpose for writing the above text?

Jack's purpose is to get Bill to trade shifts with him, so Jack can go to his previously scheduled appointment. This only becomes clear upon reading the entire note. At first it seems that Jack's main point is to tell Bill how nice it is working on the third shift. However, the last two sentences make the true intent of the note clear: Jack wants Bill to trade shifts with him on Thursday. Knowing this, it is now clear why Jack opened the note with all the information about how easy and relaxing his third-shift job is. Those first few sentences were just there to help persuade Bill to agree to the switch.

Practice problems

Solutions to the practice problems are located in the back of this book.

1. Read the following letter. Then, answer the question.

> Dear Sean,
>
> Congratulations on winning the State High School Football Player of the Year award. It is an incredible accomplishment – one that you will treasure forever. Your tremendous motivational drive and superior athletic skills were apparent to us right from the start, and we are tremendously pleased that the award voters saw exactly what we saw in you.
>
> Looking ahead, we can see even greater things in your future. Your choice of college will have a profound effect on exactly how great those things are – so we hope you're still planning to visit our campus this spring. We have a fun day of activities planned for you. By the time it's done, we think you'll agree that Eastern Reserve University is the perfect place to continue your winning tradition.
>
>
> Best Regards,
> Bill Meehan, Athletic Director
> Eastern Reserve University

What is the author's purpose for writing the above text?

2. Read the following passage. Then, answer the question.

> Mr. Grundle's New Leaf Blower
>
> Mr. Grundle purchased a new leaf blower and set the box out in his yard. He attempted to pull open the heavy packaging with his hands, but failed. Then he brought scissors, but the heavy material proved too tough for him. Finally he decided to bring out a hacksaw. When he was finished, the box lay in tatters all across the lawn.
>
> After the mess was cleaned up, Mr. Grundle set to work with his new purchase. He strapped the blower on his back, aimed at a leaf pile, and pulled the trigger. Nothing happened. He removed the leaf blower and began a 20-minute examination of the device. Finally he decided that he should probably add gasoline.
>
> Ten minutes later, Mr. Grundle's driveway was a river of spilled gasoline. He did manage to get a bit of it into the leaf blower, though. Finally he got the gasoline cleaned up, and the leaf blower strapped onto his back again. It was time for another try.
>
> This time the device roared to life, and leaves went flying every which way. Mr. Grundle was initially pleased with the effect, but less so when he noticed that the leaves were hard to control. They blew and scattered all across the lawn; he needed to be more careful about where he aimed.
>
> Finally, after pushing leaves around for half an hour and making a bigger mess than he started with, Mr. Grundle finally began to get the hang of his new machine. Unfortunately, at that very moment the blower ran out of gas.
>
> Mr. Grundle took the blower into his garage, emerged with a rake, and proceeded to rake his lawn. The next day, neighbors were surprised to see a shiny new leaf blower sitting in his trash can.

What is the purpose of this text?

Persuasive, Informative, Entertaining, and Expressive Passages

Writing usually serves a specific purpose, and that purpose usually falls into one of four categories. The writer may want to:

- *inform* the reader about some fact or event; newspaper articles often fall into this category.

- *persuade* the reader to a particular viewpoint; this sort of writing is often called *persuasive writing*.

- *entertain* the reader; for example, most fiction novels serve the purpose of entertainment.

- *express feelings*; a large amount of poetry is concerned with evoking a feeling or emotion in the reader.

One of the reader's most important jobs is figuring out this purpose (also known as the **author's intent**). By considering the author's intent, the reader gets a better understanding of what information or emotions the author intends to convey, and can better decide whether she agrees with the author, likes the writing, or believes the writing effectively did its job. See Example 1.3.

Not all writing serves only one purpose. For example, a novel that takes place in Egypt might be primarily intended to entertain the reader, but along the way it might pass along information about Egyptian geography, and might evoke certain emotions.

 Example 1.3:   *Read the following advertisement. Then, answer the question.*

> *Saturday only.*
> Giant furniture sale at Maple Furniture Depot.
> All floor models must go.
> These prices will not be seen again this year.
> Hundreds of beds, dressers, dining room tables,
> chairs, and more available.
> Take the third exit off Highway 15.
> Store hours: 10 a.m. to 8 p.m.

What is the author's intent in the advertisement above: to persuade, inform, entertain, or express feelings?

The author's intent here is to persuade. Advertisements always try to persuade the reader. In this case, the advertisement tries to persuade the reader by touting the wide variety of items on sale, and by suggesting that prices will be very low.

Advertisements also tend to inform the reader, even though this is not their main intent. This advertisement, for example, gives concrete information about when and where the sale will occur, and about what sort of items can be found there.

When a piece of writing has multiple possible intents, it is the reader's job to decide what its primary intent is. In this case, that job is quite easy. This is an advertisement for furniture, not a public service announcement; the author was clearly trying to persuade the reader to show up and buy something.

Practice problems

Solutions to the practice problems are located in the back of this book.

1. Read the following passage. Then, answer the question.

> The Dow Jones Industrial Average slid 2% Friday on fears of rising unemployment, rising inventory levels, and decreasing consumer confidence. The continued weakening of the dollar was also seen as a negative sign, raising the specter of higher commodity prices in future months. Higher oil prices, in particular, could have a chilling effect on industrial output.
>
> Interest rates held firm for the week, and a recent poll of economists predicted that they will continue to remain steady for the foreseeable future. This provided a minor bright spot in an otherwise gloomy week for investors.
>
> "We're in for a bumpy ride," said one floor trader from a major brokerage house.
>
> "Nobody's going to buy with much conviction until the unemployment numbers start to turn."

Is the intent of this text to persuade, inform, entertain, or express feelings?

2. Read the following passage. Then, answer the question.

> Graveyard Walk
>
> Steven walked through the graveyard every day on his way home from school. It was a convenient shortcut, and in broad daylight, the tombstones and dark cypress trees seemed mild and unthreatening.
>
> Things were different this evening. Steven stole through the gates as quickly as possible, fearful that he was being watched. He ran to the deep shadows of a mausoleum and caught his breath, heart pounding. He listened for ominous noises, but could hear nothing over the blood rushing through his ears.
>
> He pressed the button to light up his watch: 11:30. He must stay here a full hour to win the bet. He now wished he had never taken it.
>
> A slow scrape came from behind. Steven froze, then turned with underwater slowness. The mausoleum door was sliding open.
>
> Steven wanted to run, but could not. He could not feel his legs; he struggled to draw breath. Yellow light appeared inside the mausoleum. Shadows crept and danced as something holding the light pushed through the door. It made a terrible, guttural sound, like the groan of a dying man.
>
> The door swung fully open. In the doorway stood… an old man in a plaid shirt, a lantern in his hand, a cigarette in his mouth. He coughed again, spat, and closed the door. It was only the groundskeeper, finishing up a long day of work.
>
> The groundskeeper ambled off toward the machine shed. As soon as his back was turned, Steven left the hiding spot and ran. His friend David could keep that $5 wager. An hour in this place just wasn't worth it.

Is the intent of this text to persuade, inform, entertain, or express feelings?

Historical Context

Every piece of literature ever written – be it a great masterpiece or an amateur Web page – has a **historical context**. This means that the time and place in which the piece was written will influence the work in some way. These historical factors may affect *what* is written (the text's content), and *how* it is written (the text's style).

The medieval medical book in Example 1.4 shows how historical influences can affect content. When viewed from a modern perspective, the "four humours" theory presented in the book is laughable. But, when the historical context of the text is considered, the theory isn't quite as ridiculous: when this text was written, the theory represented cutting edge medical thinking. Thus, the time in which the text was written had a major impact on *what* was written. Such a book, if written today, would contain completely different explanations for why people become sick.

How a text is written – in other words, its style – is also part of its historical context. A novel written in the nineteenth century, for example, might use certain words that modern novels don't (like *thee* and *thine*). Or, in the case of the medical text in the next example, notice how there is no effort to be gender neutral; the text refers to *man* and *men* when it refers to people in general. A more modern text would probably try to use more gender-neutral terms (e.g., the patient).

Understanding a text's historical context is crucial to understanding the writing itself. For instance, a reader who fails to see the historical context of the medical book in the next example risks misunderstanding the text completely. Without the knowledge that the book is very old, and that the theories explained in the book were once widely believed, it might appear to the reader that the book's author was insane (or possibly just making an elaborate joke). This would be a complete misreading of the text.

Whenever an older text does something unusual, such as making a bizarre statement or putting information in a much different format from what one might expect, consider that it might not just be the work of an eccentric author; it might be part of the historical context.

(E) *Example 1.4:*   *Read the following text. Then, answer the questions.*

Medieval Medicine

The basis of all medicine is knowledge of the four humours. The humours are substances found in the body, each to a greater or lesser degree. They are: black bile, yellow bile, phlegm, and blood. The body of a normal, healthy man contains equal amounts of the four humours, whereas a sick man exhibits one or more humours that are out of balance with the rest.

Too much of one humour leads a man to exhibit a certain personality trait (or temperament), as follows: too much black bile results in a melancholic, or sad, temperament. Too much yellow bile results in a choleric, or angry, temperament. Too much blood results in a sanguine, or cheerful, temperament. Too much phlegm results in a phlegmatic, or lazy, temperament.

Each humour corresponds to one of the four elements (earth, water, fire, and air), and to a specific organ of the body. For example, yellow bile, the humour of anger, is correlated with fire, and with the gall bladder. Understanding these correlations is of great importance to the doctor. For example, a patient with an excess of yellow bile should be advised to stay away from fire (and indeed, from any hot, dry air), as it will only worsen his condition.

When a man with an imbalance of humours appears before the doctor, the proper action is to put the man's humours back in balance. There are many ways to achieve this rebalancing. For example, an excessively sanguine man can easily be put in balance by a simple bleeding. The act of bleeding reduces the patient's total amount of blood, thus reducing its proportion to the other three humours.

The situation becomes complex when the doctor is confronted with a foreign patient. Foreigners' humours are often in such imbalance that they cannot be easily diagnosed, or cured. For example, the pale men of the north tend to possess an excess of both yellow bile and phlegm, so that while sometimes they burn with hot rage, at other times they are overcome with laziness and apathy. Such problems as theirs are often not curable.

The topic of the humours is a large one, and a full explanation is far beyond the scope of this text. Suffice it to say that knowledge of the four humours is the cornerstone of all medicine, and that any man who would practice medicine must learn them intimately.

What, specifically, does the first paragraph suggest about the historical context of this text?

The first paragraph suggests that, in medieval times, people believed that illnesses automatically resulted from imbalances.

The first paragraph asserts that sick people have an imbalance of humours, whereas healthy people have balanced humours. The implication is that imbalances naturally lead to illness.

Nowadays this sort of assertion would need to be backed up with evidence. The modern reader would ask, "Assuming that these humours even exist, what does it matter if they are out of balance? How, exactly, does the imbalance make a person sick?" However, this text does not argue the point. It makes its statement and then moves on. Whenever a concept is treated this casually, it's often because the author is 100% convinced that it is true, and assumes that his readers will also believe it is true.

(P) *Practice problems*

Solutions to the practice problems are located in the back of this book.

Read the passage titled, "Medieval Medicine" in Example 1.4. Then, answer the next three questions.

1.   What, specifically, does the second paragraph suggest about the historical context of the text?

2.   What, specifically, does the third paragraph suggest about the historical context of the text?

3.   What, specifically, does the fifth paragraph suggest about the historical context of the text?

Ways That Literature From Different Cultures Presents Similar Themes

Different cultures see things in different ways. Sometimes the differences are minor and easy to ignore. Other times the differences are profound, and concern issues that people find extremely important. In such cases, these differences can provoke strong emotional reactions.

It is important to realize that cultural beliefs directly influence authors' opinions and styles. Themes such as birth and death, the role of the individual in society, the role of government, and even the customs and meanings associated with marriage (the subject of Example 1.5) are treated very differently from one culture to the next.

Individual readers will have a wide range of reactions to different cultural attitudes. Some will agree with the way certain themes are presented, while others will strongly disagree. Some will think it's okay for everyone to have a different opinion about a certain topic, while others will think that only one opinion is valid. Every reader is entitled to have a "gut reaction" to these cultural differences.

However, when trying to understand and interpret a written work, emotional reactions are not the most important things. What's most important is recognizing *when* text is written from a different cultural standpoint, and then figuring out *how* that cultural standpoint is different from one's own. Only by taking these cultural differences into account can literature truly be understood.

For instance, the passage in Example 1.5 presents a view of marriage that is completely at odds with modern American views. How should the reader interpret this text? The key is understanding that the author came from a vastly different culture. This understanding allows the reader to see the text for what it is: not a provocative essay, but instead, a simple listing of common beliefs shared by the author and his intended readership.

 Example 1.5:   *Read the following passage. Then, answer the question.*

Marriage Customs

Marriage is an important decision; it can affect the fortunes of an entire family. Young people lack experience, and do not understand the importance of making an appropriate match. This is why family elders, not the young people themselves, arrange who will marry whom.

Many factors must be considered when making a match. Astrological signs must be consulted so that bad luck is not visited upon the newlyweds. Social status and wealth must also be considered – though in some cases, exceptions can be made. For example, consider a bride that comes from a wealthy, wheat-growing family. Normally her family would only consider a wealthy groom. However, a groom whose family is poor, but owns a mill for grinding wheat, might be a good match. In this case the two businesses would help one another, providing advantages to both families.

Failure to give generous bride-gifts and groom-gifts dishonors both families. For this reason, it is suggested that every effort is made to give gifts appropriate to both families' wealth and status. The money spent on these gifts can soon be earned back, but the shame of giving inadequate gifts can last for a lifetime.

Children are of utmost importance to any marriage. This is why newlyweds must always buy a new marriage bed, and children must play upon the newly purchased bed for good luck. If many children play on the bed, a great deal of luck will grace the couple in childbirth.

Which statement best summarizes a cultural opinion held by the text's author?

A) *Marriage is an expression of love between two people.*
B) *Marriage is a sacred institution.*
C) *Marriage is mainly about giving bride-gifts and groom-gifts consistent with one's economic and social status.*
D) *Marriage is an economic, practical union between two families.*

The answer is option D: marriage is an economic, practical union between two families.

While a typical, modern American might say that love is the only reason to marry, this text treats marriage as an economic decision. The wishes of the two people being married are much less important than the practical benefits derived from families of the bride and groom.

Answers A and B are incorrect because they are attitudes likely to be held by modern Americans, not the text's author. Answer C concerns gift giving, which is mentioned in the text, but the author does not suggest that gifts are the main point of marriage. Rather, the long-term benefits derived by both families are the main point.

Ⓟ Practice problems

Solutions to the practice problems are located in the back of this book.

Read the passage in Example 1.5. Then, answer the next three questions.

1. Which of the following statements best reflects the author's culturally held beliefs about young people and their elders?

    A) Elders know what's best for young people, and should make important decisions for them.
    B) Elders should offer advice to young people about important decisions.
    C) Young people should help take care of their elders, and should help them to make important decisions.
    D) Elders should actively help young people to find a partner.

2. What specific cultural belief is suggested by the third paragraph?

3. What cultural beliefs about supernatural forces are expressed in this text?

Text Structure

Effective writing often makes use of **text structure**. A text structure is the way in which a given text is organized. Any piece of writing can include a problem and a solution to that problem, but if these thoughts are not given any structure, it may be difficult for the reader to understand that an author is even presenting a solution to a posed problem. Text structure makes text easier to read, and helps to emphasize the author's point. This can be accomplished by placing related information in close proximity or by following a pre-established layout, such as presenting a **sequence** of ideas as a bulleted or numbered list.

Formatting may be used to enhance text structure. The text's structure should be maintained, but making use of bold words, new paragraphs, and lists are some techniques that may be used to draw the reader's attention to the text structure, helping them to differentiate where a thought ends or where an important piece of information may be found. For example, a **problem-solution** structure might be illustrated by presenting the problem in one paragraph, and the solution in another. Or, the author might choose to write one solid paragraph containing both the problem and the solution, but use one font for the problem and a different font for the solution. In a **comparison-contrast** structure, the author may present two different cases with the intent of making the reader consider the differences (or similarities) between the two cases. In a **cause-effect** structure, the author normally presents an action first, and then describes the effects that result (or may result) from that action.

While formatting may sometimes give clues about a text's structure, the reader cannot rely on this method. Description, for example, is a type of text structure that almost never appears with any special formatting; it usually just appears in the middle of a paragraph. Passages that use **description** tend to describe or characterize a person, thing, or idea.

When used skillfully, text structure is invisible to the casual reader; it simply makes the information in the text easier to digest. However, a good reader should be able to identify text structure when necessary, and be able to use it in his or her own writing when appropriate. Examples 1.6 and 1.7 provide passages with two different types of text structures.

(E) Example 1.6:   *Read the following text. Then, answer the question.*

> *That old park bench is an eyesore. It used to be yellow, but rust has turned it a mottled red. The bench slats are worn and splintered, and termite holes dot their surface. When the wind blows, showers of rust and old paint fly off into the grass.*

Identify the text structure used in the passage above.

This paragraph uses a descriptive structure. After the initial sentence, which establishes the subject (the old park bench), each subsequent sentence gives an additional piece of information that helps to describe the bench. In this case, no particular text formatting was used; the description was simply placed inside a paragraph.

(E) Example 1.7:   *Read the following text. Then, answer the question.*

> *My neighbor seems to like doing everything wrong. He always leaves the garage door open, so his dog constantly escapes. He rakes leaves on a windy day, so the leaves blow right back onto his yard. He opens the window to let a wasp out of the house, and three more fly in through the gap. He tries to call his dog by yelling at it – so the dog just runs away. I sometimes wonder if the man takes pleasure in failure.*

Identify the text structure used in the passage above.

This paragraph uses a cause-effect structure. The first sentence introduces the premise (the neighbor who always does things wrong), and the last sentence sums things up. All the other sentences follow a strict cause-effect structure, first presenting a cause (like the neighbor opening a window), and then the effect (wasps fly in through the window).

Practice problems

Solutions to the practice problems are located in the back of this book.

1. Read the following passage. Then, answer the question.

    After gathering all the ingredients for the experiment:

    1. Put them all into a crucible.
    2. Heat to 500 degrees Fahrenheit.
    3. Mix until the ingredients have fully melted.
    4. Cool the mixture for 5 minutes and pour it into a holding vessel.

    Refrigerate when the mixture has cooled to near room temperature.

    What is the text structure used in the passage above?

2. Read the following passage. Then, answer the question.

    From a Web site's Frequently Asked Questions (FAQ):

    Q. Web site text is hard to read. Can I change the background color?
    A. Yes. Go to the Preferences tab in the upper right corner. Under Background, select a new color from the list.

    What is the text structure used in the passage above?

INFORMATIONAL SOURCE COMPREHENSION

Sets of Directions

Direction-following tasks require a sequence of directions to be followed explicitly. The directions may take the form of a list or may be in paragraph form. If the directions are not in the form of a list, it may be helpful to imagine that they are. Breaking a paragraph of instructions into list form can make the instructions easier to follow.

Each step in an instruction set requires remembering the results of the previous step. For a series of steps, such as those presented in Example 1.8, it may be helpful to write down the result of each step in the sequence as it is completed. This technique allows better visualization of the results of each step, and does not require remembering the details of each step. If it is not possible to write down each step (i.e., if scratch paper is not allowed), it is best to work slowly. Carefully commit the results of the current step to memory before proceeding with the next step.

E Example 1.8: *Read the following set of directions. Then, answer the question.*

1. *Start with the word "THE."*
2. *Add the letter "O" to the beginning of the word.*
3. *Add the letter "R" to the end of the word.*
4. *Add the letter "N" to the beginning of the word.*
5. *Add the letter "A" to the beginning of the word.*

Follow the numbered instructions above to transform the starting word into a different word.

What new word has been spelled?

The answer is "ANOTHER." The easiest way to get the answer is to write down (or carefully memorize) the results of each individual step before moving on to the next one. Here are the results of each step:

1. *THE*
2. *OTHE*
3. *OTHER*
4. *NOTHER*
5. *ANOTHER*

Practice problems

Solutions to the practice problems are located in the back of this book.

1. Follow the instructions below to transform the original shape into a different shape.

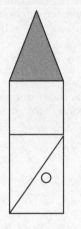

Step 1.   Start with the shape in the diagram to above.
Step 2.   Delete the right triangle that has a circle in it.
Step 3.   Rotate the shaded triangle counterclockwise 90° and move it to the left side of the square.
Step 4.   Rotate the entire shape clockwise 90°.

What does the new shape look like?

2. Follow the directions below to determine the location of the final destination from the original starting point.

Step 1.   Start off going west on Clinton Drive.
Step 2.   Turn right on Parkway Boulevard and travel 2 miles.
Step 3.   Turn left to merge onto Highway 59 and travel 5 miles.
Step 4.   Turn right onto the 151ˢᵗ Street exit.
Step 5.   Drive 7 miles and take another right at Jefferson Avenue.
Step 6.   End at 491 Jefferson Avenue immediately following the turn.

Assuming all roads traveled are either east-west or north-south roads only, which direction is the final destination relative to the starting location?

Labels' Ingredients and Directions

Nutrition labels are growing in length and complexity. Reading the ingredient list that can be found on these labels, and picking out vital information, is an important skill. This skill is useful for any consumer, as a product's ingredients may be very different from what the product's name (or advertising text) suggests.

For example, some fruit juice products contain added water or sugar, while others do not. Even a product that claims to be 100% juice may be misleading, as the juice is often a blend of less-expensive juices, or is reconstituted by adding water to concentrate. Only careful reading of the ingredient list on the nutrition label will provide this type of information.

Label reading becomes even more important when medical conditions are involved. Example 1.9 deals with the common situation of lactose intolerance; if a lactose intolerant person eats or drinks dairy products, he or she will at the very least experience discomfort. When cooking for someone who has lactose intolerance, it is more important than usual to scan labels and to know if any dairy products are going into each dish.

(E) *Example 1.9:* *Read the ingredients below. Then, answer the question.*

> No-Milk Banana Frosting
>
> 2 Bananas
> 1 cup Soymilk
> 2 Tbsp Sour Cream
> 1 cup Flour
> 2 Egg Whites
> ¼ cup Heavy Cream
> 2 Tbsp Canola Oil
> ½ tsp Vanilla

Determine whether the product above is suitable for a lactose-intolerant guest.

This frosting would not be suitable for a lactose-intolerant guest. The recipe advertises itself as "No-Milk," presumably because it uses soymilk instead of typical milk. The soymilk will not be a problem for the guest who is lactose intolerant, because it is not a true dairy product; it is created from soybeans. However, the recipe also calls for sour cream and heavy cream. Both of these are true dairy products, so the recipe is definitely not recommended for anyone who has lactose intolerance.

Of course, some conditions have much more serious consequences than lactose intolerance. A person with a severe allergy could have a serious reaction, or even die, if exposed to a high dose of an allergen. A person who has diabetes mellitus may experience similar consequences if he or she consumes too much sugar. Again, in these cases, careful label reading is more than just a handy skill – it can be a lifesaver.

Ingredient lists aren't restricted to foods or medicines. Any product that is made from several other products is likely to have an ingredient list. An example would be a computer, which often is sold with a list explaining what components the computer is made from.

(P) *Practice problems*

Solutions to the practice problems are located in the back of this book.

Read the following label. Then, answer the questions.

Nutrition Facts

Serving Size 1 cup (228 g)
Servings Per Container 2

Amount Per Serving

Calories 200   Calories from Fat 90

	% Daily Value*
Total Fat 13g	20%
Saturated Fat 5g	25%
Trans Fat 2g	
Cholesterol 30g	10%
Sodium 30mg	1%
Total Carbohydrate 31g	10%
Dietary Fiber 0g	
Sugars 5g	
Protein 5g	

Vitamin A	4%
Vitamin C	3%
Calcium	15%
Iron	4%

*Percent Daily values are based on a 2,000 calorie diet. Your Daily Values may be higher or lower depending on your calorie needs.

	Calories	2,000	2,500
Total Fat	Less than	65g	80g
Sat Fat	Less than	20g	25g
Cholesterol	Less than	300mg	300mg
Sodium	Less than	2,400mg	2,400mg
Total Carbohydrate		300g	375g
Dietary Fiber		25g	30g

1. A person who has diabetes mellitus has been advised to only consume foods that have a high fiber content. Would the product described above be a good choice to fulfill this person's dietary needs?

2. A woman is keeping a diary of her food and nutrient intake. One evening, she consumes a container of the product described above. How many calories should she note on her log?

Definitions in Context

Some words have many possible meanings. To decide which meaning the author intends, consider the word's context. A word's **context** consists of surrounding words, sentences, or paragraphs that usually help to reveal the word's meaning.

Interpreting the context of a word not only helps the reader decide which definition is correct, it can also suggest the meaning of words the reader does not understand at all. For instance, even if the reader is not familiar with some of the definitions of the word *earnest*, the word's context in Example 1.10 should allow the selection of the right definition from the available choices.

(E) *Example 1.10:*   *Read the following sentence. Then, answer the question.*

The sale of the house is likely to proceed, as the buyer has already paid $10,000 in <u>earnest</u>.

Based on the context above, which of the following definitions of the underlined word applies?

A)   seriousness of intention
B)   a token of a pledge to pay the remainder at a later date
C)   a display of emotion

While the buyer may display "seriousness of intention" (option A), and may show "a display of emotion" (option C) about buying the house, context reveals that earnest here refers to the $10,000 the buyer has already paid as a deposit on the house. In this context, option B makes perfect sense: earnest money is a pledge to pay the remaining amount.

In many test situations, it is best to put aside personal guesses and assumptions, and to work entirely with the information on the page. However, in this case, it is encouraged to use personal guesses and assumptions to guess at a word's meaning based on context. It is precisely those guesses, assumptions, and logical deductions about context and meaning that will lead to the proper definition for the unknown word.

A side note: while making a guess based on context is appropriate for an exam, it is not appropriate in real-life professional situations that demand complete understanding of written material. If it is possible to verify a word's meaning by using an outside source (a dictionary, for example), it is almost always better to do so than to simply guess about the meaning and move on.

(P) *Practice problems*

Solutions to the practice problems are located in the back of this book.

1.   Read the following sentence. Then, answer the question.

      After correcting her father about the theory of gravity, the adolescent realized that even parents are <u>fallible</u>.

      Based on the context of the sentence above, what is the definition of the underlined word?

2.   Read the following sentence. Then, answer the question.

      The old Victorian mansion was <u>tenebrous</u> until the caretaker opened the drapes, letting in light.

      Based on the context of the sentence above, what is the definition of the underlined word?

3.   Read the following sentence. Then, answer the question.

      Like the <u>waning</u> moon, hope diminished with each passing day.

      Based on the context of the sentence above, what is the definition of the underlined word?

Printed Communications

A simple, well-written document conveys information effortlessly. Well-written documents make it easy for the reader to grasp any information the author wishes to convey. Unfortunately, many real-world documents are complicated or poorly written or both. In these cases, the reader must work to uncover the meaning of the document, and to uncover important details that might supplement that meaning.

When reading to learn specific information, it may be helpful to first read the entire text quickly, without looking for anything in particular, to learn the general idea of the writing. Then, once it has been established which pieces of information are important, return to the text and look for that specific information. Finding the information should now be easy, since the overall structure of the text is known.

Example 1.11 discusses a memo that is not particularly long or complex. Still, it must be read, and possibly re-read, to extract all of its information.

 Example 1.11:   *Read the following invitation. Then, answer the question.*

Birthday Party for Bill

Time: 3 p.m. Friday
Place: Break Room

This will be a potluck. The fridge in the lower level should be open, so store anything perishable in there. We'll handle it the usual way – if your last name starts with S to Z, ask Melissa what to bring. A to G, ask Jason; H to R, ask Tom. Let's try not to skip out early this time. Plan to be there for at least an hour, if at all possible. Also, sorry to say:

No alcohol.

If an employee named Ellen Johanssen reads the office memo above, what should she do?

She should contact Tom. Any employee reading this memo needs to pay special attention to the part about whom to contact. In this case, the employee reading the memo has the last name of Johanssen, and since the letter J comes between H and R, the employee needs to contact Tom.

(P) *Practice problems*

Solutions to the practice problems are located in the back of this book.

1. Read the following memorandum. Then, answer the question.

Memorandum

TO: Spanish Club members
FROM: Lauren Fitzgerald, Spanish Club President
DATE: August 31st, 2009
SUBJECT: Annual Fundraising Event

It is that time of year again when we must start planning for our annual fundraising event. This event is one of the most important, if not the most important, events for our club, as it is the source of our funding for the entire year as well as our trip to Spain, which is scheduled for the first week of June. Due to the high level of importance associated with this event, I ask that every club member be actively involved in its planning and implementation.

We will have our first event planning meeting on Monday, September 14. At this meeting, we will be gathering ideas for event activities and assigning tasks to club members. We have set the date for the event to be Saturday, April 15. Attendance for the first meeting and all subsequent meetings is required. I look forward to seeing you all in 2 weeks and having a great start to a new year in Spanish Club.

In the memo above, what is the date of the annual fundraising event?

2. Read the following advertisement. Then, answer the question.

PUPPIES FOR SALE

4 Labrador, 6 Maltese, and 5 Yorkshire Terrier puppies need to find a good home. The Labrador pups are 8 weeks old and will be getting their first round of shots and will be ready to go at 10 weeks; they are $200.00 each. The Maltese pups are 12 weeks old, have had their shots, and are ready to go now; they are $300.00 each. The Yorkshire Terrier pups are 6 weeks old and won't be ready to go home for another 5 weeks; they are $350.00 each. All puppies have beautiful coats and are already very socialized and lovable.

In the classified advertisement above, how many weeks old do the Yorkshire Terrier puppies need to be before they are ready to take home?

Indexes and Tables of Contents

The **table of contents** provides an overview of a document, outlining its basic structure and allowing the reader to quickly look up (and skip to) the section she wants to read.

The **index** also provides a way of looking up various topics in the document. It typically consists of a list of names, topics, and ideas mentioned in a text, followed by the page number(s) where those names, topics, or ideas are mentioned. If a topic is discussed in several places, its index entry will list each page where the topic may be found.

Most long, printed, nonfiction documents have both a table of contents and an index. Short, printed, nonfiction documents may have a table of contents, but usually not an index, as short documents can be quickly read in their entirety (making an index overkill). Informational Web publications may have a table of contents, but almost never have an index, because aside from the difficulties of creating a traditional index for a collection of Web pages, search engines can easily perform the same function. Tables of contents may appear in nonfiction works, such as a software manual, or in fiction works, where, for example, the reader may find chapter names.

Though both can be used to quickly look up information, a table of contents and an index serve different functions. Whereas the table of contents is good for learning the document's overall structure, or for finding the general section where a topic may be discussed, the index is best when the reader must find a reference to a very specific detail.

(P) *Practice problems*

Solutions to the practice problems are located in the back of this book.

1. Read the following index excerpt. Then, answer the question.

> Washington, DC
>   history of, 554, 556-9
>   geography of, 552-3
>   references to, 553, 569-73
> Washington State, 219

According to the index excerpt above, on what pages of this book can one find information about the history of Washington, DC?

2. Read the following excerpt from a table of contents. Then, answer the question.

A couple is trying to decide between hiring two real estate agents, but would like to know what past clients have said about their experiences before making their decision. Which chapter would help them complete their task?

Product Information: One Product is the More Economical Buy

A number of factors influence the final cost of an item. A base price is just the starting point; anyone who has purchased a seemingly cheap item, only to find the final bill much higher due to tax, shipping and handling, and other assorted charges, can attest to this fact.

When preparing to make a purchase, it is best to collect information about all potential fees first. Calculate a grand total that includes all of those fees. Then, when comparing the item's price to prices from other stores, be sure to compare total amounts; it is not useful, for example, to compare a base price from one store against a comprehensive final bill from another store, which may include a variety of extra charges.

Sometimes choosing the best deal is not an especially difficult process. Example 1.12 displays a list of online retailers that sell a particular type of lamp. In this example, the only two factors to consider are base price and shipping cost. A little simple addition will yield the best price.

In other cases, there are more factors to consider. For example, some products can be purchased in bulk to reduce the per-unit cost. In such cases it is necessary to calculate the cost based on the number of units that will be purchased.

There are yet more considerations that can factor into making a purchase: the retailer's reliability, return policies, estimated shipping times, and more. However, the examples and questions in this section, will just focus on variables related to cost.

 Example 1.12:   *Use the table below to answer the question.*

Store	Price	Shipping and Handling
Lighting Superstore	$180	$25.00
United Lighting	$175	$30.00
A3 Furniture	$170	$20.00
Dave's Home Furnishings	$200	$0 (included in base)

A consumer wants to buy a lamp. The table above shows price quotes from four online retailers. Which retailer offers the best buy?

The best buy is from A3 Furniture. This is determined by adding the price to shipping cost for each store, and comparing the totals. Here's the math:

Lighting Superstore	180 + 25 = $205.00
United Lighting	175 + 30 = $205.00
A3 Furniture	170 + 20 = $190.00
Dave's Home Furnishings	200 + 0 = $200.00

In this case, the retailer with the lowest base price still turns out to be cheapest once shipping costs are considered. However, this is often not the case. Notice that once shipping and handling is added to base price, the prices from all four stores fall into a much narrower range than the base prices alone would suggest. Also, notice that Dave's Home Furnishings, which looks quite expensive when only the base price is considered, actually has the second-best price once all costs are totaled.

Practice problems

Solutions to the practice problems are located in the back of this book.

Use the table below to answer the questions.

Cost of Book for *Book ABC*

Store	Location	Price per book	Shipping and Handling
Company A	San Francisco, CA	$95.00	Free shipping on all orders
Company B	San Francisco, CA	$80.00	$25/book (free in-state shipping)
Company C	Chicago, IL	$90.00	$10/book
Company D	Chicago, IL	$90.00	$15/book (free shipping on all orders over $50)

1. An instructor in Nebraska is searching for a bargain on a textbook titled *Book ABC*. Which store would give her the best deal?

2. A student in San Francisco has lost her textbook and has a test the next day. Which business should she physically visit to get the least expensive book that same day?

Information From a Telephone Book

Internet searches may eventually replace the yellow pages as the preferred way to find local businesses. However, for now, telephone books are usually the best way of finding all local businesses of a given type.

Yellow pages list businesses by category. The categories are usually straightforward, but occasionally one must guess at a category name. For example, someone looking for car parts might look for a category named "Car," but the phone book may list car parts under "Automotive" instead.

Generally speaking, if there are two or more logical choices for a category name, look for the more formal one ("Automotive" instead of "Car" and "Television" instead of "TV"). If a category might logically have more than one name, there are often pointers to the proper category listed where the other names would appear. For example, looking for "Car," one might find an entry that says, "Car – *See* Automotive." This note tells the reader that the sought-after information will appear under the "Automotive" section.

Yellow book pages typically include both addresses and phone numbers. All businesses that make themselves known to the phone book publisher have a basic listing (a name and address in the small-print list). Additionally, businesses can pay for extra services, ranging from having their names appear in bold print to taking out a multi-page advertisement.

When seeking business information in the yellow pages, look both at the basic listings and at the advertisements. The basic listings will provide the most comprehensive list of possible businesses, while the advertisements may provide additional information (such as store hours, service descriptions, or alternate phone numbers) about certain businesses. The advertisements may also provide unintentional information: for example, an advertisement filled with misspellings might suggest a less-than-professional business (see Example 1.13).

(E) *Example 1.13:* *Use the yellow page excerpt below to answer the question.*

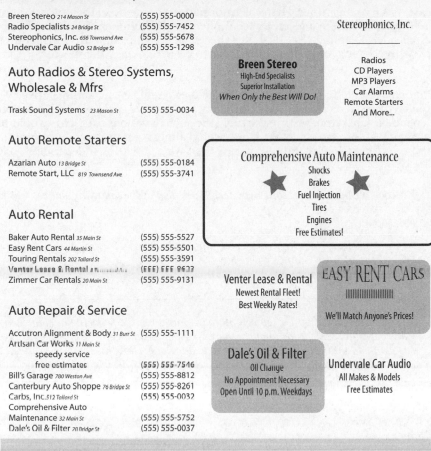

| 155 Automobile |

Auto Radios & Stereo Systems, Cont'd

Breen Stereo *214 Mason St*	(555) 555-0000
Radio Specialists *24 Bridge St*	(555) 555-7452
Stereophonics, Inc. *656 Townsend Ave*	(555) 555-5678
Undervale Car Audio *52 Bridge St*	(555) 555-1298

Auto Radios & Stereo Systems, Wholesale & Mfrs

| Trask Sound Systems *23 Mason St* | (555) 555-0034 |

Auto Remote Starters

| Azarian Auto *13 Bridge St* | (555) 555-0184 |
| Remote Start, LLC *819 Townsend Ave* | (555) 555-3741 |

Auto Rental

Baker Auto Rental *35 Main St*	(555) 555-5527
Easy Rent Cars *44 Martin St*	(555) 555-5501
Touring Rentals *202 Tallard St*	(555) 555-3591
Venter Lease & Rental *... ...*	(555) 555-9632
Zimmer Car Rentals *20 Main St*	(555) 555-9131

Auto Repair & Service

Accutron Alignment & Body *31 Burr St*	(555) 555-1111
Artisan Car Works *11 Main St*	
speedy service	
free estimates	(555) 555-7546
Bill's Garage *780 Weston Ave*	(555) 555-8812
Canterbury Auto Shoppe *76 Bridge St*	(555) 555-8261
Carbs, Inc. *512 Tallard St*	(555) 555-0032
Comprehensive Auto	
Maintenance *32 Main St*	(555) 555-5752
Dale's Oil & Filter *20 Bridge St*	(555) 555-0037

Breen Stereo
High-End Specialists
Superior Installation
When Only the Best Will Do!

Stereophonics, Inc.

Radios
CD Players
MP3 Players
Car Alarms
Remote Starters
And More...

Comprehensive Auto Maintenance
Shocks
Brakes
Fuel Injection
Tires
Engines
Free Estimates!

Venter Lease & Rental
Newest Rental Fleet!
Best Weekly Rates!

EASY RENT CARS
We'll Match Anyone's Prices!

Dale's Oil & Filter
Oil Change
No Appointment Necessary
Open Until 10 p.m. Weekdays

Undervale Car Audio
All Makes & Models
Free Estimates

A customer on Townsend Avenue wants to rent a car. Which business is likely to be most convenient for her?

Venter Lease & Rental is probably the most convenient rental service, as it is located on Townsend Avenue (the customer's street). This information may be found by looking under Auto Rental, then looking for businesses on Townsend Avenue. Venter Lease & Rental is the only one listed.

(P) *Practice problems*

Solutions to the practice problems are located in the back of this book.

Use the yellow page excerpt shown in Example 1.13 to answer the questions.

1. Business partners need to rent a car for an out-of-town meeting, but they need to make sure the cost is within their budget. Based on the yellow page excerpt, which car rental company should they contact?

2. A driver notices that his check oil light is on during his drive home from a late Thursday night dinner. Based on the yellow page except, at which auto repair location is he most likely to receive immediate attention?

Sources for Locating Information

With the rise of the Internet, the amount of information available upon demand has multiplied. The difficulty these days is not finding information – it is finding the *right* information. The first step in finding the right information is to identify appropriate sources.

Appropriate, in this case, has two meanings. First, the information should be to the point. Often, sources contain information that is *somewhat* related to a given topic. A much smaller number of sources *directly* discuss the topic in a way meaningful to the reader. Example 1.14 illustrates this concept: while all four information sources in the example have something to do with cooking, only one of them has to do with *recipes*, the specific aspect of cooking that the reader is looking for.

The second definition of *appropriate* can be roughly translated as "credible" or "authoritative." For example, consider a researcher trying to determine if a carmaker's fuel efficiency claims are accurate. This researcher might find a study published by an independent laboratory testing the fuel efficiency of various cars. This would be appropriate to the task at hand. A carmaker's Web site, on the other hand, would almost certainly not be appropriate, as that Web site is more concerned with promoting a brand and selling cars than with providing independent, scientific information.

(E) Example 1.14: *A cook wishes to learn some new recipes. Which of the following sources would provide them?*

    A) *Store Web site: "Kitchens 'n Things"*
    B) *Web site: "The Happy Baker's Culinary Reviews"*
    C) *Printed Sales Catalog: "The Savvy Chef"*
    D) *Book: "50 Delicious Southwestern Dishes"*

The answer is option D. Though all four sources relate to cooking in some way, option D is the only answer that seems to be about recipes. Answers A and C are both sales catalogs; one is online and one is printed, but both are presumably geared toward selling kitchen accessories. Answer B is a review site, not a recipe site. Option D, on the other hand, is very likely a recipe book containing 50 Southwest-themed recipes.

(P) *Practice problems*

Solutions to the practice problems are located in the back of this book.

1. A woman plans to drive from her home in Kansas to her sister's home in California. She is hoping to spend only 2 days driving in her car. What informational source could she use to help her determine if her driving goal is attainable?

2. A student is trying to find a book about civil engineering. She has been told the name of an author who is well-known for his books on this topic. She is going to the library and wants to locate any books on this topic, but specifically by this particular author. What informational source would help her locate books on civil engineering by this author?

Sample Listings of Items and Costs

Buying items can be a surprisingly complicated process. That is because many factors aside from cost enter into the decision. Retailer reliability, return policies, shipping methods, convenience, and more can affect the choice of retailer. Differences in quality, reliability, warranty, style, and more can affect the choice of product. The sheer amount of choices can be overwhelming.

A useful strategy is to identify the most important factors in a purchase, and then mentally sort each product or retailer according to those factors. For instance, the homeowner in Example 1.15 identified three qualities that she wants in an area rug. By bearing those qualities in mind while looking at a list of possible rugs, it becomes easy to sort out which rugs are suitable and which are not.

Think of any purchase as a three-stage process. The first stage is to decide what qualities are important. The second stage is to get product information to compare against the list of qualities. The third stage is to sort through the product information and decide which product or retailer best matches the desired qualities.

The information gathering stage can be problematic, as not all products and retailers have complete information published in an easy-to-find spot. Even when the right information is in plain sight, finding the most relevant points can be work. In the end, it comes down to careful reading.

If the list of potential products or retailers is long, it may help to cross out each product or retailer as soon as it fails to match any of the desired qualities. The consumer in Example 1.15 can cross off the Persian Pattern III as soon as she realizes that it costs too much. By either literally or mentally crossing off all the nonmatches, it becomes easier to find the suitable product(s) or retailer(s) left at the end.

 Example 1.15:   *Use the table below to answer the question.*

Rug name	Colors	Size	Cost
Persian Pattern III	Red, black, beige	8x10	$550.00
Checkerboard II	Black, white, blue	9x11	$400.00
Emperor William	Red, black, gold	8x10	$450.00
Crosstrends Flat Weave	Red, white, beige	8x10	$400.00

A homeowner wants to buy an area rug that includes the color black. The rug should be 8 × 10, and it cannot cost more than $500. Which product suits her needs?

Only the Emperor William rug suits the homeowner's needs. It meets all three of the listed criteria. The easiest way to arrive at this answer is to go down each row, comparing the rug's information against the consumer's specifications. As soon as a product fails to meet a specification, eliminate that row by crossing it off with a pencil or crossing it off mentally. Following this strategy, it's easy to see that each of the other three rugs has exactly one thing wrong with it. The Persian Pattern III costs more than $500. The Checkerboard II is too large (9x11, instead of the desired 8x10). Finally, the Crosstrends Flat Weave does not have the color black in it.

Ⓟ *Practice problems*

Solutions to the practice problems are located in the back of this book.

1. Use the table below to answer the question.

Theatre 10 Movie Times and Ticket Costs					
Show Times		Ticket Costs			
		Adults	Children (under 10)	Senior Citizens	Students (with ID)
Mon. – Thurs.	7:00 p.m., 9:00 p.m.	$7.00	$5.00	$6.50	$6.00
Fri. – Sat.	7:00 p.m., 9:00 p.m., 10:00 p.m.	$7.50	$5.50	$7.00	$6.50
Sunday	3:00 p.m., 5:00 p.m.	$6.00	$4.00	$5.50	$5.00

    What is the cost of a movie ticket for a student to see a movie on Friday at 9:00?

2. Use the table below to answer the question.

Greenway Golf Course Rates		
	9 Holes (With Cart/Without)	18 Holes (With Cart/Without)
Mon. – Fri.	$23.00/$15.00	$38.00/$30.00
Sat. – Sun.	$25.00/$17.00	$40.00/$32.00
Early Bird Special (everyday from 7:00 a.m. to 9:00 a.m.)	$18.00/$10.00	$33.00/$25.00

    How much does it cost to play 9 holes of golf without a cart on a Wednesday at 8:30 a.m.?

Graphic Representations of Information

While much information is presented with words, some information is represented graphically. Graphic representations of information usually come in the form of charts, graphs, or maps, though even a drawing or photograph can be considered a graphic representation of information. Of course, not all graphics are informational; some are just there for decoration. But in nonfiction works, graphics are usually informative, not decorative – in other words, they are graphic representations of information. The reader must learn how to extract the information from these graphics.

Charts and graphs come in a variety of different styles, but all of them have the same goal: they present numerical information visually, so the reader can quickly grasp a concept, or quickly compare one piece of information to another. A common type of chart is a pie chart. A **pie chart** represents a concept with a circle (or pie), and then breaks down the pie into "slices" that illustrate the pie's components. For example, in a pie chart showing how a person spent her day, the pie would represent a single day, and the slices would show the various activities that filled the day. The size of each slice would correspond to how much time was spent on each activity. As shown in Example 1.16, these types of charts are useful for showing how pieces make up a whole.

Different types of charts and graphs are used to represent different types of data. In fact, there are far too many sorts of charts and graphs to explain them all in a short space. Fortunately, it is not necessary to be familiar with each different form of chart to understand it. The reader can usually figure out a chart or graph by looking at the information presented in the key, and then carefully studying the chart.

 Example 1.16:   *Use the chart below to answer the question.*

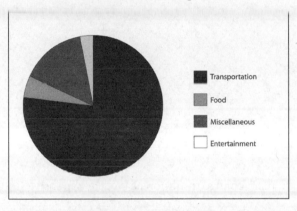

The pie chart above breaks down a businesswoman's expenses on a business trip. What was the most expensive aspect of this trip?

The most expensive part of the trip was transportation. Looking at the pie, the reader can quickly determine that the black slice is by far the biggest. Then, referring to the key, the reader can look up the color black to see what it means. In this case, black is transportation.

Some pie charts give percentages for each pie slice, so the reader can tell precisely how big the slice is. Also, some pie charts would put the key directly on the pie instead of off to the side, so that each slice would have a label on it. Expect these sorts of variations on all types of charts.

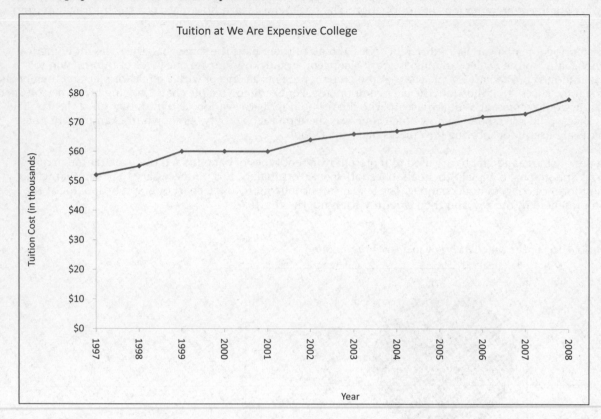

Practice problems

Solutions to the practice problems are located in the back of this book.

Use the graph below to answer the questions.

1. During what 2-year time span was there no change in tuition at We Are Expensive College?

2. During what year did tuition first reach more than $60,000?

Scale Readings

Various measurement instruments provide scale readings. A **scale**, such as that in Example 1.17, is any standard instrument of measurement that has marking at established intervals. The most common such instrument is a standard weight scale (often just called a *scale*). However, any number of other instruments, such as thermometers, blood pressure monitors, Geiger counters, and altimeters are all considered scales. Because a scale shows its results along a numerical scale (say, from 1 to 10 pounds, or from –20° to 100°), the information obtained from it is called a **scale reading**.

It is important to know the upper and lower boundaries of a scale. For example, if a thermometer only goes down to –10° Fahrenheit, and it currently seems to be showing –10°, there is a good chance that the actual temperature is *lower* than –10°. In this case, the thermometer may simply have hit its lower limit, and cannot show the actual temperature. If the type of instrument is unknown, look at the information on the instrument itself. Printed information such as numbers, labels, and indicators will usually give a clue.

 Example 1.17:   *Use the image below to answer the question.*

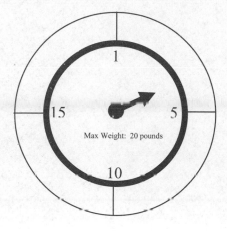

What does the instrument above measure? What is its current measurement?

This is a weight scale, and it is showing a weight of about 3½ or 4 pounds. Initially, the device may look like a clock. However, note that it has only one hand and that the numbering goes to 20, not 12. Also, if there is any confusion about what the instrument is, the label on the face, "Max Weight: 20 lb," gives an excellent clue that it is a scale. The indicator needle is pointing at a spot that is more than halfway between the one and the five; hence, the scale measurement is about 3½ or 4 pounds.

(P) *Practice problems*

Solutions to the practice problems are located in the back of this book.

Use the image below to answer the questions.

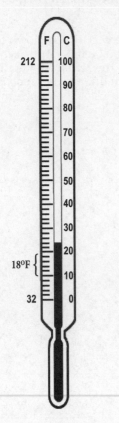

1. What is the current approximate temperature in Centigrade according to the thermometer?

2. If the current temperature were 10° Centigrade, what would be the current temperature in degrees Fahrenheit?

Legends and Keys of Maps

Maps typically show an overhead view of a specific area. Important features of the terrain may be printed on the map using lines, colors, and/or text. Additionally, various symbols and notations on the map may provide additional information.

A small portion of a typical map is devoted to a **legend**, a small area that explains the symbols and notations used on the map. The actual information provided by the legend is sometimes called the key. (In some circumstances, the terms legend and key are used interchangeably, to refer to the entire legend and its contents.)

Most legends contain a symbol that indicates the cardinal directions (north, south, east, and west) as they relate to the map. This symbol is known as a **compass rose**. If a map does not have a compass rose, it likely has an arrow pointing north, so that the map can give the reader a sense of compass direction. Usually, the top edge of a map corresponds to the direction north, but this is not always the case. The map in Example 1.18 defies this convention; on this map, the right-hand margin is actually north.

Another typical feature of maps is a **distance scale**, which is information in the legend that tells the reader how to interpret distances on the map. It usually appears as a line with a distance marking. In the map used in Example 1.18, the distance scale line represents one mile. The reader can use this information to estimate distances on the map. For example, if a road is represented by a line about five times as long as the line on the distance scale, the reader can assume that the road is five miles long.

Ⓔ *Example 1.18:* *Use the map below to answer the question.*

Map of Blackstone Recreational Area

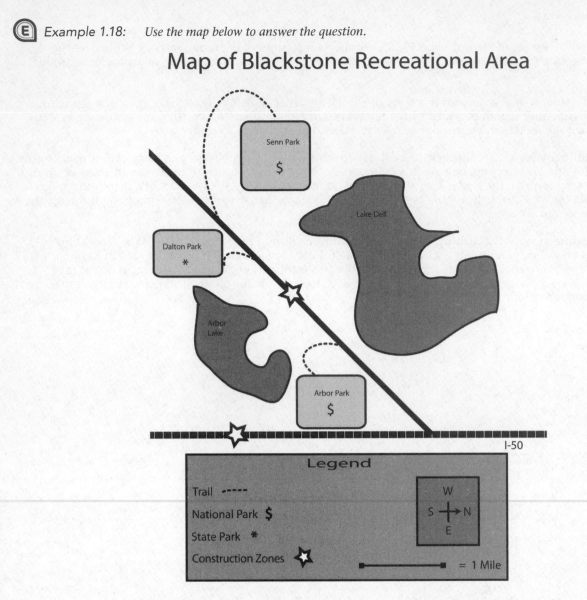

Which of the three parks on this map is farthest south: Dalton Park, Senn Park, or Arbor Park?

The answer is Dalton Park. As mentioned earlier, this map does not abide by the convention of up = *north. The reader must refer to the legend's compass rose to see that the right edge of the map is the north edge, and the left edge of the map is the south edge. With this in mind, solving the problem is as simple as deciding which park is closest to the left edge of the map. Dalton Park is farthest south.*

Ⓟ *Practice problems*

Solutions to the practice problems are located in the back of this book.

Use the map in Example 1.18 to answer the questions.

1. How many National Parks are located within the Blackstone Recreational Area?

2. What is the approximate driving distance between the two possible roadblocks?

Headings and Subheadings

Headings and subheadings organize text. **Headings** are titles that preface a section of text. Headings advertise the subject of the text that is found beneath them, making it easier to skim the text or to search for a particular topic. They also give the text extra structure. **Subheadings** are headings that appear below other headings, within the same category. Subheadings typically appear in a smaller typeface than headings, so that they may easily be distinguished. A single heading may have many subheadings, and the subheadings in turn may have their own subheadings. Headings and subheadings break the text into manageable parts, allowing the reader to skip parts that are not of interest, or to find parts that are of particular interest.

A heading or subheading always covers a *piece* of the larger topic. For instance, Example 1.19 shows a chapter from a book about philosophy. The chapter's title is "The Great Philosophers," so it is clear that the chapter will discuss a number of historical thinkers. The main headings then go on to split up the topic; each heading covers just one philosopher. This is a logical way of splitting up the larger topic of great philosophers.

 Example 1.19: *Read the following text. Then, answer the question.*

Chapter 8: The Great Philosophers
1. *Socrates*
    A. *Biography*
    B. *Major Works*
    C. *Historical Impact*
2. *Plato*
    A. *Biography*
    B. *Major Works*
    C. *Historical Impact*
3. *Descartes*
    A. *Biography*
    B. *Major Works*
    C. *Historical Impact*
4. *Kant*
    A. *Biography*
    B. *Major Works*
    C. *Historical Impact*

What is the organizational pattern exposed by the headings and subheadings above?

Each heading covers a single philosopher, and each subheading deals with a different aspect of that philosopher: his biography, major works, and historical impact. This is a very clear structure, and it's repeated several times. The reader can skim over these headings and very quickly understand the chapter's organization. If the structure were less regular, or if one of the headings were out of place, the headings would become much less useful.

Headings also tend to follow a pattern. These patterns help the reader to anticipate what comes next, and to better understand the text's structure. For example, if the first few headings in a chapter each refer to a different type of fruit (e.g., apples, pears, grapes, etc.), the reader can expect all the subsequent headings to follow the same pattern. If the next heading is titled "Grapefruit," that fits the pattern. But if the next heading is titled "Why Fruits are Delicious," the pattern is broken, and the headings become much less useful to the reader. Now the reader can no longer expect the headings to form a logical pattern, and she must read much more carefully.

Headings and subheadings are often listed in a book's table of contents, along with the chapter listings. This makes it even easier for the reader to skim the book's contents.

Headings typically only appear in nonfiction documents. A work of fiction, such as a novel, will usually have chapters, but will rarely have headings.

(P) *Practice problems*

Solutions to the practice problems are located in the back of this book.

Read the following text. Then, answer the questions.

Chapter 88: The Color Spectrum
- Red
  - Cool Reds
  - Warm Reds
- Orange
  - Light Oranges
  - Dark Oranges
- Yellow
  - Deep Yellows
  - Painting With Yellows
- Green
  - Primary Greens
  - Pastel Greens
- Blue
  - Vivid Blues
  - Faded Blues

1. What portion of this text could cause a reader confusion?

2. What is the next logical header that would come after "Blue"?

Text Features

Text features include such formatting devices as bold or italicized fonts, indented text, and bulleted or numbered lists. Text features can be meaningful (and useful) if they are used consistently to achieve a distinct purpose. For example, consider a novel that uses bold text to indicate when a character is shouting. Once the reader understands how the novel uses the feature, the bold text effortlessly conveys additional meaning: the author no longer needs to waste words explaining to the reader that a character is shouting.

Text features typically do one or more of the following things: add meaning, change meaning, or add clarity. For example, a set of instructions is formatted as a numbered list. The list does not change the meaning of the instructions, nor does it provide new information – but it does add clarity, making it easier to read the instructions. Or, consider a novel that uses italic text to mark a character's personal thoughts. The italics change the meaning of the text: the reader soon learns to interpret the italicized text as a character's thoughts. (Without italics, the reader might attribute the comments to the narrator.)

For a text feature to be useful, it must be applied consistently. A document that uses a certain feature, but does not always use the feature for the same reason, is making poor use of the feature. For example, what if a document used bold text not only to indicate book titles, but also to emphasize important words and to mark words defined in a glossary? In this case the text features would not serve their purpose, as the reader would have to decide in every case what the formatting was supposed to mean.

(P) *Practice problems*

Solutions to the practice problems are located in the back of this book.

1. Read the passage below. Then, answer the question.

    Professor Devereaux made his position clear in a 2004 interview with the Physics Review.[1] Needless to say, the results of this interview left him on the fringes of the scientific community.

    What is the purpose of using *superscript* on the number "1" in the text above?

2. Read the following excerpt from a play. Then, answer the question.

    > *Jackson enters the room and approaches Lori, who has been sitting at the kitchen table.*
    >
    > | | |
    > |---|---|
    > | **Lori** | **Hi, I didn't know you were home.** |
    > | Jackson | Just got in. |
    > | **Lori** | **Did you take care of the problem?** |
    > | Jackson | Not yet, that's why we need to talk. |

    Why has the author made part of the play's script bold?

SECTION 2: MATHEMATICS

The mathematics portion of the TEAS® covers material related to numbers and operations, measurement, data interpretation, and algebra. Calculators are not allowed on the test.

NUMBERS AND OPERATIONS

Order of Operations

Mathematical operations must be performed in the correct order when performing calculations with numbers.

- First, perform operations in parentheses. Work on the innermost set of parentheses first, then work outwards as demonstrated in Example 2.1.

 Example 2.1:   *Simplify the expression: 4 + (3 × (5 + 2)).*

$$4 + (3 \times (5 + 2)) = 4 + (3 \times 7)$$ *Simplify the expression within the innermost set of parentheses first.*
$$= 4 + 21$$ *Simplify the expression within the parentheses.*
$$= 25$$

- Second, simplify any exponents as demonstrated in Example 2.2. (An **exponent** is a number written as a superscript that is used to denote the number of times a number should be multiplied by itself.)

 Example 2.2:   *Simplify the expression: $(3 - 1)^2 + 6$.*

$$(3 - 1)^2 + 6 = 2^2 + 6$$ *Simplify the expression within the parentheses first.*
$$= 4 + 6$$ *Simplify the exponent.*
$$= 10$$

- Third, complete the multiplication and division from left to right as demonstrated in Example 2.3.

 Example 2.3:   *Simplify the expression: 2 × 8 ÷ 4 × 2.*

$$2 \times 8 \div 4 \times 2 = 16 \div 4 \times 2$$ *From left to right, 2 × 8 = 16.*
$$= 4 \times 2$$ *From left to right, 16 ÷ 4 = 4.*
$$= 8$$

Note: (2 × 8) ÷ (4 × 2) = 16 ÷ 8 = 2. This shows that multiplication in parentheses precedes the rule of multiplying from left to right.

- Finally, complete addition and subtraction from left to right.

This order can be remembered more easily using the acronym PEMDAS – **P**arentheses, **E**xponents, **M**ultiplication and **D**ivision, **A**ddition and **S**ubtraction; the order of letters indicates the order of operations.

 Practice problems

Solutions to the practice problems are located in the back of this book.

1. Simplify the expression: –2(3 – 5 + 2).

2. Simplify the expression: 2 + 6 × 3.

3. Simplify the expression: (24 ÷ 3) × 5 – 6 + 2 × 7 – 3.

Subtraction of Whole Numbers With Regrouping

When subtracting **whole numbers** (i.e., 0, 1, 2, 3, etc.) it is important to arrange the numbers in columns with like place values in each column. Subtraction is started from the ones place, then it moves to the tens place, then to the hundreds, and so on. When a larger number is subtracted from a smaller number, it is necessary to regroup, or borrow, in order to subtract. Example 2.4 applies the following steps for subtracting whole numbers:

Step 1. Arrange the whole numbers in rows with like place values in like columns.

Step 2. Subtract in the ones place, regrouping if needed.

Step 3. Subtract in the tens place, regrouping if needed.

Step 4. Subtract in the hundreds place, regrouping if needed.

Step 5. Keep moving through each place, regrouping if needed.

(E) Example 2.4: *Simplify the expression: 539 – 58.*

Step 1. *Arrange the whole numbers in rows with like place values in like columns.*

$$
\begin{array}{r}
5\ 3\ 9 \\
-\ 5\ 8 \\
\hline
\end{array}
$$

Step 2. *Subtract in the ones place. No regrouping is needed since 8 subtracted from 9 is a whole number.*

$$
\begin{array}{r}
5\ 3\ 9 \\
-\ 5\ 8 \\
\hline
1
\end{array}
$$

Step 3. *Subtract in the tens place. Regrouping is needed since 5 subtracted from 3 is not a whole number. Think of 530 as 500 + 30. Borrowing 1 from 5 (or 100 from 500) and giving it to 30 makes 400 + 130. This is shown as "4" and "13":*

$$
\begin{array}{r}
4\ \ 13 \\
\cancel{5}\ \cancel{3}\ 9 \\
-\ \ 5\ 8 \\
\hline
8\ 1
\end{array}
$$

To finish the tens column, 13 – 5 = 8.

Step 4. *Subtract in the hundreds place. No regrouping is needed since 0 subtracted from 4 is a whole number.*

$$
\begin{array}{r}
4\ \ 13 \\
\cancel{5}\ \cancel{3}\ 9 \\
-\ \ 5\ 8 \\
\hline
4\ \ 8\ 1
\end{array}
$$

Work can be checked by adding the answer with the lesser of the numbers. The solution should equal the greater number (i.e., 481 + 58 = 539).

Step 5. *Since the greatest place value is the hundreds place, Step 4 is the last step needed.*

(P) *Practice problems*

Solutions to the practice problems are located in the back of this book.

1. Simplify the expression: 1,000 – 99.

2. Subtract 98,765 from 257,143.

3. Take 4,690 away from 7,081.

One- and Two-Step Word Problems With Whole Numbers

Word problems can be solved using the following steps:

Step 1.   Read the problem carefully.

Step 2.   Determine what is being asked.

Step 3.   Read the problem again and underline important words, numbers, and keywords based on what is being asked.

Step 4.   Set up the problem.

Step 5.   Solve the problem.

Step 6.   Check your answer. Is it reasonable?

Examples 2.5 and 2.6 apply these six steps.

Example 2.5:   *A medical assistant must give a patient 100 milligrams (mg) of a medication. The medication is supplied in 50 mg tablets. How many tablets should the patient receive?*

Step 1.   Read the problem carefully.

Step 2.   How many tablets should the patient receive?

Step 3.   A medical assistant must give a patient <u>100 mg</u> of a medication. The medication is <u>supplied in 50 mg tablets</u>. How many tablets should the <u>patient receive</u>?

Step 4.   The relationship between numbers is seen here. If each tablet is 50 mg and 100 mg is ordered, that means there are 2 groups of 50 in each 100. Therefore, the patient should receive $\frac{100}{50}$ or 2 tablets.

Step 5.   Mathematical reasoning leads to the conclusion that the patient should receive 2 tablets.

Step 6.   Two tablets at 50 mg apiece does equal 100 mg.

Example 2.6:   *A man wants to fence in his garden to keep out children and dogs. The garden is a rectangle that measures 25 feet wide by 30 feet long. Fencing costs $11 per foot. How much will the fence cost to build?*

Step 1.   Read the problem carefully.

Step 2.   How much will the fence cost?

Step 3.   A man wants to fence in his garden to keep out children and dogs. The garden is a rectangle that <u>measures 25 feet wide by 30 feet long</u>. Fencing <u>costs $11 per foot</u>. <u>How much will the fence cost to build?</u>

Step 4.   Add the four sides of the garden, then multiply that sum by the cost per foot:
(25 + 25 + 30 + 30) × $11

Step 5.   25 + 25 + 30 + 30 = 110
110 × $11 = $1,210

Step 6.   Recheck the addition and then the multiplication. Yes, this answer is reasonable.

(P) *Practice problems*

Solutions to the practice problems are located in the back of this book.

1. If $637,312 was the total income that a company expected for the year, and the total expenses listed in the annual budget were $248,165, how much profit would the company expect to make?

2.

A   C   D   B

In the diagram above, the distance between A and B is 30 inches and the distance between A and C is the distance between A and B divided by 3. What is the distance between C and B?

Addition and Subtraction of Fractions or Mixed Numbers With Unlike Denominators

To add or subtract fractions, first convert any **mixed numbers** into **improper fractions**. In other words, convert any number that represents the sum of a whole number and a **proper fraction** into a fraction whose numerator is greater than the denominator. Then, determine the least common denominator (LCD) of the fractions. The **least common denominator** is the smallest common multiple of the denominators or the least number that both denominators divide into evenly. Once the LCD is determined, rewrite each fraction as an equivalent fraction with the least common denominator. Add or subtract the numerators, while keeping the common denominator the same. Check to make sure the fraction is a **simplified fraction** (i.e., in its simplest form). This means that the only common factor between the numerator and the denominator of the fraction is 1.

The flow chart shown in Figure 2.1 explains the steps for adding or subtracting two fractions or mixed numbers. Example 2.7 uses this flow chart to add two fractions together.

ADDING OR SUBTRACTING FRACTIONS

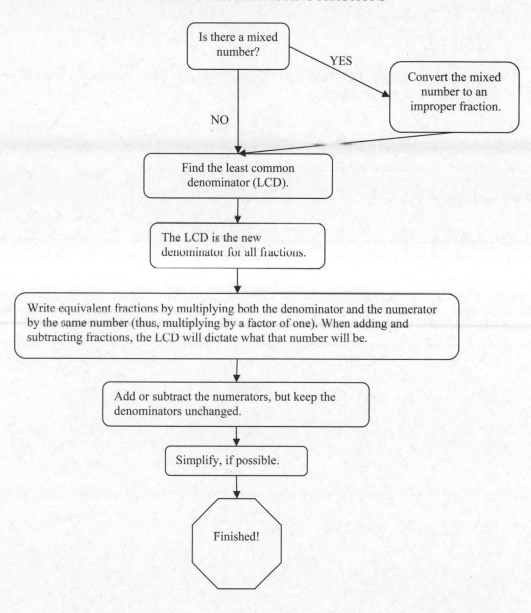

Figure 2.1 Steps for adding or subtracting two fractions or mixed numbers.

(E) *Example: 2.7*   *What is the sum of $\frac{1}{4} + \frac{1}{6}$?*

Using the flow chart:

- *There are no mixed numbers.*

- *The LCD of the denominators of 4 and 6 is 12. Therefore, each fraction needs to be changed to an equivalent fraction with a denominator of 12.*

$$\frac{1 \cdot 3}{4 \cdot 3} + \frac{1 \cdot 2}{6 \cdot 2} = \frac{3}{12} + \frac{2}{12}$$

- *Now that the two fractions have an LCD, add the numerators together, but keep the denominator unchanged:*

$$\frac{3}{12} + \frac{2}{12} = \frac{5}{12}$$

- *The final answer is $\frac{5}{12}$. This fraction is in simplest form since the numerator and denominator have no common factors other than 1.*

(P) Practice problems

Solutions to the practice problems are located in the back of this book.

1.   What is the sum of $\frac{2}{3}$ and $\frac{5}{12}$?

2.   Simplify the expression: $\frac{3}{8} + \frac{5}{6}$.

3.   Compute the difference of $3 - 5\frac{1}{3}$.

4.   Simplify the expression: $\frac{3}{15} - \frac{2}{25}$.

Division and Multiplication of Fractions or Mixed Numbers

To multiply fractions, first convert any mixed numbers into improper fractions. Then, simplify or reduce factors in the **numerator** (the top part of the fraction) with factors in the **denominator** (the bottom part of the fraction). Finally, multiply the numerators together and the denominators together. Check to make sure the fraction is a simplified fraction.

To divide fractions, first convert any mixed numbers into improper fractions. Keep the first fraction as it is written, but change the division sign to a multiplication sign, and flip the second fraction – put the numerator in the denominator and the original denominator in the numerator. Simplify or reduce factors in the numerator with factors in the denominator. Finally, multiply the numerators together and the denominators together. Check to make sure the fraction is in its simplest form.

The flow chart shown in Figure 2.2 explains these steps for dividing or multiplying two fractions or mixed numbers. Example 2.8 uses this flow chart to multiply two numbers together, and Example 2.9 uses it to divide two numbers.

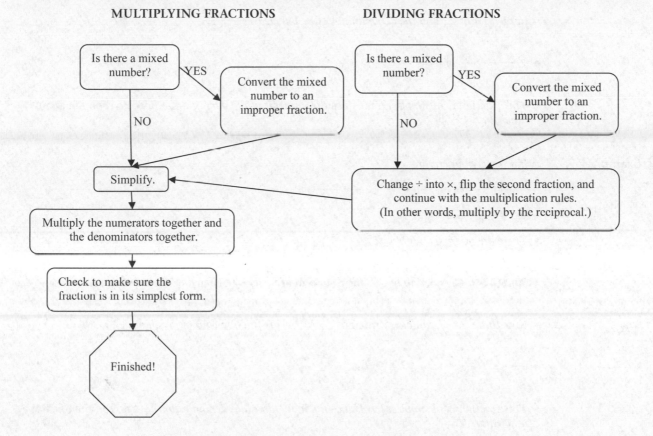

Figure 2.2 Steps for multiplying or dividing two fractions or mixed numbers.

(E) Example 2.8:   *Simplify the expression:* $2\frac{5}{8} \times 3\frac{1}{7}$.

Using the flow chart:

- *There are mixed numbers, so change them to improper fractions:*

$2\frac{5}{8} = \frac{21}{8}$ *and* $3\frac{1}{7} = \frac{22}{7}$, *so the problem becomes:* $\frac{21}{8} \times \frac{22}{7}$.

- *Note that* $\frac{21}{8} \times \frac{22}{7}$ *can be rewritten as* $\frac{21 \times 22}{8 \times 7}$. *Notice that this fraction can be simplified by dividing 7 into both the numerator of 21 and the denominator of 7 and by dividing 2 into the numerator of 22 and the denominator of 8. This leaves* $\frac{3 \times 11}{4 \times 1}$.

- $\frac{3 \times 11}{4 \times 1} = \frac{33}{4}$ *or* $8\frac{1}{4}$

- *This fraction is in simplest form since the numerator and denominator have no common factors other than 1.*

(E) Example 2.9:   *What is the quotient of* $\frac{3}{4} \div 7$?

Using the flow chart:

- *There are no mixed numbers.*

- *Since 7 is understood to be* $\frac{7}{1}$, *the reciprocal of* $\frac{7}{1}$ *is* $\frac{1}{7}$. *Therefore, the problem becomes* $\frac{3}{4} \times \frac{1}{7}$.

- *Note that* $\frac{3}{4} \times \frac{1}{7}$ *can be rewritten as* $\frac{3 \times 1}{4 \times 7}$. *This fraction cannot be simplified further.*

- $\frac{3 \times 1}{4 \times 7} = \frac{3}{28}$

- *This fraction is in simplest form since the numerator and denominator have no common factors other than 1.*

(P) Practice problems

Solutions to the practice problems are located in the back of this book.

1. What is the product of $2\frac{3}{8}$ and $\frac{2}{3}$?

2. Simplify the expression: $\frac{5}{3} \div \frac{4}{15}$.

3. Simplify the expression: $3 + \frac{2}{3} \times \frac{9}{10}$.

4. What is the quotient of $4\frac{2}{3} \div 6$?

Decimal Placement in a Product or Quotient

Multiplying and dividing decimal numbers is similar to multiplying and dividing nondecimal numbers. The main difference is that after the multiplication or division occurs in computations involving decimals, the correct placement of the decimal needs to be determined.

The process for multiplying decimals is as follows:

Step 1.   Set up the problem as if the numbers are whole numbers, without paying specific attention to the decimal points.

Step 2.   Multiply the numbers without paying specific attention to the decimal points.

Step 3.   Once the multiplication is complete, count the total number of decimal places in the factors.

Step 4.   Starting from the far right end of the product, count back (to the left) the number of decimal places you counted in step 3.

Step 5.   Put the decimal point in this spot. Finished!

Examples 2.10 and 2.11 apply these steps.

 Example 2.10:   *Multiply 5.62 and 0.3.*

Step 1.   562
          × 3

Step 2.   562
          × 3
          1686

Step 3.   *In this problem, we had 5.62 with 2 decimal places and 0.3 with just one decimal place. This is a total of 3 decimal places.*

Step 4.   *Count back 3 decimal places from the end of 1686.*

Step 5.   *The decimal belongs between the 1 and the 6. The final answer is 1.686.*

(E) *Example 2.11:*   *Simplify the expression: 11.4 cm × 7 cm × 3.06 cm.*

Step 1.

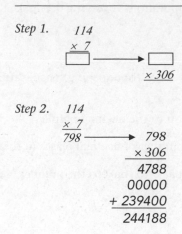

Step 2.   114
              × 7
              ─────
              798 ──────→   798
                           × 306
                           ──────
                            4788
                           00000
                         + 239400
                          ───────
                           244188

Step 3.   *In this problem, we had 11.4 with 1 decimal place and 3.06 with 2 decimal places. This is a total of 3 decimal places.*

Step 4.   *Count back 3 decimal places from the end of 244188.*

Step 5.   *The decimal belongs between the 4 and the 1. The final answer is 244.188 cm.*

The process for dividing decimals is as follows:

Step 1.   Set up the problem to be an equivalent problem in which the **divisor** (b in $\frac{a}{b}$) is a whole number by moving the decimal point in the **dividend** (a in $\frac{a}{b}$) the same number of places that the decimal point is moved in the divisor.

Step 2.   When performing long division, place the decimal point in the quotient directly above the decimal point in the dividend.

Step 3.   Divide the equation as if it were a whole number.

Example 2.12 applies these steps.

(E) *Example 2.12:*   *Simplify the expression: 0.48 ÷ 1.2.*

Step 1.   *Rewrite the problem as 4.8 ÷ 12 by moving the decimal point to the right in both the dividend and divisor. Alternatively, rewrite the problems as:*

$$1.2\overline{)0.48} \rightarrow 12\overline{)4.8}$$

Step 2.

$$12\overline{)4.8}^{\cdot}$$

Step 3.

$$\begin{array}{r} .4 \\ 12\overline{)4.8} \\ -\underline{4.8} \\ 0 \end{array}$$

Ⓟ *Practice problems*

Solutions to the practice problems are located in the back of this book.

1. Compute the product of 6.3 and 7.6.

2. Divide 0.05 into 0.710.

3. Simplify the expression: 0.3 × 0.12.

4. Simplify the expression: 0.4 ÷ 0.02.

Conversion Between Irrational Numbers and Approximate Decimal Form

Every **real number** is a number that appears on the number line as either a rational number or an irrational number. A **rational number** is any real number that can be written as a fraction, terminating (ending) decimal (e.g., 0.25), or repeating decimal (e.g., 0.212121..., which can be written as $0.\overline{21}$). **Irrational numbers** are numbers that cannot be written as fractions. Square roots, cube roots, and π are among the most common irrational numbers. Not all roots are irrational, however.

For example, $\sqrt{9}$ is a rational number (i.e., $\sqrt{9} = 3$). This is because $9 = 3^2$ and a square root is an inverse operation for squaring a number. Therefore, $\sqrt{9} = \sqrt{3^2} = 3$. When calculating the square root of a number that cannot be written as a square, such as $\sqrt{5}$ (i.e., there is no number that can be multiplied by itself to equal 5), it is possible to calculate a decimal approximation for that number. Calculators quickly and accurately give decimal approximations for irrational numbers. Without a calculator, the first digit can be approximated by thinking about what two square roots the desired root is between. For $\sqrt{5}$, the $\sqrt{5}$ is between $\sqrt{4} = 2$ and $\sqrt{9} = 3$. Therefore, $\sqrt{5}$ must be 2.___. The next digit, in the tenths place, can be estimated by reasoning that since 5 is closer to 4 than 9, it must be either 2.1 or 2.2. With the use of a calculator, it is approximately 2.236.

When given an irrational number in approximate decimal form, the process works in reverse. For example, 2.236 is greater than $\sqrt{4}$ and less than $\sqrt{9}$. Therefore, 2.236 is either $\sqrt{5}$, $\sqrt{6}$, $\sqrt{7}$, or $\sqrt{8}$. Since 2.236 is closer to 2 then 3, it is most likely the $\sqrt{5}$.

(P) *Practice problems*

Solutions to the practice problems are located in the back of this book.

1. Classify each of the following numbers as rational (Rat), irrational (Irr) or real (R).

    A) $\sqrt{36}$
    B) $-\sqrt{36}$
    C) $\sqrt{37}$
    D) $\dfrac{1}{3}$
    E) 0.6
    F) $0.\overline{66}$
    G) 0.7070007007 ...

2. What is an approximate decimal equivalent to $\sqrt[3]{10}$?

3. What irrational number can be approximated by the number 3.3166?

Calculation of Percents

Calculating percents is done by converting written statements into mathematical equations and solving for an unknown. Generically, the written statements read: "What *percent* of a *whole* is the *part*?"

There are three types of percent problems because there are three things to look for. The question many ask is to find the *part*, or the *whole*, or the *percent* (see Examples 2.13 to 2.15).

The steps for solving percent problems are the following:

Step 1.   Change the written statement into a mathematical equation.
Keep in mind:
- The word *of* translates into multiply.
- The word *is* translates into equals.
- The decimal form of the percent should be used in the equation.

Step 2.   Solve for the unknown quantity.

Step 3.   Rewrite the statement and make sure that the answer is reasonable.

(E) Example 2.13:   *15% of 500 is what number?*

Step 1. $0.15 \times 500 = \square$

Step 2. $0.15 \times 500 = 75$

Step 3.   *15% of 500 is 75. This seems reasonable since 15% of 500 should be considerably less than 500. Since 75 is less than 500, the answer is reasonable.*

(E) Example 2.14:   *25% of what number is 8?*

Step 1. $0.25 \times \square = 8$

Step 2. $\dfrac{0.25 \times \square}{0.25} = \dfrac{8}{0.25}$

Step 3.   *25% of 32 is 8. This seems reasonable since 25% of 32 should be considerably than 32. Since 8 is less than 32, the answer is reasonable.*

(E) Example 2.15:   *What percent of 250 is 10?*

Step 1. $\square \times 250 = 10$

Step 2. $\dfrac{\square \times 250}{250} = \dfrac{10}{250} = \dfrac{1}{25} = 0.04$

So, $\square = 0.04$ or 4%.

Step 3.   *4% of 250 is 10. This seems reasonable since 4% of 250 should be considerably less than 250. Since 10 is less than 250, the answer is reasonable.*

When solving a percent decrease or increase problem, the 'whole' is the original value, or the value that existed first. As shown in Example 2.16, to calculate the percent increase or decrease of a number, calculate the change between the original and new values, and divide by the original value as follows:

$$\text{percent decrease} = \frac{\text{original value} - \text{new value}}{\text{original value}} \times 100$$

$$\text{percent increase} = \frac{\text{new value} - \text{original value}}{\text{original value}} \times 100$$

 Example 2.16: *An amount goes up from 20 to 45. What is the percent increase?*

Step 1. *percent increase* $= \dfrac{\text{new value} - \text{original value}}{\text{original value}} \times 100$

percent increase $= \dfrac{45 - 20}{20} \times 100$

Step 2. *percent increase* $= \dfrac{25}{20} \times 100$

$= 1.25 \times 100$

$= 125\%$

Step 3. *125% of 20 is 25. This seems reasonable since 125% of 20 should be slightly greater than 20. Since 25 is a little greater than 20, the answer is reasonable.*

P *Practice problems*

Solutions to the practice problems are located in the back of this book.

1. What is $4\frac{1}{4}\%$ of 200?

2. What percent of 25 is 5?

3. An amount of 50 decreases by 5. What is the percent decrease?

Conversion Between Percents, Fractions, and Decimals

Conversion among percents, fractions, and decimals can be accomplished many different ways. The following diagram shows all of the possible conversions.

FRACTION ⟷ PERCENT ⟷ DECIMAL

Figure 2.3 All possible conversions among percents, fractions, and decimals.

Converting from fractions to decimals:
There are two different methods that convert fractions to decimals. One method is to divide the numerator by the denominator. This method works for all fractions. Some fractions convert to terminating decimal numbers, as shown in Example 2.17.

(E) Example 2.17: *Convert $\frac{3}{125}$ to a decimal.*

Divide the numerator (dividend) by the denominator (divisor). If using long division, be sure to place the divisor on the outside of the fraction bar and place the decimal point in the quotient directly above the decimal point in the dividend:

$$125\overline{)3.000} = 0.024$$

Some fractions convert to repeating decimal numbers, as shown in Example 2.18.

(E) Example 2.18: *Convert $\frac{1}{6}$ to a decimal.*

In the following problem, 6 repeats itself. Therefore, it may be necessary to round the answer to a certain place value. If rounded to the nearest thousandth, the answer is 0.167. Or, the exact answer could be written as $0.1\overline{6}$. The bar above the 6 means that 6 will repeat forever:

$$6\overline{)1.00000000} = 0.16666666$$

The second method for converting fractions to decimals works only for fractions whose denominators are powers of 10 (i.e., 10, 100, 1,000, etc.). In these cases, the numerators of the fractions expressed become the digits in the decimal forms of the numbers and the numbers of zeros in the denominators determine the placement of the decimal points. If a fraction had a denominator of 10, for example, then the decimal form would have one decimal place. If the fraction had a denominator of 100, then the decimal form would have two decimal places. If the fraction had a denominator of 1,000, then the decimal form would have three decimal places, etc.

When converting from fractions to decimals, it may be helpful to keep Table 2.1 in mind. This table displays fractions whose denominators are powers of 10 and the numbers written in decimal form:

Table 2.1 Fractions Whose Denominations are Powers of 10 and Equivalent Decimal Representation.

Tenths	Hundredths	Thousandths	Ten thousandths	One-hundred thousandths
$\frac{1}{10}$	$\frac{1}{100}$	$\frac{1}{1,000}$	$\frac{1}{10,000}$	$\frac{1}{100,000}$
0.1	0.01	0.001	0.0001	0.00001

(E) *Example 2.19:* *Convert $\frac{1}{5}$ to a decimal.*

$\frac{1}{5} = \frac{2}{10}$ *Since the denominator has one zero, the decimal form of the number has one decimal place.*

0.2 Both $\frac{2}{10}$ and 0.2 are referred to as two-tenths.

Converting from decimals to fractions:

To convert from decimals[1] to fractions, the decimal number expressed becomes the numerator of the fraction. The number of decimal places to the right of the decimal determines the value of the denominator. If the decimal form of a number only had one decimal place, for example, then the number would be divided by 10. If the decimal form of a number had two decimal places, then the number would be divided by 100. If the decimal form of a number had three decimal places, then the number would be divided by 1,000, etc.

The steps for converting from decimal forms to fractions are as follows:

Step 1. Write the digits of the decimal number in the numerator of the fraction.

Step 2. Write a number that is a power of 10 as the denominator. The number should have as many zeros as there are decimal places to the right of the decimal.

Step 3. Write the decimal fraction in simplest form.

Example 2.20 applies these three steps.

(E) *Example 2.20:* *Convert 0.025 to a fraction in simplest form.*

Step 1. $\frac{25}{?}$

Step 2. $\frac{25}{1,000}$

Step 3. *In this example, to rewrite this fraction in simplest form, divide both the numerator and denominator by the* **greatest common factor** *(the greatest number that will divide into both of the numbers), 25:*

$$\frac{25 \div 25}{1,000 \div 25} = \frac{1}{40}$$

Note that in words, 0.025 and $\frac{25}{1,000}$ are both read as twenty-five thousandths.

---

[1] This study guide only discusses the conversion from terminating decimals to fractions. It does not discuss converting repeating decimals to fractions.

Converting from fractions to percents:

There are two different methods that convert fractions to **percents** (ratios whose denominators are 100). Shown in Example 2.21, one method is to convert the fraction to a decimal. Then, convert the decimal to a percent.

(E) *Example 2.21:* *Convert $\frac{5}{8}$ to a percent.*

First, convert the fraction to a decimal as previously discussed:

$$\frac{5}{8} = 0.625$$

Then, convert the decimal to a percent by multiplying by 100 and adding the % symbol:

$$0.625 = 62.5\%$$

This method works for all fractions. The second method works for fractions whose denominators can be written as powers of 10 (i.e., 10, 100, 1,000, etc.). First, write the fraction as an equivalent fraction over 100. Then, write the numerator of this fraction with the % symbol, as shown in Example 2.22.

(E) *Example 2.22:* *Convert $\frac{7}{10}$ to a percent.*

First, write the fraction as an equivalent fraction over 100.

$$\frac{7}{10} = \frac{7 \times 10}{10 \times 10} = \frac{70}{100}$$

Then, write the numerator of this fraction with the % symbol:

$$\frac{70}{100} = 70\%$$

Converting from percents to fractions:

Demonstrated in Example 2.23, percents can be written as fractions by performing the following:

Step 1. Remove the % symbol.

Step 2. Write the number from step 1 in the numerator of the fraction and write 100 in the denominator.

Step 3. Simplify the fraction.

(E) *Example 2.23:* *Convert 35% to a fraction.*

Step 1.   *35*

Step 2. $\frac{35}{100}$

Step 3. $\frac{35 \div 5}{100 \div 5} = \frac{7}{20}$

Converting from percents to decimals:

Since percent literally means out of 100, converting a percent to a decimal is a process of dividing by 100. Therefore, a general rule for converting a percent to a decimal is to remove the % symbol and move the decimal point left two places, as shown in Example 2.24.

 Example 2.24:   *Convert 78% to a decimal.*

Remove the % symbol and move the decimal point left two places:
78% = 0.78

Converting from decimals to percents:

Since converting from decimals to percents is an inverse process of converting percents to decimals, multiply the decimal by 100 and add the % symbol. Stated another way, move the decimal point right two places and add the % symbol, as done in Example 2.25.

 Example 2.25:   *Convert 0.045 to a percent.*

Move the decimal point right two places and add the % symbol:
0.045 = 4.5%

 Practice problems

Solutions to the practice problems are located in the back of this book.

1. Convert 319% to a
    a. fraction.
    b. decimal.

2. Convert 0.681 to a
    a. percent.
    b. fraction.

3. Convert $\frac{3}{4}$ to a
    a. percent.
    b. decimal.

Comparison of Rational Numbers

A rational number can be either a fraction or a decimal. Ordering rational numbers by size can often be useful in solving real-world problems. To determine whether one decimal is greater than another decimal, compare the digits in each of the place values. Beginning with the digit in the greatest place value, determine which number has the greatest value. If the two values are the same, then look at the digit in the next greatest place value and compare the two. Continue in this way until all the numbers are ordered from greatest to least (see Example 2.26).

(E) Example 2.26: *Which fraction is greater: 0.778 or 0.788?*

Both numbers have a zero in the ones place. The next greatest place value is the tenths place. Both numbers have a seven in this position. The next greatest place value is the hundredths position. The number 0.778 has a 7 in this place value, while 0.788 has an 8. Since 8 is greater than 7, 0.788 is greater than 0.778.

To determine whether one fraction is greater than another, find a common denominator for the fractions. As demonstrated in Example 2.27, the fraction with the greater numerator is the greater fraction.

(E) Example: 2.27 *Which fraction is greater: $\frac{2}{3}$ or $\frac{3}{4}$?*

$$\frac{2}{3} = \frac{8}{12} \text{ and } \frac{3}{4} = \frac{9}{12}$$

Since $\frac{9}{12} > \frac{8}{12}$, then $\frac{3}{4} > \frac{2}{3}$.

The following describes another method of determining which of two fractions is greater. In the general case, let $\frac{a}{b}$ and $\frac{c}{d}$ be the fractions to compare, where a, b, c, d are integers and $b \neq 0$ and $d \neq 0$. Multiply to create a common denominator, which allows for the comparison of the numbers:

$$\frac{a}{b} \times \frac{d}{d} = \frac{ad}{bd} \text{ and } \frac{c}{d} \times \frac{b}{b} = \frac{bc}{bd}$$

Since the two fractions now have a common denominator of bd, compare $\frac{ad}{bd}$ with $\frac{bc}{bd}$. If ad is greater than bc, then $\frac{a}{b}$ is greater than $\frac{c}{d}$. Example 2.28 provides a numerical example of this procedure.

(E) Example 2.28: *Order the following fractions from least to greatest: $\frac{67}{100}, \frac{2}{3}, \frac{3}{5}$.*

The least common denominator of 100, 3, and 5 is 300. These three fractions can be rewritten as follows:

$$\frac{67}{100} = \frac{201}{300} \qquad \frac{2}{3} = \frac{200}{300} \qquad \frac{3}{5} = \frac{180}{300}$$

Based on these equivalent fractions, $\frac{180}{300} < \frac{200}{300} < \frac{201}{100}$. This means that $\frac{3}{5} < \frac{2}{3} < \frac{67}{100}$.

To compare fractions and decimals together, either convert all fractions to decimals or convert all decimals to fractions.

(P) *Practice problems*

Solutions to the practice problems are located in the back of this book.

1. Which fraction is greater: $\frac{4}{7}$ or $\frac{5}{9}$?

2. Order the following rational numbers from least to greatest: $\frac{2}{9}$, 0.222, $\frac{11}{50}$.

Estimation of the Solution to a Problem

There are many ways to calculate the approximate value, or **estimation**, of the solution to a problem; however, for clarity, only one will be presented here. Round the numbers so that there is only one nonzero digit in each number. This means that the first digit in the number will not be a zero but all the other digits will be zeros. Then perform the indicated calculations of addition, subtraction, multiplication, or division.

(E) Example 2.29: *Estimate the product: 76,899 × 634.*

Round each number so that there is only one nonzero digit in each number.

76,899 = 80,000 – 8 is the only nonzero digit in this number
634 = 600 – 6 is the only nonzero digit in this number

$$
\begin{array}{r}
80,000 \\
\times\ 600 \\
\hline
48,000,000
\end{array}
$$

The estimated product is 48,000,000.

Actual calculation:
$$
\begin{array}{r}
76,899 \\
\times\ 634 \\
\hline
48,753,966
\end{array}
$$

The estimated calculation is reasonably close to the actual answer.

(P) Practice problems

Solutions to the practice problems are located in the back of this book.

1. A trip from San Francisco, CA to Kansas City, MO is 1,865 miles. A newer car gets 32 miles per gallon of gas. Estimate how many gallons of gas it will take to make this trip.

2. Estimate the solution to 257,143 – 98,765.

Reconciliation of a Checking or Savings Account

Word problems can be solved using the following steps:

Step 1. Read the problem carefully.

Step 2. Determine what is being asked.

Step 3. Read the problem again and underline important words, numbers, and keywords based on what is being asked.

Step 4. Set up the problem.

Step 5. Solve the problem.

Step 6. Check your answer. Is it reasonable?

To balance, or reconcile, a checking or savings account, first group the deposits and add them together, then group the checks and add them together. Next, add the deposits to the previous balance and subtract the checks from that result. Finally, subtract the service charge and add the interest. Example 2.30 applies these steps.

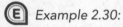 Example 2.30:   *Reconcile this checking account for the month of January 2009. The previous balance is $1,005.34. Deposits were made for $32.56, $125.42, $675.90, and $831.89. Checks were written for $85.98, $1,045.00, $16.57, $5.12, and $79.00. Interest earned is $1.79 and there is a service charge of $5.00. What is the balance after reconciling this account?*

Step 1.   *Read the problem carefully.*

Step 2.   *What is the balance after reconciling this account?*

Step 3.   *Reconcile this checking account for the month of January 2009. The previous balance is $1,005.34. Deposits were made for $32.56, $125.42, $675.90, and $831.89. Checks were written for $85.98, $1,045.00, $16.57, $5.12, and $79.00. Interest earned is $1.79 and there is a service charge of $5.00. What is the balance after reconciling this account?*

Step 4.   *Previous balance + deposits – checks – service charge + interest = reconciled account*

Step 5.   *Previous balance = $1,005.34*

Deposits = $32.56 + $125.42 + $675.90 + $831.89 = $1,665.77
Checks = $85.98 + $1,045.00 + $16.57 + $5.12 + $79.00 = $1,231.67
Service charge = $5.00
Interest = $1.79
Balance = $1,005.34 + $1,665.77 – $1,231.67 – $5.00 + $1.79 = $1,436.23

The reconciled account balance is $1,436.23 for the month of January 2009.

Step 6.   *Recheck your multiplication, addition, and subtraction. Yes, this answer is reasonable.*

Practice problems

Solutions to the practice problems are located in the back of this book.

1.

Beginning balance: $1,123.42	
Debits	Credits
$ 247.16	
$ 72.50	$ 420.00
$ 675.00	
$ 43.80	
$ 64.00	

The transactions made in a person's checking account last month are shown in the table above. What was the checking account balance at the end of the month?

2. Reconcile this savings account for the quarter ending March 2009. The previous balance is $9,369.23. Deposits were made for $156.65 and $1,316.00. Withdrawals were made for $3,500.00, $695.00, and $75.00. There is a service charge of $10.00. What is the balance after reconciling this account?

Calculation of Take-Home Pay

Word problems can be solved using the following steps:

Step 1.   Read the problem carefully.

Step 2.   Determine what is being asked.

Step 3.   Read the problem again and underline important words, numbers, and keywords based on what is being asked.

Step 4.   Set up the problem.

Step 5.   Solve the problem.

Step 6.   Check your answer. Is it reasonable?

To determine the amount of **take-home pay** for a given time period, add all of the **deductions** together and then subtract that total from the beginning salary. Example 2.31 applies the steps above to determine an employee's take-home pay.

 Example 2.31:   *A medical assistant works at a local hospital and earns $15.83 per hour. The assistant works three 12-hour shifts per week and is paid every 2 weeks. The assistant's deductions each pay period are: federal tax $116.78, federal insurance $59.28, state tax $84.68, retirement plan $75.00, and health insurance $91.23. What is the assistant's take-home pay every 2 weeks?*

Step 1.   *Read the problem carefully.*

Step 2.   *What is the assistant's take home pay every 2 weeks?*

Step 3.   *A medical assistant works at a local hospital and earns $15.83 per hour. The assistant works three 12-hour shifts per week and is paid every 2 weeks. The assistant's deductions each pay period are: federal tax $116.78, federal insurance $59.28, state tax $84.68, retirement plan $75.00, and health insurance $91.23. What is the assistant's take-home pay every 2 weeks?*

Step 4.   *Beginning salary – deductions = take-home pay.*

Step 5.   *Beginning salary = $15.83 × 36 hours × 2 weeks = $1,139.76*
Deductions = $116.78 + $59.28 + $84.68 + $75.00 + $91.23 = $426.97
Take-Home Pay = $1,139.76 – $426.97 = $712.79

The take-home pay is $712.79 every 2 weeks.

Step 6.   *Recheck your multiplication, addition, and subtraction. Yes, this answer is reasonable.*

Practice problems

Solutions to the practice problems are located in the back of this book.

1.

Expenses	Amounts
Rent	$350.00
Food	$320.00
Utilities	$215.60
Car expenses	$240.00

An employee's take-home pay from her part-time job is $1,280.50 each month. After paying the monthly expenses listed above, how much money does the employee have left from her monthly income?

2. A nurse earns $28.31 per hour at a local hospital. Deductions for each 2-week pay period are the following:
   - federal taxes = $256.18
   - federal insurance = $124.95
   - state tax = $198.12
   - retirement plan = $100.00
   - health insurance = $89.51

If the nurse works three 12-hour shifts each week, what is the take home pay every 2 weeks?

Cost of a Given Set of Items

Word problems can be solved using the following steps:

Step 1.   Read the problem carefully.

Step 2.   Determine what is being asked.

Step 3.   Read the problem again and underline important words, numbers, and keywords based on what is being asked.

Step 4.   Set up the problem.

Step 5.   Solve the problem.

Step 6.   Check your answer. Is it reasonable?

To determine the given cost of a set of items, select the items to be purchased and add their prices together, as done in Example 2.32.

(E) Example 2.32:   *A customer is shopping in a grocery store and purchases the following:*

- *1 dozen eggs for $1.19*
- *1 gallon of milk for $2.99*
- *2 steaks (2.46 pounds each) for $4.98 per pound*
- *1 loaf of bread for $2.49*
- *1 liter of soda for $0.99*

What is the total cost of the groceries before tax?

Step 1.   *Read the problem carefully.*

Step 2.   *What is the total cost of the groceries before tax?*

Step 3.   *A customer is shopping in a grocery store and purchases the following:*

- *1 dozen eggs for $1.19*
- *1 gallon of milk for $2.99*
- *2 steaks (2.46 pounds each) for $4.98 per pound*
- *1 loaf of bread for $2.49*
- *1 liter of soda for $0.99*

What is the total cost of the groceries before tax?

Step 4.   *Egg price + milk price + number of steaks × weight of steaks × steak price + bread price + soda price*

Step 5.   *Total cost* $= \$1.19 + \$2.99 + (2 \times 2.46 \times \$4.98) + \$2.49 + \$0.99$
$= \$1.19 + \$2.99 + \$24.50 + \$2.49 + \$0.99$
$= \$32.16$

Step 6.   *Recheck your multiplication, addition, and subtraction. Yes, this answer is reasonable.*

Practice problems

Solutions to the practice problems are located in the back of this book.

1.

Expenses	Amounts
Employees' Salaries	$184,000.23
Supplies and Postage	$ 9,745.17
Phone and Utilities	$ 6,300.99
Office Rent	$ 29,400.45
Travel	$ 12,570.61

The annual budget for the Problem Solving Office includes the expenses listed above. Find the total of the expenses listed in the annual budget.

2. Hot Dogs .... $1.75 each
    Hamburgers........ $2.25 each
    Sodas .... $1.19 each
    Potato Chips....... $0.99 per bag
    Sandwiches .... $2.10 each
    Cookies .... $0.65 each

The list above displays a menu at a deli. A customer bought 2 hot dogs, 1 hamburger, 2 sodas, 1 bag of potato chips, and 3 cookies. How much did the customer's purchases cost?

Materials and Costs of Planning an Event

Word problems can be solved using the following steps:

Step 1. Read the problem carefully.

Step 2. Determine what is being asked.

Step 3. Read the problem again and underline important words, numbers, and keywords based on what is being asked.

Step 4. Set up the problem.

Step 5. Solve the problem.

Step 6. Check your answer. Is it reasonable?

Similar calculations can be used to determine the quantity of material needed or the cost of planning for an event. To determine the cost of an event, for example, multiply the number of people attending by each of the items they will receive and add those results together. If everyone attending is receiving the same items, add all the items first, then multiply by the number of people attending. Example 2.33 provides an example of this computation.

Ⓔ *Example 2.33:* *A catered retirement dinner is being planned for 75 people. The catering company charges the following per person:*

- *$9.65 for a chicken entrée*
- *$10.95 for a steak entrée*
- *$2.45 for a mixed salad*
- *$3.15 for dessert*
- *$1.05 for iced tea*

Thirty-four people select the chicken entrée, and the rest choose the steak entree. If everyone is served a mixed salad, dessert, and iced tea, what is the total cost for the retirement reception?

Step 1. *Read the problem carefully.*

Step 2. *What is the cost of planning this event?*

Step 3. *A catered retirement dinner is being planned for 75 people. The catering company charges the following per person:*

- *$9.65 for the chicken entrée*
- *$10.95 for the steak entrée*
- *$2.45 for a mixed salad*
- *$3.15 for dessert*
- *$1.05 for iced tea*

Thirty-four people select the chicken entrée, and the rest choose the steak entrée. If everyone is served a mixed salad, dessert, and iced tea, what is the total cost for the retirement reception?

Step 4. *Total cost = (people × chicken entrée cost) + (people × steak entrée cost) + all people × (salad cost + dessert cost + iced tea cost)*

Step 5. *people × chicken entrée = 34 × $9.65 = $328.10*
people × steak entrée = 41 × $10.95 = $448.95
all people = 75 × ($2.45 + $3.15 + $1.05) = $498.75
Total cost = $328.10 + $448.95 + $498.75 = $1,275.80

The cost of the retirement dinner is $1,275.80.

Step 6. *Recheck your multiplication, addition, and subtraction. Yes, this answer is reasonable.*

Practice problems

Solutions to the practice problems are located in the back of this book.

1. Calla lilies and baby's breath tied together with ribbon will be used for the corsages and boutonnieres for a bridal party. Calla lilies are $2.35 per corsage or boutonniere, baby's breath is $0.95 per corsage or boutonniere, and ribbon is $0.15 per foot. There will be 15 corsages and 15 boutonnieres. Each arrangement takes 9 inches of ribbon. What is the total cost?

2.

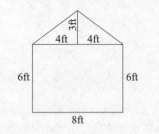

A homeowner wishes to lay down carpeting in the three areas shown in the figure above. How much carpeting is needed to cover this area?

One- and Two-Step Word Problems With Fractions or Decimals

Word problems can be solved using the following steps:

Step 1.   Read the problem carefully.

Step 2.   Determine what is being asked.

Step 3.   Read the problem again and underline important words, numbers, and keywords based on what is being asked.

Step 4.   Set up the problem.

Step 5.   Solve the problem.

Step 6.   Check your answer. Is it reasonable?

When solving addition or subtraction problems involving fractions, remember to use a common denominator (see Example 2.34). When solving addition or subtraction problems involving decimals, remember to line-up the decimal points (see Example 2.35).

Ⓔ Example 2.34:   *A coin consists of $\frac{1}{5}$ zinc, $\frac{1}{10}$ manganese, and $\frac{1}{40}$ copper. The rest of the coin is nickel. What fraction of the coin is nickel?*

Step 1.   *Read the problem carefully.*

Step 2.   *How much of the coin is nickel?*

Step 3.   *A coin consists of $\frac{1}{5}$ zinc, $\frac{1}{10}$ manganese, and $\frac{1}{40}$ copper. The rest of the coin is nickel. What fraction of the coin is nickel?*

Step 4.   *Fraction nickel = 1 – (fraction zinc + fraction manganese + fraction copper)*

Step 5.   *Fraction nickel* $= 1 - \left(\dfrac{1}{5} + \dfrac{1}{10} + \dfrac{1}{40} \right)$

$= 1 - \left(\dfrac{8}{40} + \dfrac{4}{40} + \dfrac{1}{40} \right)$

$= 1 - \dfrac{13}{40}$

$= \dfrac{27}{40}$ *of the coin is nickel.*

Step 6.   *Recheck your addition. Yes, this answer is reasonable.*

(E) *Example 2.35:* *A man works for a company that makes drinking straws. The man works in the quality control department and gets paid $10.20 per hour. He knows that each straw weighs 1.2 grams. He weighs a box marked "50 straws" and finds that it weighs 58.8 grams. Should he approve the box?*

Step 1.   *Read the problem carefully.*

Step 2.   *Should a box of 50 straws weigh 58.8 grams?*

Step 3.   *A man works for a company that makes drinking straws. The man works in the quality control department and gets paid $10.20 per hour. He knows that <u>each straw weighs 1.2 grams</u>. He weighs a <u>box marked "50 straws"</u> and finds that it <u>weighs 58.8 grams</u>. <u>Should he approve the box?</u>*

Step 4.   *Weight box should be = weight of each straw × 50 straws*
Compare this weight to 58.8 grams.

Step 5.   *Weight box should be = 1.2 × 50 = 60 grams*

The man should not approve the box since it is underweight (one straw seems to be missing).

Step 6.   *The answer is reasonable since the man should be looking for a weight of 60 grams per box.*

(P) Practice problems

Solutions to the practice problems are located in the back of this book.

1.   Juan is making a gadget that requires $3\frac{1}{2}$ feet of red wire, $5\frac{1}{3}$ feet of green wire, and $1\frac{3}{4}$ feet of yellow wire. How many total feet of wire does he need?

2.   If you purchase items that have a total cost of $42.20 before taxes, how much tax will you pay if the tax is 0.065 cents per dollar? (Round answer to the nearest cent.)

Word Problems Involving Percents

When solving an application problem involving percentages, refer to the generic statement, "What percent of a whole is the part?" The *whole* is the original value, or the value that existed first. The *part* is the new value. For example, if a test is worth 80 points and a student gets 71 correct, the *whole* is the entire value of points possible, 80, and the *part* is the portion that the student got correct, 71. The percent correct would be $71 \div 80 = 0.8875$ or 88.75%.

The first step to solving an application problem involving percentages is to rewrite the question in terms of a generic, "What percent of a whole is the part?" statement. Then, follow through with the three steps for solving percent problems as follows:

Step 1. Change the written statement into a mathematical equation.
Keep in mind:
- the word *of* translates into multiply.
- the word *is* translates into equals.
- the decimal form of the percent should be used in the equation.

Step 2. Solve for the unknown quantity.

Step 3. Rewrite the statement and make sure that the answer is reasonable.

Example 2.36 applies these three steps to a word problem involving percentages.

(E) Example 2.36: *A student needs 70% to pass a test that is worth 35 points. How many points must the student earn to pass the test?*

Step 1. $0.70 \times 35 = \square$

Step 2. $0.70 \times 35 = 24.5$

Step 3. *70% of 35 is 24.5. This seems reasonable since 70% of 35 should be slightly less than 35. Since 24.5 is less than 35, the answer is reasonable.*

(P) Practice problems

Solutions to the practice problems are located in the back of this book.

1. The enrollment at a college went up from 625 students to 710 students over a period of 1 year. What was the percent of increase? Round the answer to the nearest tenth of a percent.

2. On Monday, 3 students out of a class of 24 were absent from class. What percent of the students were absent from class?

3. The 18 students who received an A in a mathematics class made up 30% of the students in the class. Find the total number of students in the class.

Word Problems Involving Ratios, Proportions, and Rates of Change

A **ratio** is used to express a relationship between two quantities. Ratios can be written as fractions (e.g., $\frac{4}{5}$), with colons (e.g., 4:5), or with words (e.g., the ratio 4 to 5). Ratios are always written in simplest form, as shown in Example 2.37.

Example 2.37: *Express 30 minutes to 4 hours as a ratio of minutes in fraction form.*

First, change the 4 hours to minutes:

4 hours × 60 minutes = 240 minutes

Then, write the ratio in fraction form keeping the order of the ratio indicated in the problem – the number after the word "to" is the denominator of the fraction:

$$\frac{30}{240} = \frac{1}{8}$$

The ratio of 30 minutes to 4 hours is $\frac{1}{8}$.

A **proportion** states that two ratios are equal. When setting up a proportion, the numerators of both ratios must be in the same units and the denominators of both ratios must be in the same units. To solve a proportion use this formula:

$$\frac{\text{units of an item}}{\text{units of a different item}} = \frac{\text{units of an item}}{\text{units of a different item}}$$

Use the method called finding cross products to solve the equation. This means that the numerator of the ratio on the left side of the proportion is multiplied by the denominator of the ratio on the right side of the proportion. Then, the numerator of the ratio on the right side of the proportion is multiplied by the denominator of the ratio on the left side of the proportion (i.e., if you have $\frac{a}{b} = \frac{c}{d}$, then to solve it you have $ad = bc$). Example 2.38 demonstrates how to set up and solve a proportion.

Example 2.38: *Last year at the local community college 1,250 students were enrolled in 50 sections of beginning algebra. This year 1,550 students will enroll in beginning algebra. If the number of students per section is the same for each section and does not change from year to year, how many sections will need to be offered?*

First set up the proportion. Use the first sentence as the ratio on the left side of the equation and the second sentence as the ratio on the right side of the equation. Remember that the numerators of both ratios must have the same units and the denominators of both ratios must have the same units:

$$\frac{1,250 \text{ students}}{50 \text{ sections}} = \frac{1,550 \text{ students}}{a \text{ sections}}$$

Notice how the students are in the numerators of both ratios and sections are in the denominators of both ratios.

Next, use the method of cross products to solve:

1,250 × a sections = 1,550 × 50

$$\frac{1,250 \times a \text{ sections}}{1,250} = \frac{77,500}{1,250}$$

a sections = 62

62 sections of beginning algebra need to be offered.

Rate of change problems use proportions to determine the difference in completion times for a given task, as shown in Example 2.39.

 Example 2.39:   *Student A reads 10 pages an hour. Student B reads 18 pages per hour. Each has a 288 page book to complete this weekend. At this rate, how much sooner will Student B complete the book compared to Student A?*

First, set up a proportion for Student A to determine how many hours it will take to read the book:

$$\frac{10 \text{ pages}}{1 \text{ hour}} = \frac{288 \text{ pages}}{A \text{ hours}}$$

Use the method of cross products to solve:

$$10 \times A = 288 \times 1$$

$$\frac{10A}{10} = \frac{288}{10}$$

$$A = 28.8 \text{ hours}$$

It will take Student A 28.8 hours to read the book.

Now, set up a proportion for Student B to determine how many hours it will take to read the book:

$$\frac{18 \text{ pages}}{1 \text{ hour}} = \frac{288 \text{ pages}}{B \text{ hours}}$$

Use the method of cross products to solve:

$$18 \times B = 288 \times 1$$

$$\frac{18B}{18} = \frac{288}{18}$$

$$B = 16 \text{ hours}$$

It will take Student B 16 hours to read the book.

Finally, subtract Students B's hours from Student A's hours:

$$28.8 \text{ hours} - 16 \text{ hours} = 12.8 \text{ hours}.$$

Student B will complete the book 12.8 hours faster than Student A.

Ⓟ *Practice problems*

Solutions to the practice problems are located in the back of this book.

1. If John can travel 130 miles in 2 hours, how far can he travel in 5 hours if he travels at the same rate of speed?

2. A club has 9 male and 21 female members. What is the ratio of male to female members in the club?

3. The following amounts of beverages are needed to serve 72 people: 4 gallons of punch, 3 gallons of lemonade, and 2 gallons of tea. How many total gallons of these beverages are needed to serve 240 people?

Conversion Between Roman and Arabic Numerals

The **Roman numeral system** is a system of writing numbers using a combination of M, D, C, L, X, V, and I. The **Arabic numeral system** is a system of writing numbers using a combination of 0, 1, 2, 3, 4, 5, 6, 7, 8, and 9.

To change Roman numerals to Arabic numerals, as in Example 2.40, use the following rules:

1.   Write from left to right as a sum.

2.   Begin with the largest possible value: M = 1,000, D = 500, C = 100, L = 50, X = 10, V = 5, and I = 1.

3.   When I, X, or C is used to the left of a larger value, subtract its value from the larger value.

(E) *Example 2.40:*   *An antique gold coin is stamped with the date MCCXXXIV. What is this date in Arabic numerals?*

Write from left to right as a sum:

M = 1,000, so place a 1 in the thousands place.

CC = 100 + 100 = 200, so place a 2 in the hundreds place.

XXX = 10 + 10 + 10 = 30, so place a 3 in the tens place.

IV = 5 − 1 = 4, so place a 4 in the ones place.

1,000 + 200 + 30 + 4 = 1,234

The resulting Arabic numeral is 1234.

To change Arabic numerals to Roman numerals, as in Example 2.41, use the following rules:

1.   Write from left to right.

2.   Take each place value and change to a Roman numeral.

3.   I, X, and C may be written two or three times in a row as long as they are not followed by a larger value.

4.   Use I, X, and C to the left of larger values to indicate subtraction from the larger values.

5.   V, L, and D are never used to the left of a larger value.

6.   V, L, and D are never used more than one time.

(E) *Example 2.41:*   *Al Khwarizmi wrote the first book of algebra in 825 C.E. Write this date in Roman numerals.*

Write from left to right as a sum:

800 = 500 + 100 + 100 + 100, so DCCC
20 = 10 + 10, so XX
5 = 5, so V

DCCC + XX + V = DCCCXXV

The resulting Roman numeral is DCCCXXV.

P *Practice problems*

Solutions to the practice problems are located in the back of this book.

1. Convert DLIV to an Arabic numeral.

2. A museum has a piece of pottery marked MCDXLV. Write this date in Arabic numerals.

3. Convert 369 to Roman numerals.

MEASUREMENT

Estimation of Metric Quantities

The metric system is a system of measurement based on prefixes, and every prefix corresponds to a power of 10. Every unit of measure has a root word. The most common units of measure and the most common prefixes in the metric system are shown in Tables 2.2 and 2.3, respectively.

Table 2.2 Common Units of Measure in the Metric System

Type of measurement	Unit of metric measure (root words)	Abbreviation
Length	Meter	m
Volume	Liter	L
Weight	Gram	g

Table 2.3 Common Prefixes in the Metric System

Power of 10	Prefix
$10^3=1,000$	kilo (k)
$10^2=100$	hecto (h)
$10^1=10$	deka (da)
$10^0=1$	No prefix
$10^{-1}=1/10$	deci (d)
$10^{-2}=1/100$	centi (c)
$10^{-3}=1/1,000$	milli (m)

Using table 2.3, it is possible to quickly determine the relationship among metric quantities, as seen in Example 2.42.

Ⓔ *Example 2.42:*   *Which is larger: a kilometer or a meter?*

A kilometer is larger. One kilometer is equal to 1,000 meters since kilo means 1,000. Kilometer literally means 1,000 meters.

As shown in Example 2.43, estimating metric quantities given an English measurement is possible. Table 2.4 provides a few relationships between metric measurements and English measurements.

Table 2.4 Conversions Between English and Metric Measurement

Length	Weight	Volume
1 inch = 2.54 cm	1 kg = 2.2 pounds	1 L = 1.06 quarts
1 km = 1,000 m = 0.62 mile	1 ounce = 28 g	1 ounce = 30 mL
1 m = 39.37 inch	1 pound = 0.45 kg	1 teaspoon = 5 mL
1 cm = 0.394 inch		1 quart = 0.95 L
1 mile = 1.609 km		1 gallon = 3.785 L
1 yard = 0.914 m		

(E) Example 2.43: Which is an approximate metric quantity for the length of a pencil?

A)   5 m
B)   12 cm
C)   3 kg
D)   8 km

12 cm is a reasonable answer. Since 1 inch = 2.54 cm, this would make the pencil about 4.7 inches long.

5 m is not close since a meter is about the same length as a yard. This would be way too long since this is about how long a room might be.

3 kg is not a good answer, because grams are units for weight.

8 km is too long, because 1 km is even bigger than 5 m.

(P) Practice problems

Solutions to the practice problems are located in the back of this book.

1.   Is a 5-km run or a 5-mile run longer?

2.   Approximately how many inches are in 12.75 centimeters?

Conversion From One Measurement Scale to Another

Measurements may involve English or metric units. Tables 2.5 and 2.6 provide some common English and metric units of measurement, respectively. Note that the metric system is based on powers of 10.

Table 2.5 English Measurement System

Length	Volume	Weight
1 foot = 12 inches	1 cup = 8 ounces	1 pound = 16 ounces
1 yard = 3 feet	1 pint = 2 cups	1 ton = 2,000 pounds
1 mile = 5,280 feet	1 quart = 2 pints	
	1 gallon = 4 quarts	

Table 2.6 Metric Measurement System

Length	Volume	Weight
1 millimeter = 0.001 meters	1 milliliter = 0.001 liters	1 milligram = 0.001 grams
1 centimeter = 0.01 meters	1 centiliter = 0.01 liters	1 centigram = 0.01 grams
1 decimeter = 0.1 meters	1 deciliter = 0.1 liters	1 decigram = 0.1 grams
1 meter = 1 meter	1 liter = 1 liter	1 gram = 1 gram
1 dekameter = 10 meters	1 dekaliter = 10 liters	1 dekagram = 10 grams
1 hectometer = 100 meters	1 hectoliter = 100 liters	1 hectogram = 100 grams
1 kilometer = 1,000 meters	1 kiloliter = 1,000 liters	1 kilogram = 1,000 grams

Although the English and metric systems are two separate measurement systems, the two systems can be compared using the approximations given in Table 2.7.

Table 2.7 English Versus Metric Measurement System

Length	Volume	Weight
1 inch ≈ 2.54 centimeters	1 quart (1.06 quarts) ≈ 1 liter	2.2 pounds ≈ 1 kilogram
1 yard (1.09 yards) ≈ 1 meter		1 ounce ≈ 28 grams

As seen in the Examples 2.44 and 2.45, proportions are commonly used to convert between the different measuring scales.

(E) Example 2.44: *How many centiliters are in 10 liters?*

Setup this proportion: $\dfrac{1\ liter}{100\ centiliters} = \dfrac{10\ liters}{x}$, *so x = 1,000 centiliters.*

(E) Example 2.45: *How many inches are in 4 yards?*

Setup this proportion: $\dfrac{1\ yard}{3\ feet} = \dfrac{4\ yards}{x}$, *so x = 12 feet.*

Use this solution to setup this proportion: $\dfrac{1\ foot}{12\ inches} = \dfrac{12\ feet}{y}$, *so y = 144 inches.*

The solution is 144 inches.

Ⓟ *Practice problems*

Solutions to the practice problems are located in the back of this book.

1. How many milligrams are there in 5 grams?

2. If 1 kilogram is approximately 2.2 pounds, how many pounds are there in 6 kilograms?

3. Complete the following: 3 pounds = _____ ounces.

4. Complete the following: 20 cups = _____ quarts.

Appropriate Units of Measure and Measurement Tools

There are many different tools that are used for measurement. It is important to understand which tool is most appropriate to use for any given measurement. Table 2.8 shows some of the most common tools used for measurement.

Table 2.8 Common Tools Used for Measurement

Types of measurement	Appropriate units of measure	Appropriate measurement tools
Length or Height	Inches (in) Feet (ft) Yards (yd) Miles (mi) Meters (m) with or without any of the metric prefixes	Calipers – a caliper is used to measure very small lengths, usually 6 inches or fewer with greater precision than a ruler. Rulers – used for measurements no longer than 12 inches. Yard Sticks – used for measurements no longer than 1 yard, 3 feet, or 36 inches. Meter Sticks – used for measurements no longer than 1 meter. Tape Measures – used for larger measurements (e.g., taking measurements of rooms in a house) that are usually no more than 50 feet long.
Weight	Pounds (lb) Ounces (oz) Grams (g) with or without any of the metric prefixes.	Scales are used to measure weight. There are many types of scales. Some are digital and some are not. Some scales are used to weigh only small amounts and some are used to weigh larger amounts.
Volume	Teaspoons (tsp) Tablespoons (Tbsp) Pints (pt) Quarts (qt) Gallons (gal) Liters (L) with or without any of the metric prefixes.	Beakers Graduated Cylinders Measuring Cups Pipettes Measuring Spoons (for medication)

(P) *Practice problems*

Solutions to the practice problems are located in the back of this book.

1. A pharmacist must measure out exactly 20 grams of a cream. What would be an appropriate measurement tool for this task?

2. A carpenter has a 3-foot long piece of plywood from which two smaller sections must be cut: one 11 inches long and the other 13 inches in length. What would be the appropriate tool(s) for measuring out each section length, respectively?

Determination of a Measurement Based on Given Measurements

Due to the fact that the world and the universe are very large, there must be methods that will allow measurement of these very long distances. The method that is used is called scaling. Using scaling, very long distances can be scaled down to very small lengths that will fit on paper, such as a map. For instance, one inch on a map may represent 10 miles. There are two ways that this may be represented. One way is with a ratio. A ratio might say 1:10, in this case meaning 1 inch to 10 miles. As done in Example 2.46, a ratio reading would require the map reader to use a ruler to measure the desired distance.

The scale may also be represented graphically. With a graphical representation, there would be a line on the map indicating the length of the line that represents 10 miles. A graphical representation requires the reader to use either a ruler or a piece of paper marked with the length of the line to measure the desired distance.

(E) *Example 2.46:*   *Suppose that 1 inch on a map represents 15 miles on the ground. If a desired distance measures 6.5 inches on the map, how far is this distance on the ground?*

Start with the length measured on the map, and then multiply by the ratio given on the map. Be sure to set up the ratio so that the desired unit (in this case, miles) is on top. Then, multiply.

$$6.5 \text{ inches} \times \frac{15 \text{ miles}}{1 \text{ inch}} = 97.5 \text{ miles}$$

Scaling is also used in countless other applications. A blueprint of a house may be scaled so that the reader can measure the blueprint to figure out how long certain walls in the house are. Model cars are often scaled down from the real version of the car. Model cars are often scaled as 1:24, which means that every 1 inch on the model car is equal to 24 inches on the real vehicle.

(P) *Practice problems*

Solutions to the practice problems are located in the back of this book.

1.   On a blueprint of a house, every 1 inch equals 1 foot of actual linear footage. If a wall for the dining room measures 16 inches long on the blueprint, how long is the actual wall?

2.   On a scaled model of our solar system, 1 inch equals 100,000 miles. If the actual distance between the Sun and the Earth is 93,000,000 miles, how many inches does this distance represent in the model?

DATA INTERPRETATION

Dependent and Independent Variables

Every set of data has a dependent and an independent variable. The **independent variable** is the variable that is put *into* the set of data, or the *in*put. The **dependent variable** is the output based on the input (see Example 2.47).

 Example 2.47:   *A worker gets paid by the hour.*

In the sentence above, which variable is the dependent variable: the amount of money earned or the number of hours worked?

_____

To find the correct amount of pay, the boss would put in the number of hours worked and get out the amount earned. Since hours go in, the hours worked is the independent variable.

Another way to determine which variable is the dependent variable is to determine which variable depends on the other. The variable that depends on the other is the dependent variable (see Example 2.48).

 Example 2.48:   *A person exercises to control their blood pressure.*

In the sentence above, which variable is the independent variable, and which dependent variable?

_____

The blood pressure changes depending on the amount of exercise. Therefore, blood pressure is the dependent variable and exercise is the independent variable. In this case, it would not make sense to say that the amount of exercise depends on the blood pressure.

In a situation in which the data are graphed on an xy-plane, the independent variable is most often the x values and the dependent variable is most commonly the y value.

Practice problems

Solutions to the practice problems are located in the back of this book.

1.   "The amount of studying she did for the TEAS® test impacted her score on the test."

    In the sentence above, what is the dependent variable?

2.   "What effect is the treatment having on the two groups?"

    In the question above, what is the independent variable?

Interpretation of Data From Line, Bar, and Circle Graphs

There are many types of graphs used to solve problems. Graphs are visual summaries of data. Three common types of graphs are:

Line graphs – A line graph is a graph that shows changes over a period of time or compares the relationship between two quantities (see Example 2.49). Line graphs are created on coordinate axes. The horizontal axis is typically referred to as the *x*-axis and the vertical axis is typically referred to as the *y*-axis. To denote any point given, either on one of the axes or in one of the quadrants created by the two axes, write the *x*-coordinate and then the *y*-coordinate as an **ordered pair** (*x,y*). (Tip: One way to remember this is that an ordered pair is in *alphabetical* order, × then *y*.) As seen in Example 2.49, the point (8:00, 50) indicates that at 8:00 a.m., the temperature was 50°F.

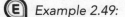 *Example 2.49:*

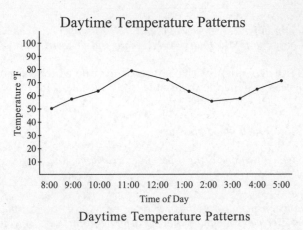

Daytime Temperature Patterns

The line graph above compares the time of day to the temperature. What conclusions can be drawn from this graph?

There are numerous possible answers. Here are two possibilities:
- *The warmest time of day was around 11:00 a.m.*
- *The greatest difference in temperature between 8:00 a.m. and 5:00 p.m. was 30° F (80° F at 11:00 a.m. and 50° F at 8:00 a.m.).*

Circle (or pie) graphs – A circle (or pie) graph is a circular graph divided into sectors representing the frequency of an event. As seen in Example 2.50, sectors on these types of graphs often represent a percentage of the whole, where the whole circle or pie equals 100%. A circle (or pie) graph shows how much of the whole each part represents.

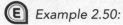 *Example 2.50:*

Grade Distribution for Health Class

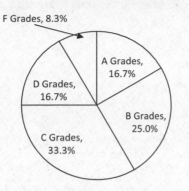

The circle graph above depicts the grade distribution for the students in a health class. If there are 24 students in the class, how many students received each letter grade?

Grade	Calculation	Number of students
A	24 × 16.7%	4
B	24 × 25.0%	6
C	24 × 33.3%	8
D	24 × 16.7%	4
F	24 × 8.3%	2
Total	24 × 100.0%	24

Histograms and **bar graphs** – A histogram is a graph used to compare the frequencies of an event. The frequencies are displayed as vertical touching bars. A bar graph is a graph used to compare the frequencies of an event. The frequencies are displayed as nontouching, horizontal or vertical bars. Histograms and bar graphs both display the frequencies of an event. Histograms often display the frequency of continuous data (data that can assume any value), while bar graphs measure the frequency of noncontinuous data, such as the number of times an event occurs. Although histograms and bar graphs are both created on coordinate axes, the bars on a histogram *must* touch other. The bars do not have to and often do not touch in a bar graph, as seen in Example 2.51.

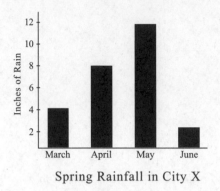

Example 2.51:

Spring Rainfall in City X

The bar graph above shows the number of inches of rain that fell in a certain city in the months of March, April, May, and June. What conclusions can be drawn from this graph?

There are several possible answers. Here are two possibilities:
- *Four inches of rain fell in March.*
- *May had the greatest amount of rain, and June had the least amount of rain.*

ⓟ *Practice problems*

Solutions to the practice problems are located in the back of this book.

1) Refer to the line graph in Example 2.49. The temperature on the given day varied throughout the day from 8:00 a.m. to 5:00 p.m. When did the temperature decrease?

Use the graph below to answer the following three questions.

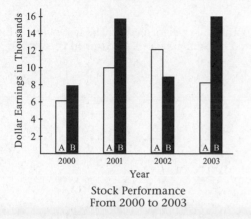

Stock Performance
From 2000 to 2003

2) The graph above shows the performance of Stock A and Stock B from 2000 to 2003. In what year were the earnings for stock A the greatest?

3) How much more did Stock B earn than Stock A in the year 2003?

4) In what year did the earnings of stock A exceed the earnings of stock B?

Use the graph below to answer the following two questions.

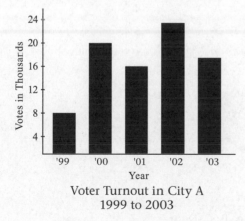

Voter Turnout in City A
1999 to 2003

5) The graph above shows the number of people in City A who voted during the years 1999 to 2003. The city has 80,000 eligible voters. What percent of the eligible voters voted in 1999?

6) According to the graph above, what was the decrease in voters from 2002 to 2003?

Organization of Data Using Tables, Charts, and Graphs

Data can be organized in many different ways. Depending on the type of data, one type of table, chart, or graph may be more desirable than another. When organizing data, it is also important to keep the audience in mind. Some audiences will be more receptive to a table with more specific data in it than to a pie graph with a generic type of information.

Tables are helpful for organizing raw data. Here is a list of 20 test scores from a math class:

98, 77, 65, 76, 82, 99, 91, 55, 43, 61, 73, 88, 86, 82, 92, 93, 76, 63, 100, 45

As a list, these scores are difficult to look at and understand exactly how the class performed on the test overall. Table 2.9 organizes the data into categories, showing how many students scored in each category. Organized this way, a teacher can see how the grades were dispersed.

Table 2.9 Number of Students Earning A, B, C, D, or F

Grade category	Number of students
90-100, A	6
80-89, B	4
70-79, C	4
60-69, D	3
59 and below, F	3

A chart serves as a visual picture of the information given in the table. Figure 2.3 illustrates how a teacher can quickly see which letter grades the students had most frequently. It is important to keep in mind that not all charts are easy to read. Sometimes the exact number in each category is difficult to read, but can be easily estimated based on the scale on the vertical side of the chart. A chart should be chosen over a table when the visual presentation of the information is most important.

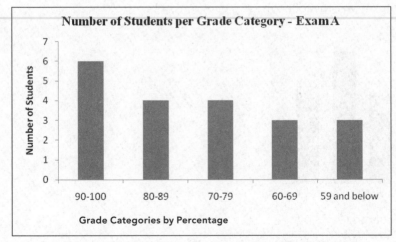

Figure 2.3 Number of students earning A, B, C, D, or F.

Graphs can also show this information visually. One of the most common graphs is a line graph, as shown in the Figure 2.4. Just like a chart, a graph should be used when it is desired to visually present information to an audience. Graphs, like the one shown, are more often used to show change over a period of time.

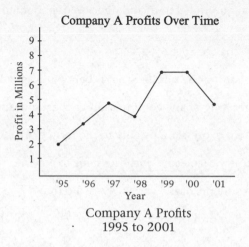

Figure 2.4 Line graph comparing Company A's profit over time.

Ⓟ *Practice problems*

Solutions to the practice problems are located in the back of this book.

1. The line graph shown in Figure 2.4, shows the profits of Company A for 6 years, from 1995 through 2001. List three conclusions that can be drawn from this graph.

2.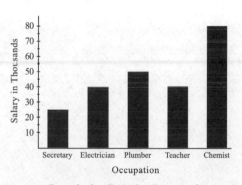

    The graph above shows the average salaries of people in certain occupations in a given town. List three conclusions that can be drawn from this graph.

3.

Grade	Number of students
A	4
B	5
C	12
D	6
F	3

The grade distribution on an examination for a class of 30 students is shown above. If a circle (pie) graph is used to represent the grade distribution for students in the class, what fraction of the circle would be needed to represent the number of students who received a B on the exam?

ALGEBRAIC APPLICATIONS

Addition, Subtraction, Multiplication, and Division of Polynomial Terms

In order to discuss addition, subtraction, multiplication, and division of polynomial terms, there are some definitions that should be known:

- **Constant** – A quantity that does not change.

- **Coefficient** – The numerical part of a term; the number that is being multiplied to the variable.

- **Expression** – One or more terms consisting of any combination of constants and/or variables.

- **Variable** – An unknown quantity in an expression, usually in the form of a letter such as x, y, or z.

- **Like terms** – Terms that have the same variable and with the same exponent.

- **Degree** – The exponent or sum of exponents of the variable(s) of a term.

- **Divisor** – The denominator in a division problem; for example, in $\frac{14}{2}$, 2 is the divisor.

- **Dividend** – The numerator in a division problem; for example, in $\frac{14}{2}$, 14 is the dividend.

- **Quotient** – The answer to the division problem; for example, in $\frac{14}{2}$, 7 is the quotient.

A **term** is a constant, a variable, or a product of a constant and a variable. Terms in an expression are separated by a plus or minus sign. A **polynomial** is a term or combination of terms. A **monomial**, for example, is a polynomial with one term. A **binomial** is a polynomial with two terms.

When adding (or subtracting) like terms in a polynomial, add (or subtract) the coefficients and keep the variables the same. Examples 2.52 and 2.53 simplify the addition and subtraction, respectively, of two expressions.

 Example 2.52: *Simplify the expression:* $(8x^2 - 7x + 3) + (3x^2 - 2x - 1)$.

When adding two polynomials, remove the parentheses and collect the like terms.
$8x^2 - 7x + 3 + 3x^2 - 2x - 1$.

The like terms are grouped together: $\underline{8x^2 + 3x^2} \underbrace{- 7x - 2x} \underbrace{+ 3 - 1}$.

Add the like terms by adding their coefficients and keeping the variables the same: $11x^2 - 9x + 2$

 Example 2.53: *Simplify the expression:* $(8x^2 - 7x + 3) - (3x^2 - 2x - 1)$.

When subtracting two polynomials, distribute the minus to the second polynomial. It may help to write a 1 in front of the second polynomial.
$(8x^2 - 7x + 3) - 1(3x^2 - 2x - 1)$

Distribute the –1 to $3x^2 - 2x - 1$. Notice how this changes the signs of each term in the second polynomial: $8x^2 - 7x + 3 - 3x^2 + 2x + 1$

The like terms are grouped together: $\underline{8x^2 - 3x^2} \underbrace{- 7x + 2x} \underbrace{+ 3 + 1}$.

Add the like terms by adding their coefficients and keeping the variables the same: $5x^2 - 5x + 4$

When multiplying polynomials, multiply the coefficients and multiply the variables. When multiplying common variables (such as × times x), add the exponents on the common variables. Example 2.54 uses the **distributive property** (a property that usually removes parentheses in an expression, such as $a(x + y) = ax + ay$).

(E) Example 2.54: *Simplify the expression: $-5y (7y^2 - 4y - 2)$.*

Since one of the factors being multiplied is a monomial $(-5y)$, distribute the monomial to $7y^2 - 4y - 2$.

$-5y (7y^2) - 5y (-4y) - 5y (-2)$
$-35y^3 + 20y^2 + 10y$

Combine like terms, if possible. The terms in the product above are not like, so the problem is complete.

Example 2.55 uses the FOIL process to determine the product of two binomials. **FOIL** standards for "First, Outer, Inner, Last." This means to multiply the first term within each set of parentheses first. Then, multiply the outer terms within each set of parentheses together, followed by multiplying the inner terms together. Finally, multiply the last terms within each set of parentheses together. Once the multiplication is complete, combine like terms.

(E) Example 2.55: *Simplify the expression: $(3x - 1)(2x + 5)$.*

The FOIL process can be used to multiply two binomials.

$$\overset{F}{\overbrace{(3x)(2x)}} + \overset{O}{\overbrace{(3x)(5)}} - \overset{I}{\overbrace{(1)(2x)}} - \overset{L}{\overbrace{1(5)}}$$
$$6x^2 + 15x - 2x - 5$$

Add like terms and the problem is complete: $6x^2 + 13x - 5$

When dividing polynomials, the divisor can be a monomial or binomial. Division problems with monomial divisors are usually much simpler than those with multinomial divisors; the latter usually requires factoring or long division. Example 2.56 has a monomial divisor.

(E) Example 2.56: *Simplify the expression: $(24x^2 y + 14xy - 8xy^2) \div (-4xy)$.*

When dividing two polynomials in which the divisor is a monomial, create fractions by dividing each term in the dividend by the divisor.

$$\frac{24x^2y}{-4xy} + \frac{14xy}{-4xy} - \frac{8xy^2}{-4xy}$$

Reduce each fraction that was created.

$$-6x - \frac{7}{2} + 2y$$

Make sure there is nothing else that simplifies.

The quotient is $-6x - \frac{7}{2} + 2y$.

Ⓟ *Practice problems*

Solutions to the practice problems are located in the back of this book.

Simplify each expression.

1. $(6x^2 - 5x + 8) - (x^2 + 7x - 1)$

2. $(5x - 4)(5x + 4)$

3. $(24x^2y - 6xy + 12xy^2 - 4) \div (12xy)$

Translation of Word Phrases and Sentences Into Expressions, Equations, and Inequalities

A phrase in words can be translated into a mathematical expression. (Note: Expressions do not contain an equal sign or inequality sign.) A statement or sentence can be translated into an **equation** or **inequality**. Statements and sentences contain verbs such as *is*, *was*, or *becomes*, and use symbols such as =, <, ≤, >, and ≥. Expressions usually do not contain such verbs and do not use such symbols. Table 2.10 provides some basic translations of the symbols. Keep in mind that the order in which the words appear in this table may be slightly rearranged in a problem. Examples 2.57 to 2.59 illustrate how to translate word phrases and sentences into expressions, equations, and inequalities, and vice versa.

Table 2.10 Mathematical Symbols and Their Translations

Symbol	Reads as
=	is, was, measures, becomes
<	is less than, is no greater than
≤	is less than or equal to, is at most
>	is greater than, is more than
≥	is greater than or equal to, is at least
–	less than
+	more than
2	twice

Ⓔ *Example 2.57:* *Translate the following phrase into a mathematical expression:* Five less than twice the length.

The unknown is the length, so let length be some variable such as L. Less than *means to subtract and* twice *means "two times." The expression is*

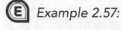

$$2\ (L) \underbrace{-\ 5}_{\text{5 less than}} \text{ which is } 2L - 5$$

$\underbrace{2\ (L)}_{\text{twice the length}}$

Ⓔ *Example 2.58:* *Translate the following sentence into an equation:* A number is five less than the sum of the number and four.

The unknown is the number, which can be defined as n. *The equation is*

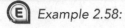

$$\underbrace{n}_{\text{a number}} \underbrace{=}_{\text{is}} \underbrace{(n\ +\ 4)}_{\text{the sum of number and 4}} \underbrace{-\ 5}_{\text{5 less than}} \text{ which is } n = (n+4) - 5$$

(E) Example: 2.59: *Translate the following equation into a sentence. More than one answer is possible.*

$$9(n-4) = \frac{n}{2}$$

The unknown is the number, which can be defined as n. First, translate parts of the equation:

4 less than a number
$$\overbrace{n-4}$$

the quotient of the number and 2 OR half a number
$$\overbrace{\frac{n}{2}}$$

Now, 9 is being multiplied to the quantity :

product of 9 and 4 less than a number
$$\overbrace{9(n-4)}$$

Finally, the two expressions are equal to each other so use "is" or "is equal to" in the translation. The sentence could be:

"The product of 9 and 4 less than a number is the quotient of the number and 2," or "The product of 9 and 4 less than a number is equal to half a number."

(P) Practice problems

Solutions to the practice problems are located in the back of this book.

1. Translate the following sentence into an inequality: *Five is less than half a number.*

2. Translate the following inequality into a sentence: $4n \geq n + 10$.

Equations with One Unknown

The addition principle and the multiplication principle may be applied when solving an equation with one unknown. The **addition principle** is a rule that makes it possible to move terms from one side of an equation to the other by adding opposites to each expression. The **multiplication principle** is a rule that makes it possible to isolate the variable in an equation by multiplying both expressions by the reciprocal of the variable's coefficient. (Note: The **reciprocal** of a number is the multiplicative inverse of the number. For example, the reciprocal of $\frac{1}{2}$ is 2 and the multiplicative inverse of -4 is $-\frac{1}{4}$.)

An equation can be solved using the following steps:

Step 1. Use the distributive property (e.g., $a(x + y) = ax + ay$) to remove any parentheses.

Step 2. If there are fractions present, remove them by multiplying each term by the least common denominator (LCD).

Step 3. Use the addition principle to move like terms together on both sides of the equation.

Step 4. Use the multiplication principle to isolate the variable by multiplying both sides of the equation by the reciprocal of the coefficient of the variable.

Step 5. Check the solution. Substitute the answer into the original equation to make sure both expressions result in the same value.

Examples 2.60 and 2.61 use these steps to solve an equation.

Example 2.60: *Solve the following equation for x: $2(3x - 1) = 4x - 14$.*

Step 1. *Use the distributive property to remove any parentheses.*

$$2(3x - 1) = 4x - 14$$
$$6x - 2 = 4x - 14$$

Step 2. *There are no fractions, so there is no need to multiply terms by the LCD.*

Step 3. *Use the addition principle to move like terms together.*

$$6x - 2 \underset{\sim}{+ 2} = 4x - 14 \underset{\sim}{+ 2}$$
$$6x = 4x - 12$$
$$6x \underset{\sim}{- 4x} = 4x \underset{\sim}{- 4x} - 12$$
$$2x = -12$$

Step 4. *Use the multiplication principle to isolate the variable by multiplying both sides of the equation by the reciprocal of the coefficient of the variable.*

$$2x = -12$$
$$\left(\frac{1}{2}\right)(2x) - \left(\frac{1}{2}\right)(-12)$$
$$\left(\frac{1}{\cancel{2}}\right)(\cancel{2}x) = \left(\frac{1}{2}\right)(-12)$$
$$x = -6$$

The solution is $x = -6$.

Step 5. Check the solution.

$$2(3(-6) - 1) = 4(-6) - 14$$

$$2(-19) = -24 - 14$$

$$-38 = -38$$

Since this is a true statement, the solution is correct.

(E) Example: 2.61: Solve the following equation for x: $\dfrac{x}{6} - \dfrac{1}{3} = \dfrac{x}{2} + \dfrac{2}{3}$

Step 1. There are no parentheses to remove, so move to step 2.

Step 2. If there are fractions present, remove them by multiplying each term by the LCD.

The LCD of all four terms is 6. When multiplying by the LCD, distribute the LCD to both sides:

$$6\left(\frac{x}{6} - \frac{1}{3}\right) = 6\left(\frac{x}{2} + \frac{2}{3}\right)$$

$$6\left(\frac{x}{6}\right) - 6\left(\frac{1}{3}\right) = 6\left(\frac{x}{2}\right) + 6\left(\frac{2}{3}\right)$$

$$x - 2 = 3x + 4$$

Step 3. Use the addition principle to move like terms together.

$$x - 2 \underline{+ 2} = 3x + 4 \underline{+ 2}$$

$$x = 3x + 6$$

$$x \underline{- 3x} = 3x \underline{- 3x} + 6$$

$$-2x = 6$$

Step 4. Use the multiplication principle to isolate the variable by multiplying both sides of the equation by the reciprocal of the coefficient of the variable.

$$\left(-\frac{1}{2}\right)(-2x) = \left(-\frac{1}{2}\right)(6)$$

$$x = -3$$

The solution is $x = -3$.

Step 5. Check the solution.

$$\frac{x}{6} - \frac{1}{3} = \frac{x}{2} + \frac{2}{3}$$

$$6\left(\frac{-3}{6} - \frac{1}{3}\right) = 6\left(\frac{-3}{2} + \frac{2}{3}\right)$$

$$6\left(\frac{-3}{6}\right) - 6\left(\frac{1}{3}\right) = 6\left(\frac{-3}{2}\right) + 6\left(\frac{2}{3}\right)$$

$$-3 - 2 = -9 + 4$$

$$-5 = -5$$

Since this is a true statement, the solution is correct.

(P) *Practice problems*

Solutions to the practice problems are located in the back of this book.

1. Solve the equation for y: $3(4y - 1) = 16y + 5$.

2. Solve the equation for x: $\dfrac{x}{10} = \dfrac{5}{12}$.

3. Solve the equation for x: $\dfrac{x}{4} - \dfrac{1}{6} = \dfrac{x}{3} + 1$.

Equations or Inequalities Involving Absolute Values

The **absolute value** of number n, written $|n|$, is the distance between the number n and zero on the number line. This means:

- $|n| = n$ when n is a positive number
- $|n| = -(n)$ when n is a negative number

In order to solve an absolute value equation with the variable x, use the above definition to get rid of the absolute value symbols. In other words:

$|x - n| = x - n$ when $x - n$ is positive
$|x - n| = -(x - n)$ when $x - n$ is negative

To solve an absolute value inequality such as $|x - n| < a$, $|x - n| \leq a$, $|x - n| > a$, or $|x - n| \geq a$, Table 2.11 can be used to remove the absolute value signs and solve for the variable (x):

Table 2.11 Absolute Value Equations

To solve	Create the equation/inequality
1. $|x - n| = a$	$x - n = a$ or $x - n = -a$
2. $|x - n| < a$	$-a < x - n < a$
3. $|x - n| \leq a$	$-a \leq x - n \leq a$
4. $|x - n| > a$	$x - n > a$ or $x - n < -a$
5. $|x - n| \geq a$	$x - n \geq a$ or $x - n \leq -a$

Note: Beware of absolute value equations and inequalities in which one of the expressions, or sides, contains zero or a negative number. This usually results in infinite solutions or no solution. Table 2.12 lists the types of equations and inequalities that can result in such solutions.

Table 2.12 No Solution and All Real Numbers as a Solution for Equations Involving Absolute Values

Words of caution: Equations and inequalities that have *no solution* or *all real numbers* as a solution	
If $|x - n| =$ negative number	then there is *no solution*, or $\varnothing$*
If $|x - n| < 0$	then there is *no solution*, or $\varnothing$
If $|x - n| <$ negative number	then there is *no solution*, or $\varnothing$
If $|x - n| \leq$ negative number	then there is *no solution*, or $\varnothing$
If $|x - n| > 0$	then the solution is *all real numbers*, or $\Re$
If $|x - n| >$ negative number	then the solution is *all real numbers*, or $\Re$

*The symbol $\varnothing$ refers to the "empty set" meaning there is no solution.

Examples 2.62 to 2.64 demonstrate how to solve equations or inequalities involving absolute values.

(E) *Example 2.62:*   *Solve the equation: $|x - 3| = 5$.*

According to #1 in Table 2.11, two equations can be created to solve for x:
   $x - 3 = 5$ or $x - 3 = -5$

Solve the equations:
   $x - 3 + 3 = 5 + 3$ $x - 3 + 3 = -5 + 3$
       $x = 8$ $x = -2$

So, the solutions are $x = 8$ and $x = -2$.

Give both solutions as the answer. Also, verify that the solutions are correct:
$|8 - 3| = |5| = 5$ and $|-2 - 3| = |-5| = 5$.

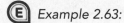 **Example 2.63:**   Solve the inequality: $|3y - 2| \geq 7$.

According to #5 in Table 2.11, a compound inequality can be created to solve for y:

$3y - 2 \geq 7$ or $3y - 2 \leq -7$

Solve the inequalities by isolating y in each one.

$$3y - 2 \geq 7 \text{ or } 3y - 2 \leq -7$$
$$3y - 2 + 2 \geq 7 + 2 \text{ or } 3y - 2 + 2 \leq -7 + 2$$
$$3y \geq 9 \text{ or } 3y \leq -5$$
$$\frac{3y}{3} \geq \frac{9}{3} \text{ or } \frac{3y}{3} \leq \frac{-5}{3}$$
$$y \geq 3 \text{ or } y \leq -\frac{5}{3}$$

The solution includes all real numbers greater than or equal to 3, or numbers that are less than or equal to $-\frac{5}{3}$.

Give both solutions as the answer. Also, verify that the solutions are correct:
$$3(3) - 2 \geq 7$$
$$7 \geq 7$$

And any number greater than 3 will result in an expression greater than 7:
$$3(-5/3) - 2 \leq -7$$
$$-5 - 2 \leq -7$$
$$-7 \leq -7$$

Any number less than −5/3 will result in an expression less than −7.

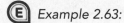 **Example 2.64:**   Solve the inequality: $|3y - 2| + 5 \leq 1$.

Isolate the absolute value before attempting to solve the inequality.

$$|3y - 2| + 5 - 5 \leq 1 - 5$$
$$|3y - 2| \leq -4$$

Caution! This is an absolute value with a negative number on the opposite side. Since an absolute value can never be less than or equal to a negative number, this inequality has no solution (or $\varnothing$).

(P) **Practice problems**

Solutions to the practice problems are located in the back of this book.

1.   Solve the inequality: $|8x - 3| + 4 > 2$.

2.   Solve the inequality: $|3y - 2| < 7$.

SECTION 3: SCIENCE

The science section is divided into four categories: scientific reasoning, human body science, Earth and physical science, and life science.

SCIENTIFIC REASONING

Reasons for Conducting Investigations

Proper scientific investigations involve critical thinking. Such investigations are used to establish sound procedures in a variety of areas, such as the workplace. Investigations are conducted to identify potential problems and to create solutions to those problems before they actually occur. For example, it may be beneficial for a company to investigate procedures for emergency situations before an emergency occurs. If such investigations are not conducted, trial-and-error solutions in a time of emergency can be both costly and time intensive. In addition, if emergency staff (e.g., medical personnel or nuclear engineers) is involved, then the effective implementation of procedures that are in effect before the emergency occurs may save lives.

In addition, the results of an investigation may also be of great value if existing procedures fail to solve a technical problem. A systematic inquiry into a technical problem may establish an entirely new method of solution not previously considered (consider living in outer space). As a result, new innovations may arise that not only solve a problem, but may lead to the creation of consumer products that provide a greater standard of living. Proper investigations have led to radically new designs that improved the quality of life.

(P) *Practice problems*

Solutions to the practice problems are located in the back of this book.

1. Identify two reasons for conducting scientific investigations.

2. Give an example of an investigation that has led to radically new designs that improve the quality of life.

Questions and Concepts That Guide Scientific Investigations

Scientific investigations begin with a curiosity about the environment in which we live. The most basic questions regarding nature are sufficient to inspire scientific inquiry. Such inquiry or investigation starts with the desire to carefully define the terms of the question. For example, "Why is the sky blue?" is a common question posed by many children. A natural starting point is encapsulating a **quantitative** (or numerical) understanding of the words *sky* and *blue* that extends beyond their commonly understood meanings. For instance, the term *sky* might be defined as a certain extent of atmosphere above the Earth's surface, and the term *blue* may be defined as a certain range of wavelengths within the electromagnetic spectrum. The precise construction of definitions allows for subsequent evaluation of the question itself.

The formulation of a **hypothesis,** or an explanation formulated to answer the questions being investigated, has at its essence a statement that can be tested. The steps for forming a hypothesis are the following:

Step 1. Identify the problem: Observe and determine the problem to be investigated.

Step 2. Ask questions: Ask questions and attempt to formulate a solution to the problem.

Step 3. Formulate a hypothesis: Formulate explanations (i.e., hypotheses) to answer the questions. This involves making predictions that follow from the initial statement of the problem. The language used within the hypothesis must be well-defined, such that any subsequent testing of the hypothesis is not subject to erroneous interpretation.

Testing the hypothesis involves systematically identifying the variables involved, followed by creating a plan of action that involves observation and experimentation. If no reasonable test can be designed, it becomes necessary to reformulate the hypothesis. It is of little value to quantitatively pursue the validity of a statement without any ability to measure an outcome.

(P) Practice problems

Solutions to the practice problems are located in the back of this book.

Four clinical protocols to test the hypothesis below are presented in questions 1 to 4. For each protocol, determine whether or not it is a good protocol to follow.

Good cholesterol (HDL) flushes out bad cholesterol (LDL) from the arteries of humans.

1. One patient is administered a single dosage of HDL medication, followed by periodic blood tests.

2. Each individual in six groups (10 patients/group) is administered the same dosage of HDL medication, followed by a single blood test per patient.

3. Each of six groups (10 patients/group) is administered a different dosage of HDL, followed by periodic blood tests.

4. Each person in a group of 10 patients is administered a different dosage of HDL, followed by periodic blood tests.

Communication and Defense of Scientific Arguments

Strict scientific arguments rely on the rules of logic that govern the scientific method. To effectively communicate such an argument, the information must be formally presented in the proper order:

1) Problem identification
2) Question asking
3) Hypothesis development
4) Data collection and experimentation
5) Analysis
6) Conclusion

The first three steps have already been defined. The remaining steps are defined here:

Data collection: Collect data throughout the scientific process to test the hypotheses or predictions in a controlled environment. During this process, scientists gather as much information as possible in an attempt to answer the originally posed question as well as to create new questions. Data collection uses four main steps:

Step 1. Observation: Scientists use the five senses to learn as much as possible during data collection. Observation can be direct, such as listening to a bird call, or indirect, such as observing qualities of planets.
Step 2. Measurement: Measuring allows for collection of quantitative data.
Step 3. Samples: Data typically cannot be collected from every member of a population. Thus, scientists collect information from a representative sample of the population. This means that scientists obtain data from a subset of the population that looks like the population, but is small and more manageable.
Step 4. Organization: The data should be organized. This may involve placing information in tables and/or charts.

Experimentation: Experimentation involves comparing a control group and an experimental group. The two groups both equally represent the population. The difference is that the experimental group is different from the control group based on one variable. Both groups are compared to understand what effect the variable has on the experimental group. That is, the experiment tests the question, "What effect does the independent variable have on the dependent variable?"

When writing the methods for the data collection and experimentation step of an investigation, the methods used to collect the data must be adequately described to avoid misunderstanding. The techniques used to analyze the data, including the use of all controls and variables, must be clearly explained.

Analysis: Scientists must analyze data collected during experimentation. The researchers must determine if the data is reliable (consistent with past results) and whether or not it supports the hypothesis.

Conclusion: The purpose of the scientific process is to develop a conclusion. Scientists produce models to represent the explanations supported by the data. A scientist should carefully word his or her conclusion in a manner that is consistent with the hypothesis.

In scientific research, inference is used often as a way of drawing conclusions without direct observation. In addition, after many experiments and the development of many models, it is possible to develop a theory about an event. This is a broad statement of what is thought to be true. Note that it is always possible to find information that may refute a theory; therefore, a theory that is thought to be true may be proven incorrect when technology enables better data collection.

In general, the defense of a scientific argument is largely dependent on the strength of the data and its analysis. An argument gains merit after it has been reviewed by experts in the field of science. Over time, an argument may lose merit. During the review process, for example, any subjective bias (intentional or unintentional) found within the argument must be removed. If the bias compromises the conclusion, the argument must be discarded. In addition, any scientific argument is subject to repeatability. If the results cannot be duplicated, then an argument loses its credibility. Based on continuous scrutiny and review, the highest confidence in a theory comes with the test of time.

(P) *Practice problems*

Solutions to the practice problems are located in the back of this book.

1. List the six parts of a scientific argument.

2. How does a scientific argument change over time?

Reasons to Include Technology and Mathematics in Science Research

Proper scientific research would not exist without the associated language of mathematics. The description of science is quantitatively accomplished through the use of differing levels of mathematics (e.g., algebra, geometry, and calculus). Data is recorded in numerical form using specified measurements. Highly advanced, modern instruments are used as measuring devices to obtain the most precise data. These data are then related to one another through relationships often established by graphs and empirical formulas. Advanced technology is used to generate these graphs, as well as to provide numerical models to describe mathematical relationships. It is precisely this type of analysis that provides the basis for logically sound conclusions.

If mathematics was not used, the best scientific descriptions would be purely qualitative in nature. No modern conveniences could exist without mathematics, because the creation of all technology is ultimately mathematical. It is scientific research that allows humanity to advance beyond the most primitive of conditions. The continuing interplay of technology and mathematics provides the basis for cutting-edge scientific research.

(P) *Practice problems*

Solutions to the practice problems are located in the back of this book.

1.   Give two reasons why scientific research is dependent on technology.

2.   Without mathematics, scientific research would not be possible. Explain why this is true.

Use of Technology and Mathematics to Improve Investigations

Individuals in technical fields (e.g., detectives, medical personnel, engineers) are interested in finding solutions to problems within a given time frame. Subsequent investigation in a precise and timely manner is highly dependent on the application of various mathematical and technological skills. Throughout recent history, the increased rigor of mathematics and the advent of new technologies have improved the success rate within these technical fields, and have often fueled the creation of entirely new fields of investigation. Consider the technological advances in forensics that have been invaluable aids to criminal science, or the use of satellites that have improved data available to cosmologists.

Quantitative investigations using numerical information (or data) begin with careful record keeping. Data management through the use of software programs improves the efficiency of an investigation. The subsequent manipulation of data may require different branches of mathematics (e.g., algebra, geometry, or calculus) depending on the rigor of the technical field. In addition, Example 3.1 shows how a visual representation of data in graphical form allows the technician to grasp overall trends (or patterns) within the data, itself. The ability to graphically model data has been advanced with computer programs that create spreadsheets. If a high-powered numerical solution is sought (as with hurricane tracking), the continuing advancement of computing power and computing speed provide the means for improved manipulation of data.

(E) *Example 3.1:*

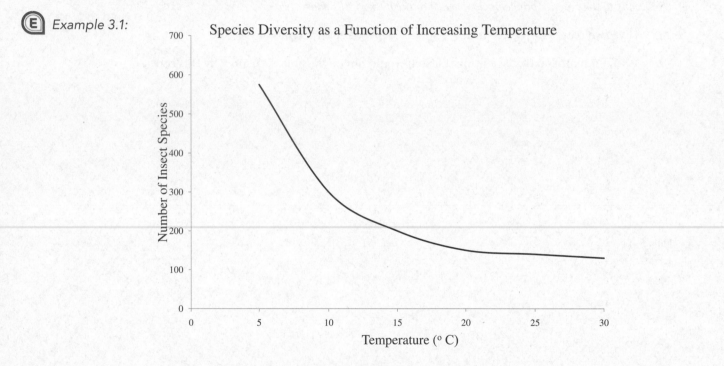

What does the diagram above suggests about insects and temperature?

The curve in the graph suggests that the largest number of insect species adapt to cold temperatures and fewer to warmer temperatures.

Communications are also improved through the use of mathematics and technology. The sharing of information within corporate entities (or across vast distances) has been revolutionized with modern technology and is experiencing continual growth of intranet (and Internet) capabilities. The transfer of such information has also been vastly improved with the mathematical software of binary digital technology. In addition, the hardware of fiber optics has improved the processing rate of communication.

(P) *Practice problems*

Solutions to the practice problems are located in the back of this book.

1. Describe how mathematics and science have increased communication in the corporate world.

2. List two industries that benefit from the advancement of mathematical and technological skills.

Alternative Explanations and Models

Scientific explanations (or models) are offered as direct results of the evidence that currently supports them. This evidence is gathered using the methods, techniques, and technologies of a particular era. However, as improvements are made, collection of new data often leads to more refined, alternative explanations. Measuring and observational devices have been developed so that smaller increments of time and length have become accessible. Small-scale behaviors have been observed to differ from large-scale behavior; therefore, more precise data often lead to further understanding (consider the advent of microscopes that assist in visualizing cellular structure). As a result, a more refined model is a better fit for new data. In addition, the observation of the small-scale behavior of atomic processes has led to the support of theories of relativity and quantum mechanics that extend beyond ordinary human existence.

Technology improvements on a large scale have also led to model refinements. Greater computing power and processing speeds have enabled details of weather patterns to be studied that were not known until recently (consider hurricane modeling). In addition, the large-scale observations of our most powerful telescopes have led to refinements in galactic modeling.

An explanation of natural law may not only require refinement, but may require an entirely new paradigm shift. Alternative explanations that are in direct opposition to previous understanding have been documented. For example, before the era of Copernicus and Galileo, it was widely believed that the Sun revolved around the Earth. As early telescopic observations became commonplace, the revolutionary explanation of planetary orbits around the Sun became the dominant explanation.

Ⓟ *Practice problems*

Solutions to the practice problems are located in the back of this book.

1. Explain how improved technology leads to better scientific explanations.

2. Apply the advancement of technology to our understanding of the solar system through history.

Formulation and Revision of Scientific Explanations and Models

Any scientific investigation demands that a logical procedure be followed. A reasonable explanation of an event can only occur after gathering sufficient evidence to support (or refute) that explanation. Logic follows rules that are independent of the subjective fallacies of the investigator. Rules of logic typically follow deductive or inductive reasoning. **Deductive reasoning** is a method whereby conclusions follow from general principles. **Inductive reasoning** is a method of arriving at general principles from specific facts. As seen in Examples 3.2 and 3.3, while deductive reasoning leads to a specific conclusion, inductive reasoning relies heavily on a preponderance of information that leads to a certain degree of confidence in a conclusion.

Ⓔ *Example 3.2:*

    (1)   All men are mortal.
    (2)   Sultan is a man.

    Based on these two statements, what conclusion may be drawn?

    Since statement 2 says that Sultan is a man and statement 1 says that all men are mortal, deductive reasoning can be used to conclude that Sultan is mortal.

Ⓔ *Example 3.3:*

    (1)   I observed the Sun setting this evening.
    (2)   I have observed the Sun set daily, hundreds of times in my lifetime.

    Based on these two statements, what general conclusion can be drawn?

    Inductive reasoning can be used to conclude that the Sun must set every day. Although there seems to be tremendous evidence from statement 2 to support this conclusion, the conclusion is not certain (even though it is highly likely).

The evidence that eventually may support (or refute) a scientific model (or conclusion) must be gathered in such a way as to control the variables in a systematic way. If available, a controlled laboratory setting allows for careful analysis of each dependent variable's change under the influence of an independent variable change. However, scientific explanations are always subject to change in light of new information. This is not a fault of the scientific method, but rather a reflection on its evolutionary nature. Scientific theories have been revised throughout history as new methods and techniques of investigation have become available. For instance, the ability to study planetary details with a telescope allowed Galileo and his followers to use evidence to conclude that the Earth revolves around the Sun, not the Sun around the Earth.

Ⓟ *Practice problems*

    Solutions to the practice problems are located in the back of this book.

    1.

Temperature (K)	Volume (L)
2.0×10^2	20
4.0×10^2	40
6.0×10^2	60
8.0×10^2	80

    A cylinder with an airtight piston was heated in a laboratory where the internal temperature and volume were recorded as shown in the table above. The hypothesis is that volume increases proportionally with temperatures when pressure is held constant. Is this hypothesis supported or refuted by the data?

    2.   Define deductive and inductive reasoning.

HUMAN BODY SCIENCE

Anatomy and Physiology

Human body science can be divided into two subjects: anatomy and physiology. **Anatomy** is the study of the structure of organs and body systems, and **physiology** is the study of the function of the organs and body systems.

Anatomy
The human body is a complex structure. As shown in the hierarchy displayed in Figure 3.1, **atoms**, the smallest parts of elements that still retain all the original properties of the element, combine to form a **molecule** (a chemical bonding of atoms that possesses its own characteristics independent of the atoms themselves). Specific molecules combine to form **cells**, the basic unit of all life. Cells combine in terms of function and type to form **tissues**. At the **organ** level, two or more tissue types work together to perform a specific function. At this level, it is possible to perform extremely complex functions. When organs work together to perform a task the result is an **organ system**. There are 11 organ systems in the human body. The highest level of organization is the **organism**. The organism is the result of all organ systems working together within the body. The following explanation discusses the four tissue types, 11 organ systems, and ways in which the organ systems interact.

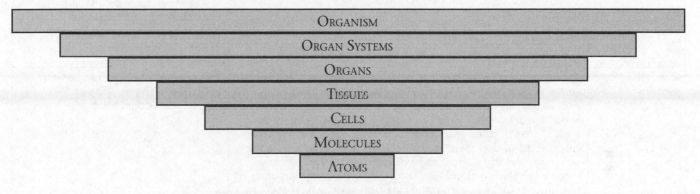

Figure 3.1 Hierarchy of the structure of the human body.

There are four basic tissue types in humans: epithelial, connective, muscular, and nervous. Table 3.1 describes each of these types. Table 3.2 describes each of the 11 organ systems in the human body and how these systems work together. Table 3.3 defines common anatomical terms used when discussing anatomy.

Table 3.1 Tissue Types and Their Descriptions

Tissue type	Description
Epithelial tissue	Epithelium serves two functions. It can provide covering (such as skin tissue) or produce secretions (such as glandular tissue). Epithelial tissue commonly exists in sheets and does not have its own blood supply. Subsequently, epithelium is dependent on diffusion from the nearby capillaries for food and oxygen. Epithelial tissue can regenerate easily if well nourished. Epithelial tissues are classified according to two criteria: number of cell layers and cell shape. Simple and stratified epithelial tissues vary in relation to the number of cell layers. Simple epithelium contains one layer of cells. It is found in body structures where absorption, secretion, and filtration occur. Stratified epithelium has more than one layer of cells and serves as protection. The shape of epithelial cells includes squamous, cuboidal, and columnar.
Connective tissue	Connective tissue is found throughout the body; it serves to connect different structures of the body. Connective tissue commonly has its own blood supply; however, there are some types of connective tissue, such as ligaments, that do not. The various types of connective tissue include bone, cartilage, adipose (fat), and blood vessel.
Muscle tissue	Muscle tissue is dedicated to producing movement. There are three types of muscle tissue: skeletal, cardiac, and smooth. Skeletal muscle supports voluntary movement since it is connected to bones in the skeletal system. Voluntary movements are consciously controlled by the brain. Smooth muscle is under involuntary control, which means it cannot be consciously controlled. It is found in the walls of hollow organs, such as intestines, blood vessels, bladder, and uterus. Like smooth muscle, cardiac muscle movement is involuntary. Cardiac muscle is found only in the heart.
Nervous tissue	Nervous tissue provides the structure for the brain, spinal cord, and nerves. Nerves are made up of specialized cells called neurons that send electrical impulses throughout the body. Support cells, such as myelin, help protect nervous tissue.

Table 3.2 Organ Systems

Organ system	Description	Relationships with other organ systems
Circulatory system	The circulatory system (also called the cardiovascular system) consists of the heart, blood vessels (e.g., arteries, veins, and arterioles), and blood. It supports the circulation and distribution of various substances throughout the body. Oxygen, hormones, and nutrients from food are some of these substances.	• Hormones released from the endocrine system influence blood pressure. • The urinary system helps regulate blood volume and pressure by adjusting urine volume. • The nervous system controls the blood pressure, heart rate, and distribution of blood to various parts of the body. • In women, estrogen helps preserve vascular health. • The integumentary system allows heat to escape by dilating superficial blood vessels. • Blood cells are formed in the marrow of the bones in the skeletal system.
Digestive system	The digestive system consists of all the organs from the mouth to the anus involved in the ingestion and breakdown or processing of food. The organs along this path include the esophagus, stomach, small and large intestines, rectum, and anus. The digestive system manufactures enzymes that break down food so that the nutrients can be easily passed into the blood for use throughout the body. Any food that is not digested is expelled through the anus. The absorption of nutrients actually occurs in the small intestine, which consists of the duodenum, jejunum, and ileum. After that, the colon removes water from the waste that remains. Two other organs included in the digestive system are the liver and pancreas. The liver produces bile that helps break down fats, and the pancreas delivers enzymes to the small intestine that aid in digestion.	• Increased skeletal muscle activity increases the motility of the gastrointestinal tract.
Endocrine system	The endocrine system serves to controls body functions. Glands in the endocrine system secrete hormones that travel through the blood to organs throughout the body. Glands such as the pineal, pituitary, thalamus, hypothalamus, thyroid, thymus, and adrenal regulate processes such as growth and metabolism. The pancreas, testis, and ovaries also have endocrine functions, even though they are part of other body systems.	• The lymphatic system provides a means of transportation for some hormones. • The muscular system provides protection for some endocrine glands. • The nervous system controls the secretion of hormones from the pituitary gland.
Integumentary system	The integumentary system consists of the skin, mucous membranes, hair, and nails. It protects internal tissues from injury, waterproofs the body, and helps regulate body temperature. This system also serves as a barrier to pathogens (microorganisms capable of producing disease).	• The respiratory and digestive systems provide oxygen and nutrients to the skin to help it remain healthy. • Oxygen and nutrients for the skin travel through blood vessels in the cardiovascular system. • The lymphatic system picks up excess fluid from the skin to avoid swelling. • The skeletal system provides shape and support. • Hormones from the endocrine system regulate hair growth and hydration. • The skin serves to protect internal organs, including those in the reproductive system.

Organ system	Description	Relationships with other organ systems
		• The muscular system generates heat that is expelled through the skin as sweat. • The urinary system activates vitamin D. • The nervous system regulates the production of sweat, interprets stimuli, and adjusts the diameter of blood vessels in the skin.
Lymphatic system	The lymphatic system consists of lymph nodes, lymph vessels that carry lymph (a clear fluid rich in antibodies), the spleen, the thymus, and the tonsils, which are made of lymphoid tissue. It supports the immune system by housing and transporting white blood cells to and from lymph nodes. The lymphatic system also returns fluid that has leaked from the cardiovascular system back into the blood vessels.	• The urinary system helps with proper lymphatic functioning by helping to maintain proper water/acid-base/electrolyte balance of the blood. • The brain helps control the immune response. • Acidic secretions in both the reproductive and integumentary systems prevent bacterial growth.
Muscular system	The muscular system consists of skeletal muscles, tendons that connect muscles to bones, and ligaments that attach bones together to form joints. The cardiac and smooth muscles are not included in this organ system.	• The endocrine system releases hormones that influence muscular strength. • The nervous system regulates and coordinates muscle activity. • The reproductive system encourages larger muscle size in men. • The bones provide levers for muscular activity.
Nervous system	The nervous system consists of the brain, spinal cord, and nerves, and it serves as the body's control system. Sensory receptors detect stimuli that can occur both inside and outside the body. The conduction of nervous impulses along nerves is extremely fast, making it possible for immediate reflexive responses to protect the body from threats. Once a threat is detected, the nervous system activates the appropriate muscles or glands to respond.	• The endocrine system releases hormones that regulate the activity of neurons. • The urinary system helps dispose of metabolic wastes and maintains the correct electrolyte balance for proper nerve function.
Reproductive system	The main purpose of the reproductive system is to produce offspring. This system consists of the testes, penis, ovaries, vagina, and breasts. The reproductive system is specialized in men to produce sperm and in women to produce eggs (or ova). The reproductive organs also house hormones that encourage or suppress activities within the body (e.g., libido and aggression) and influence the development of masculine or feminine body characteristics.	• The lymphatic system transports sex hormones. • The muscular system is involved in childbirth. • The respiratory rate increases during pregnancy.
Respiratory system	The respiratory system keeps the body's cells supplied with oxygen and removes carbon dioxide as it is released from cells. It consists of the nasal cavity, pharynx, larynx, trachea, bronchi, and lungs. The lungs house tiny air sacs called alveoli. It is through the walls of alveoli that oxygen and carbon dioxide move in and out of the lungs via small blood vessels called arterioles.	• The muscular system aids in breathing by producing volume changes (the diaphragm and intercostal muscles). • The nervous system regulates breathing rate and depth.
Skeletal system	The skeletal system provides support and protection for the body and its organs and supplies a framework that, when used in conjunction with the muscles, creates movement. It consists of bones, cartilage, ligaments, and joints. The skeletal system also serves as storage for minerals such as calcium and phosphorus.	• The endocrine system releases hormones that regulate growth and the release of calcium. • The digestive system provides nutrients necessary for the mineralization of bones. • The urinary system activates vitamin D, which is necessary for calcium absorption into bone.

Organ system	Description	Relationships with other organ systems
		• The muscular system helps place stress on the bones during exercise, which increases the deposit of calcium into bones. • The nervous system recognizes painful stimuli in the bones and joints. • The cardiovascular system supplies oxygen and nutrients while removing wastes, such as lactic acid. • The reproductive system influences the shape of the skeletal form. • The integumentary system provides vitamin D necessary for absorbing calcium into bone.
Urinary system	The urinary or excretory system helps maintain the water and electrolyte (sodium, chloride, and potassium are electrolytes) balance within the body, regulates the acid-base balance of the blood, and removes all nitrogen-containing wastes from the body. The nitrogen-containing wastes are by-products of the breakdown of proteins and nucleic acids.	• The endocrine system helps regulate the reabsorption of water and electrolytes in the kidneys. • The liver (digestive system) synthesizes urea that must be excreted by the kidneys.

Table 3.3 Common Terms Used When Discussing Anatomy

Anatomical term	Definition
Anatomical position	a standard position in which the body is facing forward, the feet are parallel to each other, and the arms are at the sides with the palms facing forward
Superior	toward the upper end of the body or body structure
Inferior	toward the lower end of the body or body structure (opposite superior)
Anterior	toward the front of the body or body structure
Posterior	toward the back of the body or body structure (opposite of anterior)
Medial	toward the middle of the body or body structure
Lateral	toward the outer sides of the body or body structure (opposite of medial)
Intermediate	between medial and lateral
Proximal	close to the origin of the body part or point of attachment
Distal	away from the origin of the body part or point of attachment (opposite of proximal)
Superficial	toward or at the body surface
Deep	away from or below the body surface (the opposite of superficial)
Sagittal section	cut made along a longitudinal plane dividing the body into right and left parts
Midsagittal section	sagittal section made down the median of the body
Transverse section (cross section)	cut made along a horizontal plane to divide the body into upper and lower regions
Frontal section (coronal section)	cut made along a longitudinal plane that divides the body into front and back regions
Dorsal body cavity	contains the cranial cavity and spinal column
Ventral body cavity	contains all the structures within the chest and abdomen; diaphragm divides the ventral cavity into the thoracic cavity (superior to the diaphragm); below the diaphragm are the abdominal and pelvic cavities

Functions of the human body: Each individual begins as a single cell that multiplies to form distinct patterns or groupings of cells called tissues. Tissues grow and mature to form specific organs, and organs develop into systems that carry out body functions. Subsequently, the human body is an integrated structure designed to carry out the functions of life. Table 3.4 displays some of these functions.

Table 3.4 Functions of the Human Body

Function	Description
Adaptation	receive, interpret, and respond to internal and external stimuli via the nervous system
Circulation	transport oxygen and other nutrients to tissues via the cardiovascular system
Elimination	remove metabolic wastes from the body via the renal system
Locomotion	allow voluntary and involuntary movement of body via the musculoskeletal and neurological systems
Nutrition	take in and break down nutrients to be used for metabolism via the digestive system
Oxygenation	take in oxygen and expel carbon dioxide via the respiratory system
Regulation	hormonal control of body functions via the endocrine system
Self-duplication	production of offspring via the reproductive system

Ways in Which the Organ Systems Interact: The 11 organ systems in the human body work together to carry out the functions necessary for life. There are several functions that are common among all complex, higher level animals. These include maintaining boundaries, responding to environmental changes, moving about, ingesting and digesting nutrients, reproducing, growing, removing waste, and producing energy through metabolism. Each of these functions, as well as some of the organs used for these functions, is discussed in Table 3.5. When all the needs of the body are met and all of the organ systems are working properly, the body is in a stable state known as **homeostasis**.

Table 3.5 Ways in Which the Organ Systems Interact

Function	Description
Maintaining boundaries	The cells in the human body are eukaryotic cells, which means they are surrounded by a membrane as are the organelles inside the cells. The membrane, which is semipermeable, allows some substances to pass through while restricting others. The integumentary system that surrounds the entire body protects it from environmental stimuli and pathogens.
Responding to environmental changes	The human body has the ability to sense and respond to environmental stimuli, both voluntarily and involuntarily. An individual's ability to physically move away from danger is an example of a voluntary response. The hand's ability to withdraw from painful stimuli before the brain perceives the pain is an example of an involuntary reflex response.
Moving	The primary purpose of muscular tissue is to support movement of the body. The muscular system moves the bones in the skeletal system and this movement is voluntary. The muscular tissues in the cardiovascular, digestive, reproductive, urinary, and respiratory systems also support movements, and this movement is involuntary.
Ingesting and digesting	The organs in the digestive system work to remove nutrients from food and transport those nutrients to other parts of the body using the cardiovascular system.
Reproducing	The reproductive system plays a key role in reproduction, and hormones regulate this process.
Growing	Growth occurs due to changes in several body systems. The skeletal and muscular systems change shape. The digestive system removes needed nutrients from food. The cardiovascular system transports these nutrients to the cells. The endocrine system releases hormones that signal when and how much growth should occur.
Excreting	Once nutrients have been removed from food in the digestion system, the waste that remains is excreted from the body using organs in both the digestive system and the urinary system.
Metabolizing	Metabolism is the use of energy by cells as a result of chemical reactions within the cells. The digestive and respiratory systems supply the nutrients and oxygen that the body needs to support metabolism. The blood distributes these materials throughout the body and hormones secreted by the glands of the endocrine system regulate the body's metabolism.

ⓟ *Practice problems*

Solutions to the practice problems are located in the back of this book.

Indicate where each of the tissue types can be found in the human body by matching the type of tissue to the human body part.

1. A) Connective tissue   _____ i. Bone

    B) Epithelial tissue   _____ ii. Brain

    C) Muscle tissue   _____ iii. Heart

    D) Nervous tissue   _____ iv. Skin

Match the body function with the body part to which it correlates.

2. A) Circulatory system   _____ i. This system breaks down food so that the nutrients can be easily passed into the blood and circulated throughout the body.

    B) Digestive system

    C) Endocrine system   _____ ii. This system helps cleanse the blood and houses the white blood cells that are involved in protecting the body from environmental pathogens.

    D) Integumentary system

    E) Lymphatic system   _____ iii. This system helps maintain the water and electrolyte balance within the body, regulates the acid-base balance in the blood, and removes all nitrogen-containing wastes from the body.

    F) Muscular system

    G) Nervous system

    H) Reproductive system   _____ iv. This system keeps all the cells in the body supplied with oxygen and removes the carbon dioxide.

    I) Respiratory system   _____ v. This system produces movement through contractions.

    J) Skeletal system   _____ vi. This system produces offspring.

    K) Urinary system   _____ vii. This system protects internal tissues from injury, waterproofs the body, and helps regulate body temperature. This system also serves as a barrier to foreign substances.

_____ viii. This system provides support and protection for the body, supplies a framework used to create movement, and serves as storage for minerals, such as calcium.

_____ ix. This system acts as the body's control system and is necessary to protect the body from changes in the internal and external environment.

_____ x. This system controls body functions.

_____ xi. This system works as the transportation system for substances such as oxygen, carbon dioxide, and nutrients in the body.

Circulatory System

The circulatory system, also known as the cardiovascular system, is the transportation highway for the entire body. It consists of the heart, blood, and blood vessels. The **heart** is an organ that contracts and pumps blood throughout the body. Rhythmic contractions of the heart enable blood to be transported throughout the body. **Arteries** are blood vessels that transport blood away from the heart to the capillaries. **Veins** are blood vessels that transport blood from the capillaries back to the heart. The **capillaries** are tiny blood vessels that transport blood from arteries to veins within the body. Capillaries also serve as the location for the exchange of oxygen, carbon dioxide, fluid, and nutrients within the body. Figure 3.2 displays how arteries, capillaries, and veins interact.

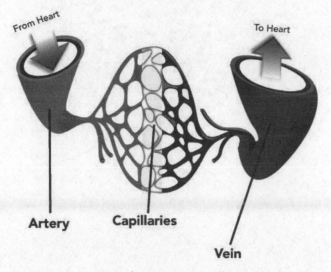

Figure 3.2 Picture of an artery, capillaries, and a vein.

The heart consists of four chambers: the right and left atriums and the right and left ventricles. It also has four valves that prevent the flow of blood back into the heart's chambers after a contraction. The valves include the tricuspid and pulmonary on the right side of the heart and the mitral and aortic on the left side of the heart. The following description, accompanied by Figure 3.3, details the flow of blood through the heart.

Deoxygenated blood enters into the heart through the superior and inferior vena cava. The blood travels into the right atrium and, during contraction of the atrium, flows through the tricuspid valve into the right ventricle. The blood is pushed through the pulmonary valve into the pulmonary artery and lungs when the right ventrical contracts. Here, it picks up oxygen. The oxygenated blood is then carried back to the heart (by the pulmonary veins), into the left atrium, through the mitral valve, and into the left ventricle. Contraction of the left ventricle forces the blood through the aortic valve, through the aorta, and out to the entire body.

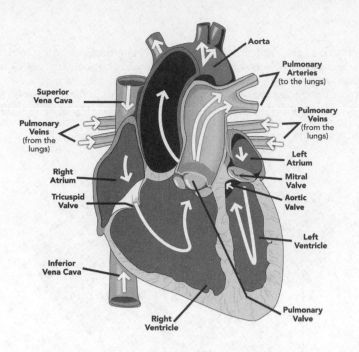

Figure 3.3 Flow of blood through the heart.

P *Practice problems*

Solutions to the practice problems are located in the back of this book.

1. Using Figure 3.3, if the mitral valve is damaged, which of the following problems may occur?

    A) Backflow of blood into the left atrium
    B) Backflow of blood into the right atrium
    C) Incomplete emptying of the right ventricle
    D) Incomplete emptying of the left ventricle

Identify whether the following statements are TRUE or FALSE.

2. Blood that passes through the tricuspid valve enters the left ventricle.

3. Blood that passes through the mitral valve enters the pulmonary artery.

4. After contraction of the left ventricle, blood enters the aorta.

5. After contraction of the right ventricle, blood enters the pulmonary artery.

6. After contraction of the right atrium, blood enters the right ventricle.

7. The pulmonary valve ensures that blood stays in the aorta.

Respiratory System

The respiratory system provides for air exchange and supplies tissues with oxygenated blood. The primary function of the **lungs** is breathing in oxygen and exhaling carbon dioxide. As shown in Figure 3.4, this process begins as air is inhaled through the nose into the **trachea**, passing into the right and left **bronchial tubes**. Within the bronchial tubes are tiny hairs called **cilia**, which keep the airway clear by removing unwanted matter from the lungs. After leaving the bronchial tubes, air travels into the **alveoli**, which are tiny air sacs that are surrounded by capillaries. The alveoli permit the exchange of oxygen and carbon dioxide to occur. The oxygen is then transported by red blood cells into the bloodstream. This process begins when the **diaphragm**, an abdominal muscle that contracts, pulls air into the lungs during **inspiration** (the act of taking in oxygenated air). When the diaphragm relaxes, carbon dioxide is forced out of the body through **expiration**.

Pulmonary function decreases with age, smoking, and exposure to pollutants and irritating chemicals. Although the normal aging process is unavoidable, exercising and keeping active assist with maintaining adequate lung function. Smoking, pollutants, and chemical exposures should be avoided.

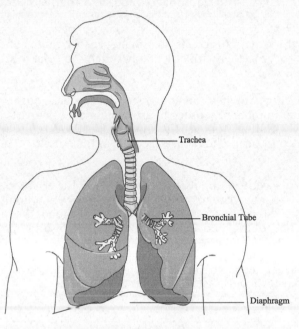

Figure 3.4 Diagram of the respiratory system.

(P) *Practice problems*

Solutions to the practice problems are located in the back of this book.

Complete the statements below.

1. The respiratory system supplies the body with _____ and removes _____.

2. It is through the walls of the _____ that oxygen and carbon dioxide move in and out of the capillaries in the lungs.

3. Which of the following happens during inspiration?

    A) Carbon dioxide enters the lungs from the arterioles around the alveoli.
    B) Oxygen leaves the lungs through the arterioles around the alveoli.
    C) The diaphragm contracts.
    D) The diaphragm relaxes.

Nervous System

The nervous system contains the central nervous system (CNS) and the peripheral nervous system (PNS). The brain and spinal cord are part of the **central nervous system**. Cranial and spinal nerves that extend beyond the CNS make up the **peripheral nervous system**. The PNS is divided into the autonomic nervous system and the sensory-somatic nervous system. The **autonomic nervous system** controls automatic body functions, like heartbeat and digestion. This system includes both **sympathetic nerves** (which are active when a person is excited or scared) and **parasympathetic nerves** (which are active when a person is eating or at rest). These two types of nerves have opposite effects on the body, which helps to maintain a balanced internal environment. The **sensory-somatic nervous system** consists of 12 pairs of cranial nerves and 31 pairs of spinal nerves and associated **ganglia** (collections of nerve cell bodies). This system controls voluntary actions, like talking and walking.

Nerve cells have **dendrites** that receive stimuli from the internal and external environment and bring those stimuli to the **neurons** (specialized cells that make up the nervous system and transmit messages) for interpretation. The **axon** of nerve cells connects one neuron with another neuron over a fluid filled gap called a **synapse.** Chemical neurotransmitters pass through the synapse to transmit an impulse to another neuron. This transmission happens at about 90 meters per second.

Overall, the nervous system has three main functions: to provide sensory, motor, and integrative functions within the body. All of these functions work together with other body systems to react to **stimuli** and maintain homeostasis within the body.

The sensory function includes feeling pain, heat, and other stimuli. The face, fingers, and toes are more sensitive to stimuli because they have a greater number of **sensory neurons** than do other parts of the body. When the body senses pain, it may automatically withdraw from it. This response is called a **reflex** and occurs when neurons transmit a message to the spinal cord, which in turn sends a message back to the muscles to react before the message is transmitted to the brain.

The motor function serves to carry electrical impulses from the CNS to the **effectors**, which are most commonly the glands and muscles. In this way, decisions that are made in the integrative function are acted upon by other parts of the body. For example, if a person who is hungry sees a table of available food, the integrative function of the brain tells the body's muscles to move toward the food and the salivary glands begin to produce saliva.

The integrative function uses sensory information to make decisions by joining together sensory input with memories already stored within the brain. The integrative function also uses sensory information to develop thoughts and feelings upon which decisions may be based at a later time.

(P) *Practice problems*

Solutions to the practice problems are located in the back of this book.

Identify whether the following statements are TRUE or FALSE.

1. The nervous system directs bodily defenses against external stimuli.

2. The nervous system regulates heart and breathing rates.

3. The nervous system supplies the body with oxygen and removes carbon dioxide.

4. The nervous system releases heat built up by the muscular system.

Digestive System

The digestive system is composed of the alimentary canal and accessory structures. It includes the mouth, esophagus, stomach, small intestine (which is made up of the duodenum, jejunum, and ileum), large intestine (or colon), and anus (see Figure 3.5). Accessory structures include the teeth, salivary glands, pancreas, liver, and gallbladder. The gastrointestinal tract (stomach and intestines) is a long, muscular tube lined with smooth muscle in which **peristalsis**, rhythmic contractions that propel food towards the colon and anus, occurs. These contractions move food along the gastrointestinal tract as the food is mechanically and chemically broken down.

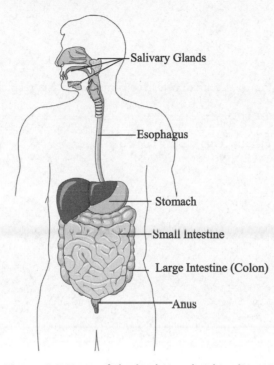

Figure 3.5 Parts of the body involved in digestion.

There are several parts of the body involved in digestion. During the process of **digestion** (the mechanical and chemical breakdown of foods), teeth grind, chew, and tear food into smaller pieces to increase the surface area upon which enzymes can act. **Enzymes** are chemicals that break down proteins, carbohydrates, and fats into nutrients that can be absorbed through the wall of the intestine into the bloodstream. Salivary amylase, an enzyme from the parotid salivary glands, begins chemical digestion of carbohydrates. Once swallowed, the bolus of food passes through the esophagus and into the stomach. Cells in the stomach lining secrete mucus for lubrication, an enzyme to begin protein digestion (protease), hydrochloric acid, and intrinsic factor, which increases the stomach's absorption of vitamin B12. Mechanical churning of the stomach also continues to break the food down into smaller pieces.

At this point, fat-laden **chyme** (the mixture of food, chemicals, and enzymes in the stomach) remains in the stomach longer than carbohydrate-laden chyme, which advances more quickly into the small-intestine (duodenum) through the **pyloric sphincter.** This sphincter releases chyme from the stomach into the small intestine. The first section of the small intestine, called the **duodenum**, releases two hormones: secretin and cholecystokinin (CCK). Secretin travels to the pancreas to trigger release of bicarbonate, which neutralizes the stomach acid entering the duodenum. In addition, secretin triggers the release of pancreatic enzymes that further aid chemical digestion in the small intestine. CCK is released from the duodenum as well and initiates bile release from the gallbladder, while decreasing motility and acid production by the stomach. Additional enzymes needed to complete the digestion of fats, proteins, and carbohydrates are released. Absorption of the nutrients occurs in the small intestine through finger-like projections called **villi**. Villi and **microvilli** increase the surface area within the small intestine, increasing the area from which absorption can take place. Each villus contains arterioles and lymphatic vessels through which absorption occurs.

The remaining products of digestion that are not absorbed are transported to the colon. Absorption of water, which affects water and electrolyte balance, occurs in the colon, and the storage and formation of feces also occurs.

(P) *Practice problems*

Solutions to the practice problems are located in the back of this book.

1. The digestion of carbohydrates begins in the _____.

2. The propulsion of food through the gastrointestinal tract is called

   A) chemotaxis.
   B) digestion.
   C) peristalsis.
   D) metabolism.

3. The surface area for absorption in the small intestine is increased as a result of

   A) enzymatic action on nutrients.
   B) villi and microvilli.
   C) mechanical breakdown that occurs during chewing.
   D) the parasympathetic nervous system.

Immune System

The **immune system** (tissues, cells, and organs that fight off illness and disease) is composed of both innate (nonspecific) and adaptive (specific) defenses that are designed to protect the body from **pathogens** and other foreign invaders.

Innate immune functions provide a nonspecific type of defense. These defense mechanisms occur the same way every time, regardless of the type or number of pathogens that are present. Innate defenses include a first line of defense, which includes both physical and chemical barriers (skin, mucous membranes, and digestive enzymes).

Innate defenses also include a second line of nonspecific defenses. These include fever, inflammation, **phagocytosis** (engulfing of pathogens by white blood cells), natural killer cells, interferons, chemotaxis, and release of cytokines. Mild to moderate fevers benefit the body by killing pathogens that grow better at a lower body temperature. Inflammation occurs as a response to irritating chemicals, heat, trauma, or infection by pathogens. Redness, heat, swelling, and pain are the four cardinal signs of inflammation. Natural killer cells, or NK cells, produce **perforins** (pore-forming proteins) that target cancer and virus cells. Perforins cause these cells to **lyse**, or rupture. **Interferons** are the body's response to a viral infection and prevent replication of the virus after 7 to 10 days. They also activate macrophages and NK cells. **Chemotaxis** is the method by which the **leukocytes** (white blood cells) respond to damaged body tissues. This is accomplished in part through **cytokines**, chemical messengers that are released by damaged tissues. **Diapedesis**, which is the process of white blood cells squeezing through capillary slits in response to cytokines, occurs, followed by cellular adhesion molecules (CAMs) guiding the white blood cells to the site of damage or infection.

Adaptive responses are known as the third line of defense, or the specific defenses. These include both the humoral, or antibody-mediated, and the cell-mediated responses. In the antibody-mediated branch, **antibodies** are produced that are specific for the invading **antigen**. The antigen binds to **B cells** (types of lymphocytes or small leukocytes) followed by binding with T-helper cells. This activates the B cells to produce antibodies. In active immunity, an individual receives a **vaccine** that simulates an actual infection by a pathogen, stimulating the body to produce antibodies for future protection. In passive immunity, an individual does not produce his or her own antibodies, but rather receives them directly from another source, such as mother to infant through breast milk. Once the immune system has produced antibodies against a pathogen, it is able to recognize that pathogen in the future and destroy it more effectively.

In cell-mediated immunity, T cells are primarily responsible for recognizing nonself cells. A **T cell** is a lymphocyte that triggers the action of other lymphocytes. In a three-step process, macrophages capture the nonself cell, a T-helper cell binds to it and secretes a cytokine that signals the cytotoxic T cell. The cytotoxic T cell responds through chemotaxis and actively destroys the nonself cell.

(P) *Practice problems*

Solutions to the practice problems are located in the back of this book.

1. What kind of immunity is produced by a vaccine?

   A) Naturally acquired passive immunity
   B) Artificially acquired passive immunity
   C) Naturally acquired active immunity
   D) Artificially acquired active immunity

2. Which of the following are released by damaged cells in an effort to draw white blood cells to the area of damage?

   A) Phagocytes
   B) Cytokines
   C) Interferons
   D) Leukocytes

3. What is the physiological benefit of a mild to moderate fever?

   A) Warns individual that body is under attack by a pathogen
   B) Stimulates release of macrophages
   C) Decreases metabolism
   D) Enhances destruction of pathogens

Factors That Influence Birth and Fertility Rates

Fertility rates refer to the average number of children a woman will have during her childbearing years, which occur between the ages of 15 and 44. Fertility rates are significant because they coincide with the replacement rate, which is the number of births needed to maintain the population at its current number. The replacement rate in developed countries is approximately 2.1, while the replacement rate in less-developed countries is approximately 2.3, mainly due to higher infant, child, and adult death rates. However, the current fertility rate in less-developed countries is much higher than 2.3 and the fertility rate in developed countries is lower than 2.1. For example, the fertility rate of Africa is 7 children per woman, while the fertility rate in eastern European and developed Asian countries is closer to 1. The implication of these numbers is that the population in less-developed countries will continue to rise, straining the resources in each particular country. In contrast, developed countries that have a fertility rate of less than 2 will see a decrease in the number of their population. For countries such as China, which has a policy of one child per household, this may be desirable due to overcrowding and strain that currently exists.

Various factors affect birth and fertility rates including religion, culture, economy, employment, government, education, literacy, infant mortality rates, abortions, and accessibility of family planning. Each of these factors must also be considered when exploring the birth and fertility rates of a population.

(P) *Practice problems*

Solutions to the practice problems are located in the back of this book.

1. Fertility rates are higher in which of the following types of countries?

   A) Less developed
   B) More developed
   C) Countries in equatorial geographic regions
   D) Countries in temperate geographic regions

2. Which of the following are factors that may affect birth rates? (Select all that apply.)

   A) Religion
   B) Culture
   C) Economy
   D) Taxes
   E) Government
   F) Transportation
   G) Literacy
   H) Infant mortality rates
   I) Abortions
   J) Accessibility of family planning

Population Growth and Decline

The growth and decline of a population in a country is a result of the difference between that population's birth and death rates as well as the number of people who immigrate to or emigrate from that country. **Crude birth rate** is defined by the number of births per 1,000 people per year, while **crude death rate** is defined by the number of deaths per 1,000 people per year. **Immigration** is the act of an individual moving into a region or country to live (migrate into), while **emigration** is the act of an individual moving out of one region or country to live in another (migrate out of). Changes in any of these numbers greatly impact the population. If a country's birth rate is higher than its death rate the population in that country will grow unless emigration occurs. If population growth occurs in a country that currently does not have enough resources for its residents, a greater shortage of resources will occur. If a country's birth rate is lower than its death rate the population in that country will decrease unless immigration occurs.

Changes in a population are also affected by the country's economy, politics, medical care, natural resources, food, land, water, and climate. Each of these factors must also be considered when exploring the implications of the decline or growth of a population.

(P) *Practice problems*

Solutions to the practice problems are located in the back of this book.

Use the diagram below to answer the questions.

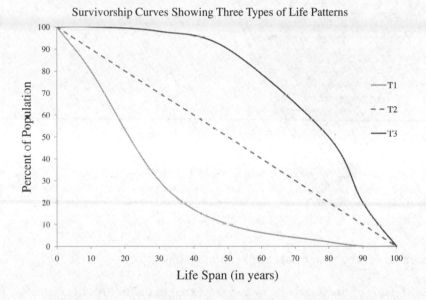

Survivorship Curves Showing Three Types of Life Patterns

1. Which of the survivorship curves demonstrates a long life expectancy for adults over 50?

2. Which of the survivorship curves demonstrates the highest mortality rate shortly after birth?

LIFE SCIENCE

Biological Classification System

The biological classification system was developed by biologists to name, organize, and categorize organisms. Early classification was accomplished by comparative anatomy. Recently, modifications to the system have taken place to improve the classification so as to reflect common descent rather than physical similarities.

Currently, DNA sequence similarities are major factors used in the classification of organisms. After it was discovered that bacteria consist of two distantly related groups, archaea and eubacteria, an eighth taxonomic rank, that of domain, was added to the hierarchy of biological classification. The eight levels in the **taxonomy** hierarchy are as follows: domain, kingdom, phylum, class, order, family, genus, and species. Although the root of the tree of life is controversial, one interpretation of the tree has the taxonomy hierarchy starting at the broad domain level, with Archaea, Eubacteria, and Eukarya. There are six kingdoms; Animalia, Fungi, Plantae, and Protista are all members of the Eukarya domain. Eubacteria is the only kingdom in the Eubacteria domain, and Archaebacteria is the only kingdom in the Archaea domain. The system ends at the species level, which contains millions of unique entries. Figure 3.6 shows this specificity range as an upside down triangle, with the domain at the top and the species at the bottom point of the triangle:

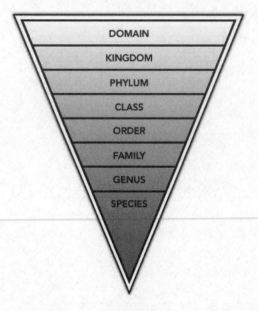

Figure 3.6 Hierarchy of the biological classification system.

When classifying individual species, the Latin name of the genus and species is written in italics with the genus capitalized and the species not capitalized. For example, the **binomial nomenclature** for humans is *Homo sapiens*, and the common fruit fly is classified as *Drosophila melanogaster*.

Ⓟ *Practice problems*

Solutions to the practice problems are located in the back of this book.

1. Match the letter on the left with the Roman numeral on the right.

A)	Species *Ursus arctos*	_____ i.	grizzly bear and brown bear
B)	Genus *Ursus*	_____ ii.	grizzly bear, brown bear, spectacled bear, and lion
C)	Family *Ursidae*	_____ iii.	grizzly bear
D)	Order *Carnivora*	_____ iv.	grizzly bear, brown bear, spectacled bear, lion, and mule deer
E)	Class *Mammalia*	_____ v.	grizzly bear, brown bear, and spectacled bear
F)	Phylum *Chordata*	_____ vi.	grizzly bear, brown bear, spectacled bear, lion, mule deer, and fire-bellied toad
G)	Kingdom *Animalia*		
		_____ vii.	grizzly bear, brown bear, spectacled bear, lion, mule deer, fire-bellied toad, and jellyfish

Natural Selection and Adaptation

Charles Darwin was the first to study and write about species adaptation. In 1859, Darwin wrote *On the Origin of Species*, after spending time in the Galapagos Islands studying the native wild life. He was the first to coin the term "natural selection." **Natural selection** occurs when some individuals of a species are better able to survive in their environment and reproduce than others. This is also known as *survival of the fittest*. Some of the characteristics that enable those individuals to survive and reproduce are inherited and can be passed on to offspring and then to future generations. Darwin did not know the mechanism of heredity, but today we know that **genes** (stretches of DNA on a chromosome that provide information for an organism's characteristics) are responsible for heredity. Every gene exists in different forms called **alleles**. Some alleles contain one or more **mutations**, which are changes in the DNA that affect the way a gene functions. Through mutations and combinations of alleles, some individuals of a species are better able to survive and adapt to the environment in which they live. This process is called **adaptation.**

Mutations are permanent changes in DNA sequences. They can also be thought of as species variations that can be passed down from generation to generation. Organisms have environmental pressures, like avoiding predators and competing for food, water, and space, as demonstrated in Example 3.4. If a variation/mutation causes a positive result that makes it easier for the organism to withstand environmental pressures, it is said to be an adaptation.

(E) *Example 3.4:*   *Darwin found a large variety of finches on the Galapagos Islands. A faster finch may get away from predators more effectively than slower finches. A stronger finch may get more food than weaker finches. These finches are more likely to survive and pass on their traits to the next generation of finches.*

Likewise, finches naturally have variations in their beak shapes. A finch with a pointed, thin beak may be able to catch and eat insects in his environment efficiently, while a finch with a blunt, rounded beak may be able to eat only fruit. The organism with the best adaptation to a particular environment is likely to survive and pass on his traits to the next generation. Over time, natural selection causes changes in the traits of a species.

Although adaptation is the end result, the process of natural selection produces it. The variability among individuals is caused by mutation and different combinations of alleles. Individuals with mutations that are best suited to a particular environment are more likely to reproduce and pass along their mutations. As a result, more favorable genes are passed to future generations, and as time passes, the species becomes better suited to its environment. This is the process known as natural selection. As this process repeats itself in a species, that species evolves, or changes genetically over time. A good example of this process is resistance to antibiotics amongst certain bacterial strains. One individual had a mutation allowing it to survive in the presence of an antibiotic, and it passed its mutation along to future generations.

(P) *Practice problems*

Solutions to the practice problems are located in the back of this book.

1.   Two strains of yeast are placed in a hot environment. Strain A has a mutation in a gene that results in an ability to tolerate and grow at the high temperature. Strain B does not have a mutation in the same gene and is unable to survive as well in the hot environment. The yeast strains are allowed to grow and reproduce for a time. After a number of generations, a sample is tested and only Strain A is found. This is an example of what?

2.   Identify whether the following statement is TRUE or FALSE.

The action of natural selection is due to the presence of mutations in DNA that are passed on from generation to generation.

Nucleic Acids

Before discussing the structures and functions of different cell parts, it is important to understand the structure and function of nucleic acids; specifically, **DNA** (deoxyribonucleic acid) and **RNA** (ribonucleic acid). The job of **nucleic acids** is to store and transmit hereditary information. Structurally, a nucleic acid is a chain of **nucleotides** that consists of a pentose, a phosphate group, and a nitrogenous base. A **pentose** is a type of sugar. A **phosphate group** is a molecule in the backbone of DNA and RNA that links adjoining bases together. A **nitrogenous base** is a molecule found in DNA and RNA that encodes the genetic information in cells. There are five types of nitrogenous bases: adenine, cytosine, guanine, thymine, and uracil. Adenine, cytosine, and guanine are found in both DNA and RNA, while thymine is unique to DNA and uracil to RNA.

Shown in Figure 3.7, DNA is most often seen in a structure known as the double helix. This complex is able to form because weak bonds are able to form between the hydrogen atoms and oxygen or nitrogen atoms between bases in the complementary strands of DNA. This kind of weak bond is called a hydrogen bond because one partner in the bond is always a hydrogen atom. In DNA, adenine (A) always pairs with thymine (T), and guanine (G) always pairs with cytosine (C).

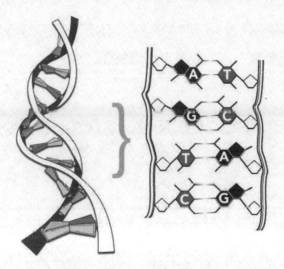

Figure 3.7 DNA's double helix structure.

Notice in the enlarged section of the DNA's double helix that adenine and guanine have two rings (they are classified as **purines**) and that thymine and cytosine only have one ring (they are classified as **pyrimidines**).

In RNA, the pyrimidine base of uracil is used instead of the thymine base found in DNA. Cytosine, adenine, and guanine are still present in RNA. Unlike the double-helix structure of DNA, for the most part, RNA exists as a single-stranded string of nucleotides.

Aside from the differences in the pyrimidine bases, the other fundamental difference between the two nucleic acids of DNA and RNA is their pentose component, which is deoxyribose in DNA and ribose in RNA. The basic components of the nucleic acids are shown in Figure 3.8. Notice that both nucleic acids include the elements of hydrogen, oxygen, nitrogen, carbon, and phosphorus:

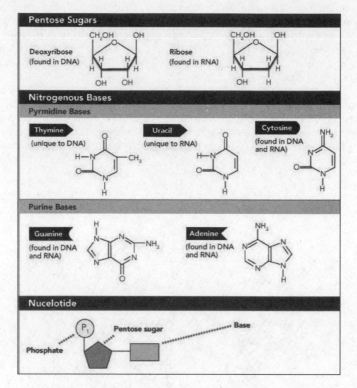

Figure 3.8 Basic components of nucleic acids.

If DNA is the genetic blueprint of the cell, then RNA can be thought of as the messenger within the cell. The message stored in the bases of DNA must be transferred to the ribosomes to make proteins. So, cells copy the instructions in the DNA into RNA (**transcription**) and send the messenger RNA to the ribosomes. Then, proteins are made by ribosomes from the information and sent out to the entire cell. This process of protein production from messenger RNA is called **translation**. DNA, RNA, and ribosomes work hand in hand to produce the proteins necessary for life in cells.

Ⓟ *Practice problems*

Solutions to the practice problems are located in the back of this book.

1. Identify whether the following statement is TRUE or FALSE.

    RNA is the messenger between DNA and protein production.

2. Indicate whether the following bases are found in DNA only, RNA only, or both DNA and RNA.

    A) Adenine
    B) Cytosine
    C) Guanine
    D) Thymine
    E) Uracil

Parts of a Cell

Bacteria (both Eubacteria and Archaebacteria) have the most basic types of cells that can exist independently of other cells. This type of cell is called **prokaryotic.** Prokaryotic cells contain the following parts and organelles (refer to Figure 3.9 for a diagram of a prokaryotic cell):

- An outside, rigid layer called the **cell wall** that helps separate the inside and outside of the cell, and an inside plasma membrane that is semipermeable, allowing certain substances in and out of the cell as needed.

- An inner layer called the **cytoplasm** is a rich protein fluid with gel-like consistency that houses **organelles**, or "tiny organs." Each organelle serves a unique function within the cell. The **nucleoid** is the condensed DNA of the cell. It contains genes and the genetic blueprints for the formation of proteins that make up the machinery of the cell. **Plasmids** are small, circular portions of DNA not associated with the nuceloid. They contain a small number of genes compared to the DNA in the nucleoid. RNA is copied from the DNA to take the instructions from the nucleoid to the rest of the cell. It is chemically similar to DNA. **Ribosomes** manufacture proteins for the cell from the RNA messages. They are very small bodies that are free-floating within the cytoplasm. Proteins do most of the work in the cells.

- Certain prokaryotic cells contain a flagellum for cellular movement. **Flagella** are long and whip-like and project outward from the cell. Bacteria also have pili that allow communication and transfer of information between two cells.

Eukarya have eukaryotic cells, which are not only more complex than prokaryotic cells, but are also many times larger. Some eukaryotic cells live as single cells, but many exist as part of a larger complex of cells comprising a multicellular organism. There are numerous organelles inside the cell, each with specialized roles. Eukaryotic cells contain the following parts and organelles (refer to Figure 3.10 for a diagram of a eukaryotic cell):

- A plasma membrane envelops the cell and is semipermeable to allow certain substances and water in and out. The cytoplasm inside the cell contains the cell contents and the organelles and is gel-like.

- Ribosomes in eukaryotic cells function like ribosomes of prokaryotic cells to make proteins based on RNA messages from the cell's genes.

- The **endoplasmic reticulum** (ER) is a tubular transport network within the cell. It appears as a stack of flattened membranous sacs. There are two types of endoplasmic reticulum: smooth and rough. The rough ER is studded with ribosomes – causing it to have a rough, gritty appearance – while the smooth ER is not. The smooth variety of endoplasmic reticulum is important for numerous metabolic processes in the cell. The ER is responsible for moving proteins from one part of a cell to another and for moving proteins to the outside of a cell (a process called **secretion**).

- The **Golgi apparatus** is involved in the packaging and transport of proteins in the cell, including protein secretion. The Golgi apparatus is composed of layers of membranes and has multiple functions: it refines proteins that have been manufactured by the ribosomes, it sorts the proteins and prepares them for transport to other parts of the cell or to the cell membrane for secretion, and it works hand in hand with the ER in protein movement and processing.

- **Vesicles** are small membrane-bounded sacs within the cytoplasm. Vesicles are used to transport proteins or other substances in or out of the cell. There are many types of vesicles. Three common types are vacuoles, lysosomes, and peroxisomes. The **vacuole** is a basic storage unit of the cell that can hold various compounds; the **lysosome** contains digestive enzymes that are capable of disposing of cellular debris and worn cellular parts; and the **peroxisome** functions to rid the body of toxic components, such as hydrogen peroxide. Peroxisomes are also major sites of oxygen use and energy production. The liver contains many peroxisomes because toxic substances build up here.

- **Mitochondria** are the powerhouses of the cell because they are the locations where the cellular fuel **ATP** (adenosine triphosphate) is produced. The mitochondria are large, kidney-bean shaped organelles surrounded by membranes. They also have membranes inside in series of folds called **cristae** (singular: *crista*) in which enzymes are found. The enzymes on the cristae help convert sugar into ATP to power the cell.

- **Microtubules** are cellular tracks that, during mitosis, form the mitotic spindle. The spindle helps organize and segregate the chromosomes during cell division. **Centrosomes** are microtubule-organizing centers that help to form and organize the mitotic spindle during mitosis.

- The **nucleus** is a very large organelle in the central portion of the cell that is enclosed by a double membrane with pores in it. It is the control center of the entire cell because it contains the cell's genetic material and directs all of the activities of the cell.

- The **nucleolus** is a small body within the nucleus and functions to produce ribosomes that get moved to the cytoplasm to make cell proteins.

- Some eukaryotic cells have whip-like projections called flagella (singular: flagellum). If there are more than a few, the projections are called cilia. These structures can beat with movements that allow the cells to move. The flagella and cilia of eukaryotic cells are much larger than prokaryotic flagella and are completely different organelles from those found in bacteria.

Plant cells and a variety of eukaryotic cells contain many of the same features as the eukaryotic cell described above with the following exceptions (refer to Figure 3.11 for a diagram of a plant cell):

- Plants contain **chloroplasts**, which are organelles that contain chlorophyll. Chlorophyll allows the capture of sunlight to be used for production of glucose during photosynthesis. Chloroplasts have many structural similarities to mitochondria, but plant cells need both mitochondria and chloroplasts.

- Plant cells have much larger vacuoles (that contain water) than eukaryotic cells have. The cells use the water in the vacuoles to maintain proper cell pressure.

- On the outside of the cell, plants have a solid cell wall that acts as a barrier to the outside and gives structure to the cell.

(P) *Practice problems*

Solutions to the practice problems are located in the back of this book.

1. Identify whether the following statement is TRUE or FALSE.

   The nucleus is the site of ATP production in cells.

A scientist wishes to construct a synthetic cell and wants to make sure it has the proper organelles for protein production, transport, and secretion. Given this situation, identify whether the following statements are TRUE or FALSE.

2. Chloroplasts are needed.

3. A Golgi apparatus is needed.

4. Ribosomes are needed.

Cellular Organelles

The previous section described the parts of a cell and their functions. This section provides diagrams to help visualize the structure of these parts (refer to the previous section for details on the parts' functions). The most basic of cell types, the prokaryotic cell, is shown in Figure 3.9. Notice that the nucleoid contains the DNA, the cytoplasm contains the ribosomes and plasmid, and the surface is layered first by the plasma membrane, then the cell wall, and finally the capsule.

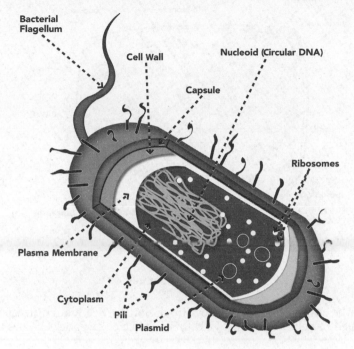

Figure 3.9 Prokaryotic cell.

More complex than the prokaryotic cell is the eukaryotic cell. The eukaryotic cell is shown in Figure 3.10:

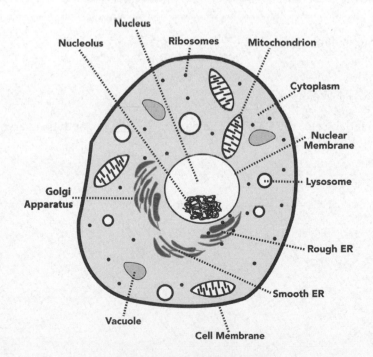

Figure 3.10 Eukaryotic cell.

Notice that the nuclear membrane encases the nucleus (which contains DNA); the cytoplasm surrounds the ER, ribosomes, Golgi apparatus, mitochondria, vacuoles, and lysosomes; and the surface is a cell membrane.

Similar to the eukaryotic cell, the plant cell is shown in Figure 3.11. Again, important parts are highlighted:

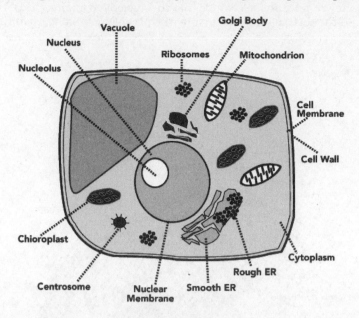

Figure 3.11 Plant cell.

Notice that the plant cell and the eukaryotic cell are structurally similar. Two main differences between these two types of cells are that a plant cell has chloroplasts and a cell wall and a eukaryotic cell does not.

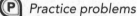 *Practice problems*

Solutions to the practice problems are located in the back of this book.

1. Which of the following is present in eukaryotic and prokaryotic cells?

    A) Golgi apparatus
    B) Endoplasmic reticulum
    C) Mitochondrion
    D) Cytoplasm

2. Complete the following sentence.

    In prokaryotic (bacterial) cells, the DNA is located in the _____, and in eukaryotic (animal/plant) cells, the DNA is found in the _____.

Chromosomes, Genes, Proteins, RNA, and DNA

Chromosomes contain sections called genes, which contain information that specifies the production of proteins. Genes send messages within the cell and to other cells in the form of a code, which is made possible through complementary base pairing. Within the genes are double-stranded molecules of DNA that are composed of the nitrogenous bases: four chemical groups that always match up in pairs. Adenine pairs with thymine and guanine pairs with cytosine. Thus, chromosomes consist of subunits of genes, and genes consist of DNA.

To translate the complementary code on DNA into a protein, RNA is required. The code on the DNA strand is copied into RNA within the cell nucleus and transported to the ribosome. One main difference between DNA and RNA is that one base is different between the two: thymine does not exist in RNA. Uracil is used instead. At the ribosome, the RNA code is translated into an amino-acid chain. A chain of amino acids results in a **protein**.

Thus, a protein consists of information derived from DNA and RNA. Proteins play a vital part in the body's functioning. Chromosomes, genes, DNA, and RNA are the substances that preside over protein production. In the cell, information flows from DNA to RNA to proteins.

(P) *Practice problems*

Solutions to the practice problems are located in the back of this book.

Complete the statements below.

1. _____ are large structures of DNA that contain the _____, the blueprints for making an individual.

2. The central dogma of biology states that _____ gives rise to RNA, which gives rise to protein.

Cell Differentiation

Differentiation produces a more-specialized cell from a less-specialized cell. To form an **embryo** (an animal or a plant in the early stages of development after fertilization), a fertilized egg begins dividing and becomes a mass of cells called a **zygote**. The most critical stage of development is called gastrulation, in which individual tissue layers begin to form. The genes of each cell regulate the process of differentiation during all stages of development.

Differentiation determines what cell type each cell will become. In humans, there are hundreds of cell types. The genes that control differentiation direct each cell when to form the particular proteins and structures that make it a specific cell type.

The process of differentiation occurs with cells in the developing embryo but can also occur in adults. Cells can divide and remain undifferentiated. This produces **stem cells**. Totipotent, pluripotent, and multipotent cells are three types of stem cells.

(P) *Practice problems*

Solutions to the practice problems are located in the back of this book.

1. Identify whether the following statement is TRUE or FALSE.

   Cellular differentiation may occur in a developing embryo or in an adult.

2. What is an embryo?

RNA and DNA Involvement in Cell Replication

Mitosis is the process of cell duplication in which two daughter cells receive exactly the same nuclear material as the original cell. Prior to mitosis, the cell must make an exact copy of all of its DNA to have complete DNA for both new cells. The synthesis of the new DNA occurs in the S phase (S stands for synthesis). Before and after synthesis, there are gap periods referred to as G_1 and G_2. During the gaps between mitosis and DNA synthesis, the cell's DNA is available for transcription into RNA, which is necessary for the cell machinery to be able to make proteins and perform other cellular functions. The S phase, G_1, and G_2 are all classified as **interphase**, as seen in Figure 3.12.

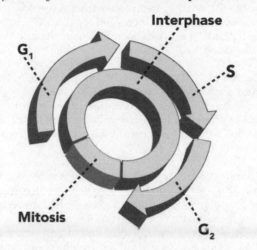

Figure 3.12 Three phases of interphase and mitosis.

In G_1, the DNA double helix unwinds to expose the bases. RNA bases pair with their complementary partners on the DNA to form the messenger RNA strand. Once an entire gene is copied into the complementary messenger RNA (mRNA), the DNA double helix closes and the mRNA exits the nucleus, taking the information it contains to the ribosome.

In the S phase of interphase, the DNA double helix unwinds with the help of enzymes (proteins that increase the speed of reactions). This breaks the hydrogen bonds between the base pairs and separates the bases from their complementary partners, but does not remove the bases from the backbone of their half of the double helix. The exposed bases pair with new complementary bases that are then synthesized into a new complementary strand with the help of an enzyme called DNA polymerase. At the same time, the other strand from the original double helix is going through the same process. Thus, two new strands of identical DNA form where only one strand previously existed. Each of the two strands has one strand from the original double helix and one strand that was newly synthesized.

The G_2 phase of interphase includes continued protein synthesis and cell growth in preparation for cell division.

Ⓟ *Practice problems*

Solutions to the practice problems are located in the back of this book.

1. Identify whether the following statement is TRUE or FALSE.

   There are three steps of the cell cycle during interphase.

2. Explain briefly (in 1 to 2 sentences) how the DNA double helix can be released to allow replication.

Mitosis and Meiosis

Mitosis occurs to replace old and dying cells with genetically identical ones. During mitosis, the cells have to double their DNA content to pass one complete copy to each daughter cell. For example, mitosis occurs among cells of the skin, the liver, and other organs in the digestive system.

Sexual reproduction works differently from mitosis. The cells that form a new organism via sexual reproduction are called **gametes**. During sexual reproduction, a gamete from one individual combines its DNA with the DNA of a gamete from another individual. The combining of DNA from two gametes would produce too much DNA if gametes did not reduce their DNA content. The process by which gametes reduce their DNA content is called **meiosis**. Meiosis occurs only in gametes or fertilized eggs, depending on the species. One of the additional benefits of meiosis is that it results in extra genetic variability, as will be described below.

The purpose of meiosis is to halve the number of chromosomes (individual units of DNA comprised of several genes). Cells that contain two sets of chromosomes are known as **diploid cells**. In mammals, all cells but gametes are diploid cells. Cells that contain a single set of chromosomes are known as **haploid cells**. In mammals, only gametes are haploid cells, but in some organisms, most cells are haploid cells and only the fertilized egg is a diploid cell. In a diploid cell, each individual chromosome has a twin chromosome called a **homologous** chromosome; it is almost identical in size, function, and genes.

In mitosis, the individual chromosomes duplicate during the S phase and condense into chromosomes that have both copies of the individual chromosome attached at one spot to form sister **chromatids**. Next, during metaphase of mitosis, chromosomes with their sister chromatids line up on a plate (called a **metaphase plate**) down the middle of the nucleus. On that plate, the chromosomes line up in no particular order. Spindle fibers form between the centrosomes (there is one centrosome on either side of the nucleus) and attach to the chromosomes on the metaphase plate. The sister chromatids separate and each one moves toward a different centrosome. At the end of metaphase, one chromatid from each chromosome is near each centrosome. The new nuclei that form around each group of chromosomes get one chromatid from each chromosome. In mitosis, **cytokinesis** begins at this point, separating the two sets of chromosomes into different cells. Mitosis is complete.

In meiosis, when the chromosomes line up at the metaphase plate, each chromosome searches out its homologous chromosome. In a meiotic metaphase plate, the chromosomes are lined up in pairs of two homologous chromosomes, each one containing two sister chromatids. In this tangle of chromatid arms, some genetic material gets traded between sister chromatids, leading to some extra genetic variability. The formation of the meiotic spindle and the separation of the chromosomes into two groups proceeds just as in mitosis, but in meiosis, it is the homologues that separate rather than the sister chromatids. The result is two cells, each new cell having only one set of chromosomes. The first stage of meiosis (referred to as Meiosis I) is now complete, and the result is two haploid cells. However, during meiosis I, the sister chromatids did not separate, so each cell still has two copies of its haploid set of chromosomes. The cells do not go into interphase but immediately start meiosis II. During meiosis II, each of the chromosomes (remember they are still duplicated) lines up on the metaphase plate and the sister chromatids separate, as in mitosis. The result of the two meiotic divisions is four haploid cells. Figure 3.13 and Table 3.6 illustrate the differences between mitosis and meiosis:

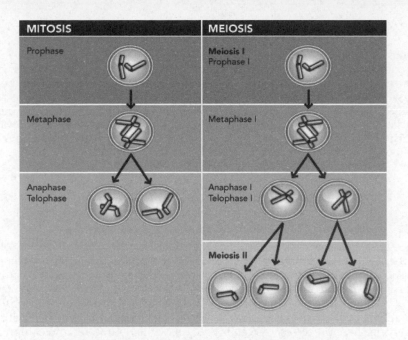

Figure 3.13 Comparison of mitosis and meiosis.

Table 3.6 Stages of Mitosis and Meiosis

Mitosis	Meiosis
Prophase – The spindle fibers form and the centrioles moves to opposite sides of the cell. The nuclear membrane disappears.	**Prophase I** – Homologous chromosomes condense and link in the process-forming tetrads. This allows crossing over or recombination to occur.
Metaphase – The chromosomes align midway along the spindle fibers.	**Metaphase I** – Homologous chromosomes move to the metaphase plate.
Anaphase – The chromosomes begin to separate from their daughters. Cytokinesis begins.	**Anaphase I** – Homologous chromosomes separate, but the sister chromatids stay together.
Telophase – Identical sets of chromosomes are at opposites ends of the cell. Spindle fibers disappear, nuclear membranes reappear, and cytokinesis completes.	**Telophase I** – Cytokinesis has occurred and two haploid daughter cells are the result.
	Prophase II –A brief stage in which spindle fibers begin to reappear and centrioles move to opposite poles.
	Metaphase II –Sister chromatids align at a new metaphase plate.
	Anaphase II – Sister chromatids separate again.
	Telophase II –Four haploid cells result after cytokinesis.

(P) *Practice problems*

Solutions to the practice problems are located in the back of this book.

1. Complete the following sentence.

   During meiosis, a _____ cell will give rise to four _____ cells.

2. Identify whether the following statement is TRUE or FALSE.

   Mitosis and meiosis occur in all types of cells.

Photosynthesis and Respiration

Both photosynthesis and cellular respiration result in the formation of cellular energy for an organism, yet the two processes differ in their end results. **Photosynthesis** is the process carried out by green plants, green algae, and certain bacteria, in which the energy from sunlight is trapped by the green pigment **chlorophyll** and used for synthesis of glucose. These organisms are able to carry out photosynthesis due to the specialized organelle called a chloroplast. In the chloroplast, carbon dioxide, water, and energy from the Sun are used to produced adenosine triphosphate (ATP), which is a cellular fuel that provides the energy to produce glucose from carbon dioxide and water, liberating oxygen in the process. An organism that is able to produce its own food is termed an **autotroph**, and most autotrophs use photosynthesis to live. Figure 3.14 is a graphical representation of this equation:

$$6CO_2 \quad + 6H_2O + Energy \rightarrow C_6H_{12}O_6 + 6O_2$$
$$Carbon\ dioxide + Water + Sunlight \rightarrow Glucose + Oxygen$$

Figure 3.14 The chemical equation for photosynthesis.

In contrast to photosynthesis, cellular respiration uses one of the end products of photosynthesis, glucose, to produce ATP for cells. Cellular respiration is used by **heterotrophs**; heterotrophs are organisms that cannot produce their own food. During **cellular respiration**, glucose is broken down by the process of glycolysis, which transfers some of the energy in glucose to ATP. The end-products of glycolysis are fed into the citric acid cycle (Krebs cycle), to produce even more ATP. Together, glycolysis and the citric acid cycle constitute cellular respiration. Cells use mitochondria to carry out this cycle. During these processes, oxygen is used up, while both water and carbon dioxide are formed as by-products. This carbon dioxide is expelled, but can be used by autotrophs during photosynthesis. The chemical equation for cellular respiration is the reverse of that of photosynthesis. Figure 3.15 is a graphical representation of this equation:

$$C_6H_{12}O_6 + 6O_2 \quad \rightarrow 6CO_2 \quad + 6H_2O + Energy$$
$$Glucose + Oxygen \rightarrow Carbon\ dioxide + Water + Energy$$

Figure 3.15 The chemical equation for cellular respiration.

Ⓟ *Practice problems*

Solutions to the practice problems are located in the back of this book.

1. A new type of algae has been discovered. To determine whether or not this algae is an autotroph, the scientists should observe for which of the following?

   A) Chloroplasts
   B) Mitochondria
   C) Glucose
   D) ATP

2. Complete the following sentence.

   The organelle in plants that allows photosynthesis to occur is the _____, which contains the chemical _____ to trap energy from the sun.

Storage of Hereditary Information

Chromosomes are located in the nucleus of a cell and contain stretches of DNA called genes. Genes contain coded information that controls the heredity of particular traits, such as eye and hair color. This code is made up of the sequences of the nitrogenous bases of DNA: adenine (A), thymine (T), cytosine (C), and guanine (G). Each piece of the code is called a **codon** and is composed of three of the bases. There are 64 codons, because 64 different 3-letter combinations can be formed from A, T, C, and G. Each codon matches to a specific **amino acid**. There are 20 different amino acids, so some codons match to the same amino acid. A chain of amino acids then forms a protein. Proteins are the workhorses of the cell, and one gene matches to one protein. It is the proteins that are responsible for the expression of genetic traits.

When organisms pass genes from one generation to the next they are spreading such traits. Each gene contains different information for influencing a trait of an organism. The sum of all the proteins directed by the genes of an individual are responsible for the inherited differences between one person and another.

Ⓟ *Practice problems*

Solutions to the practice problems are located in the back of this book.

1. Complete the following sentence.

    Chromosomes contain stretches of DNA called _____, which contain the information that controls particular traits for an individual.

2. Identify whether the following statement is TRUE or FALSE.

    Genetic traits are expressed through the actions of proteins.

Changes in DNA and Mutations in Germ Cells

Mutations in the **genome** (a complete set of DNA for an individual that contains all genes) occur primarily by two mechanisms: errors during DNA replication or via a **mutagen**, a substance that induces mutations. Cells have back-up plans in place for both of these possibilities, which greatly reduces the overall rate at which mutations arise.

During DNA replication, a cell must double its DNA and make a duplicate copy of the entire genome, a task not accomplished without mistakes. Synthesis of the complementary strand of DNA could occur solely through base pairing, but this would be exceptionally slow. Cells speed up the process of DNA synthesis by using an enzyme called DNA polymerase. As DNA polymerase makes its way down a DNA strand, spontaneous errors may occur. When DNA polymerase adds DNA bases along a strand, errors may occur. In humans, errors can occur in 1 out of every 1,000 genes during each replication cycle, or up to 5% of the genes in the human genome. However, DNA repair mechanisms exist to reduce this error rate down to less than one DNA base in every 10^9 to 10^{12} bases. That is less than 0.3% of genes in the human genome and often far less. To accomplish this task, DNA polymerase performs proofreading of the newly synthesized strands. If it recognizes a mispairing of bases, it attempts to correct the problem by insertion of the proper base. Although this reduces the overall error rate, the cell has another back-up plan in place: **mismatch repair**. After the new DNA has been replicated, this mechanism scans over the DNA to find any mismatches of bases. If mismatches are found, it repairs the mismatch by removing the incorrect base and replacing it with the proper one. If a mutation is able to pass through the cracks of these systems, the DNA sequence from then on is altered. Certain forms of cancer arise because of failure in mismatch repair.

During its life, a cell may be exposed to certain substances capable of damaging DNA. These mutagens can be anything from harmful chemicals to ultraviolet rays from the Sun. **Excision repair** mechanisms inspect the DNA for these types of damage and attempt to repair it. Since modification by mutagens often occurs over a section of DNA, as opposed to individual bases, the excision repair mechanism will cut the defective strand of DNA, remove those bases that are near, including the mutated ones, and allow DNA polymerase to generate a new, correct piece of DNA. Certain skin diseases are a result of this excision repair mechanism not functioning properly.

Even though an individual may accumulate mutations over his or her lifetime that lead to certain diseases, disorders, or cancers, those mutations will only pass on to future generations if they are present in the DNA of **germ cells** (reproductive cells that give rise to sperm and ovum). For example, an individual may develop skin cancer due to excess sun exposure, but that individual's offspring will not also have skin cancer unless those mutations are also found in the gametes. The vast majority of these mutations will arise spontaneously due to replication errors and may then be passed on to future generations. Certain families carry mutations in their germ cells that routinely get passed to offspring and confer certain diseases or disorders, and only those individuals in the family that receive that particular mutation or set of mutations will develop a particular disease or disorder.

Ⓟ *Practice problems*

Solutions to the practice problems are located in the back of this book.

1. Name the major enzyme responsible for DNA replication in cells.

2. Identify whether the following statement is TRUE or FALSE.

   DNA in gametes is the DNA passed on to future generations.

Phenotypes and Genotypes

Phenotypes are the physical expressions of genetic traits. In some organisms, such as pea plants, phenotypes include seed color, pod shape, or flower color. In organisms like humans, a phenotype may be a body characteristic, such as brown hair or blue eyes.

A **genotype**, on the contrary, is an organism's underlying genetic makeup or code. It is a blueprint for building and maintaining all structures within the cells of the body, from small proteins to metabolic activities. The DNA within genes codes for proteins that determine hereditary traits that will be passed on between generations. Interactions between the genotype and the environment affect the phenotype of the organism.

Note that organisms can have different genotypes, but the same phenotype, that is, the organisms look the same.

(P) *Practice problems*

Solutions to the practice problems are located in the back of this book.

1. Complete the following sentence.

   _____ are the entire set of genes in organisms, while _____ are the characteristics and traits that are expressed by those genes.

2. Different coat colors between cat breeds are examples of genotype or of phenotype?

Mendel's Laws of Genetics and the Punnett Square

Genetics is the study of heredity or how traits are passed on from parent to offspring. Gregor Mendel began researching how characteristics of pea plants were passed to offspring from parent plants in the 1800s. He studied seven characteristics that occurred in contrasting traits. He looked at plant height (long or short stems), flower position along stem (axial or terminal), pod appearance (inflated or constricted), pod color (green or yellow), seed color (green or yellow), flower color (purple or white), and seed texture (smooth or wrinkled). He collected seeds from various plants and recorded the characteristics of each plant from which he took a seed. He planted the seeds the next year and noticed that it was possible for different traits to occur other than those shown by the parent plant. Mendel went further than these first observations. He also cross-pollinated plants showing pure traits. A plant shows a pure trait if its offspring always have the same trait.

Mendel noticed that when he crossed a short pea plant with a tall pea plant, the short trait seemed to disappear in the first generation of offspring. He called the tall trait dominant because it seemed to dominate over the short trait. The short trait that disappeared was called the recessive trait.

In the second generation of offspring, the short trait (recessive trait) occasionally occurred again. This is how we know that an organism can carry a gene without showing the physical characteristics of that gene in its phenotype.

A gene is a piece of DNA on a chromosome that controls a particular genetic trait, and as just discussed, there are multiple forms of a gene. These alternative forms are called alleles. Alleles are represented using letters. Dominant alleles are represented by capital letters, and recessive alleles are represented by lowercase letters. The genotype (genetic makeup) of an organism consists of alleles inherited from both parents. The appearance of an organism resulting from its genotype is the phenotype. When both parents give the offspring the same allele, the offspring is **homozygous** for that particular trait. If each parent gives the offspring a different allele for a particular trait, the offspring is **heterozygous** for that trait.

To predict what characteristics will occur in offspring, a Punnett square can be used. The **Punnett square** is a graphical way to show all the possible combinations of alleles given the two parents' genotypes.

Example 3.5 illustrates why the offspring of one parent homozygous for a dominant allele and one parent homozygous for a recessive allele always have the phenotype of the parent that has the dominant alleles. One parent's possible gametes are in Column 1. The other parent's possible gametes are in Row 1.

(E) *Example 3.5:*   *Draw a Punnett square for the following cross:*

Homozygous rose with thorns (T) x Homozygous rose without thorns (t)

A rose that is homozygous for thorns is denoted TT.
A rose that is homozygous for no thorns is denoted tt.

A Punnett square illustrates the crossing of these two parents as follows:

	T	T
t	Tt	Tt
t	Tt	Tt

All offspring will have thorns because all offspring will inherit at least one dominant allele.

Also, this Punnett square represents the Law of Dominance, which states that if two parents are pure for contrasting traits, only one form of the trait will appear in the offspring. Therefore, if you have a mother and a father who are pure for that trait, all of the offspring will show the dominant trait and all will be heterozygous.

As seen in Example 3.6, when a homozygous parent is crossed with a heterozygous parent, there is a 50% chance that an offspring will be homozygous for the same gene as in the homozygous parent and a 50% chance that the offspring will be heterozygous.

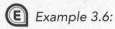 Example 3.6: *What are the possible offspring of the following crossing:*

Homozygous rose with thorns (T) × Heterozygous rose with thorns (Tt)

A rose that is homozygous for thorns is denoted TT.
A rose that is heterozygous for thorns is denoted Tt.

A Punnett square illustrates the crossing of these two parents as follows:

	T	*T*
T	*TT*	*TT*
t	*Tt*	*Tt*

In this case, all offspring will show the dominant trait because all will inherit at least one dominant allele. The recessive alleles that were inherited will not appear.

When two heterozygous plants are crossed, two of the possible offspring will be homozygous. In Example 3.7, there is a 25% chance that one offspring will be homozygous for the dominant trait and a 25% chance that one offspring will be homozygous for the recessive trait. There is a 50% chance that the two other possible offspring will be heterozygous. Another way of looking at this particular case is that 75% of the possible offspring will have thorns and 25% will not.

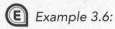 Example 3.7: *What are the possible offspring of the following crossing:*

Heterozygous rose with thorns (Tt) × Heterozygous rose with thorns (Tt)

A rose that is heterozygous for thorns is denoted Tt.

A Punnett square illustrates the crossing of these two parents as follows:

	T	*t*
T	*TT*	*Tt*
t	*Tt*	*tt*

Based on this square, it is clear that an offspring has a 25% chance of being homozygous for thorns, a 50% chance of being heterozygous with thorns, and a 25% chance of being homozygous for no thorns.

Sometimes, an organism can display incomplete dominance. **Incomplete dominance** is when the dominant and recessive genotypes interact to produce an intermediate phenotype, a mix of the two traits. For example, sickle-cell disease is a genetic disease affecting red blood cells. Homozygous recessive individuals have this disease, while homozygous dominant individuals are normal. Heterozygous individuals have a very mild case of the disease.

 Practice problems

Solutions to the practice problems are located in the back of this book.

1. What are the possible offspring of the following crossing:

   Homozygous rose without thorns (tt) × Heterozygous rose with thorns (Tt)?

2. In humans, a hypothetical disease, allomentia, is carried on the allele *a*, which is recessive to *A* (the absence of allomentia). Someone who has the genotype *Aa* does not have allomentia but can be considered a carrier of the disease, since he or she can contribute an *a* allele to his or her offspring. If a carrier of allomentia (*Aa*) mates with another carrier of allomentia, what is the chance that an offspring will be a carrier of allomentia?

EARTH AND PHYSICAL SCIENCE

Periodic Table of the Elements

1 IA	2 IIA												13 IIIA	14 IVA	15 VA	16 VIA	17 VIIA	18 0
1 H																		2 He
3 Li	4 Be	3	4	5	6	7	8	9	10	11	12		5 B	6 C	7 N	8 O	9 F	10 Ne
11 Na	12 Mg	IIIB	IVB	VB	VIB	VIIB	[	- VIIIB -	]	IB	IIB		13 Al	14 Si	15 P	16 S	17 Cl	18 Ar
19 K	20 Ca	21 Sc	22 Ti	23 V	24 Cr	25 Mn	26 Fe	27 Co	28 Ni	29 Cu	30 Zn		31 Ga	32 Ge	33 As	34 Se	35 Br	36 Kr
37 Rb	38 Sr	39 Y	40 Zr	41 Nb	42 Mo	43 Tc	44 Ru	45 Rh	46 Pd	47 Ag	48 Cd		49 In	50 Sn	51 Sb	52 Te	53 I	54 Xe
55 Cs	56 Ba	71 Lu	72 Hf	73 Ta	74 W	75 Re	76 Os	77 Ir	78 Pt	79 Au	80 Hg		81 Tl	82 Pb	83 Bi	84 Po	85 At	86 Rn
87 Fr	88 Ra	103 Lr	104 Unq	105 Unp	106 Unh	107 Uns	108 Uno	109 Une										

Lanthanide Series	57 La	58 Ce	59 Pr	60 Nd	61 Pm	62 Sm	63 Eu	64 Gd	65 Tb	66 Dy	67 Ho	68 Er	69 Tm	70 Yb
Actinide Series	89 Ac	90 Th	91 Pa	92 U	93 Np	94 Pu	95 Am	96 Cm	97 Bk	98 Cf	99 Es	100 Fm	101 Md	102 No

Figure 3.16 Periodic table.

The Sun

Energy sources that are found beyond our Earth are immediately evident in the day and night sky. During the day we recognize the largest celestial objects as being the Sun and the Moon (at certain times). However, the Moon does not provide its own source of energy. Our vision of the Moon is only a reflection of the Sun's light toward our direction. During the night, if the sky is clear, we are able to see stars of varying brightness. While these stars do have internal sources of energy, their distance from us (measured in **light-years**, or the distance that light will travel within 1 year of time) is so vast that Earth receives only a tiny fraction of light from them in comparison to what the Sun (only light-minutes away) provides. Even though the Sun is only an average star in terms of energy output, its near proximity means that the light Earth receives from it is far dominant in relation to what the Earth receive from other stars. The energy itself reaches Earth in several forms of electromagnetic waves, primarily within the visible, ultraviolet, and x-ray bands. **Electromagnetic waves** are waves of radiation that are characterized by electric and magnetic fields. Such waves are members of a spectrum, distinguished by wavelengths ranging from very short (a trillionth of a meter) to very long (kilometers). The spectrum is divided into bands of wavelengths, ordered from short to long: gamma ray, x-ray, ultraviolet, visible, infrared, microwave, and radio waves. The visible part of the spectrum can be further subdivided by color bands from long to short: red, orange, yellow, green, blue, indigo, and violet.

The energy from the Sun supports almost all life on Earth by the process of photosynthesis, which converts carbon dioxide and water into organic compounds (usually sugars) and oxygen. The organic compounds, rich in carbon, act as a major source of biomass on Earth. The Sun is also primarily responsible for driving weather and climate conditions on Earth.

Ⓟ *Practice problems*

Solutions to the practice problems are located in the back of this book.

1. Order the following forms of electromagnetic radiation from short to long wavelengths: infrared, x-ray, radio, and ultraviolet.

2. Order the 7 visible forms of electromagnetic radiation from short to long wavelengths.

Kinetic, Potential, and Other Energies

Energy and its ability to do **work** (the results of any change in energy) are often quantified in units of the metric system called **Joules** (J) or **calories**. Although Joules are the larger of the 2 units, both are considered small quantities in most real-world applications. It is often more useful to refer to kilojoules (or kilocalories), which are larger by a factor of one thousand.

The amount of energy associated with an object's motion may be quantified through a calculation of its **kinetic energy** (KE), or energy of motion. Any increase in an object's velocity (in units of meters per second in the metric system) will result in a dramatic increase in the object's KE. Specifically, any doubling of the velocity will cause the KE to increase by a factor of four times, as seen in Example 3.8.

(E) *Example 3.8:*   *KE can be calculated using the equation: $KE = \frac{1}{2} mv^2$, where m = the mass of an object and v = the velocity of an object. Using this equation, a 1-kilogram (kg) mass traveling at 2 meters/second (m/s) yields 2 J of energy:*

$$KE = \frac{1}{2} mv^2 = \frac{1}{2} \times 1\ kg \times (2\ m/s)^2 = 2\ J$$

When the velocity of this 1-kg mass is doubled to 4 m/s, the total amount of KE yields 8 J of energy:

$$KE = \frac{1}{2} mv^2 = \frac{1}{2} \times 1\ kg \times (4\ m/s)^2 = 8\ J$$

The amount of stored energy in an object may be quantified through a calculation of its **potential energy** (PE), or stored energy. Energy may be stored in several ways, as in a common battery cell or the gasoline in a fuel tank. The Earth's gravity may also store energy when an object is held at a certain height. Specifically, any doubling of the height will also double the PE. Example 3.9 illustrates this concept:

(E) *Example 3.9:*   *PE can be calculated using the following equation: PE = mgh, where m = the mass of an object, g = standard gravity constant, and h = the height at which an object is located. Using this equation and letting g = 10 m/s², a 1-kg mass at a height of 1 meter stores 10 J of energy:*

$$PE = mgh = 1\ kg \times 10\ m/s^2 \times 1\ m = 10\ J$$

When the height of this 1-kg mass is doubled to 2 meters, the total amount of PE yields 20 J of energy:

$$PE = mgh = 1\ kg \times 10\ m/s^2 \times 2\ m = 20\ J$$

KE and PE have a unique connection. PE can be used to produce an object's motion, which is KE. Both forms of energy have a dynamic interplay through the conservation of energy. Conservation of energy occurs when a total constant energy is maintained by the conversion of energy between kinetic and potential. If a system is considered closed and isolated (no mass or energy is entering or leaving), then energy may only be converted from one form of energy to another. Generally, the energy of motion (KE) may be increased, but only at the expense of converting stored energy (PE). The reverse conversion may also occur (kinetic to potential), but the total energy for the system must remain fixed. In short, the **Law of Conservation of Energy** says that energy is not lost but rather transferred back and forth between KE and PE. Given a fixed amount of total energy in a system, an increase in KE will result in a decrease in PE (and vice versa), but the total amount of energy will remain the same.

(P) *Practice problems*

Solutions to the practice problems are located in the back of this book.

1.   Suppose a 5-kilogram object is held at a height of 6 m. What is the object's potential energy at this height? Assume g = 10 m/s².

2.   Suppose an object possesses a total energy of 100 J when held at a height of 10 m. If the object is then released, how much kinetic energy and potential energy will the object have at a height of 2 m?

Measurable Properties of Atoms

Matter is anything that takes up space and has mass. Remember, mass is not the same as weight. **Mass** is the quantity of matter an object has. Substances that cannot be broken into simpler types of matter are called **elements**. All known elements are arranged in a specific order on the periodic table (see Figure 3.16). An atom is the smallest part of an element that still retains all the original properties of the element.

Since ancient Greece, an atom has been defined as the smallest piece of indivisible matter. However, modern physics (within roughly the last 100 years) has shown that an atom has smaller components within its confines. These smaller bits of matter, called protons, neutrons, and electrons, contribute to an atom's mass and charge in quantifiable ways. **Protons** are positively charged subatomic particles found in the nucleus of an atom. It has been determined that the number of protons distinguishes one atom from another. In addition, the number of protons in the nucleus of an atom of an element is the **atomic number** of the element (see Example 3.10). The atomic number serves as an ordering device for the periodic table. **Neutrons** are neutral subatomic particles found in the nucleus of an atom. **Electrons** are negatively charged subatomic particles found in various energy levels (orbital shells) around the nucleus.

An atom's charge is uniquely identified by its protons and electrons (neutrons do not contribute to the charge, as they are neutral). As long as the positive contribution (+1) from each proton in an atom is balanced by the negative contribution (–1) from each electron, an atom is said to be electrically neutral. However, a **chemical reaction**, or a dynamic event that alters the chemical makeup of an atom, may cause an imbalance in the charge, resulting in excess protons (or electrons). The imbalance produces a positively or negatively charged atom called an **ion**.

An atom's mass, while not directly measurable, can be determined using modern statistical techniques. All three components of an atom each contribute to the overall mass in a unique way. While a proton and a neutron have approximately the same mass, an electron's mass contributes much less to the atom (about 2,000 times less). Therefore, the total mass of an atom is driven primarily by its number of protons and neutrons according to the mass number. As demonstrated in the next example, the **mass number** is the total number of protons and neutrons found within the nucleus of an atom. While larger atoms have larger mass numbers, a given atom may also have several versions called isotopes that also differ by mass number. The **atomic mass** is the average mass of all of the known isotopes of an element. In most cases, it represents the most common isotope when rounded to a whole number (the mass number of that isotope).

Ⓔ *Example 3.10:*

8

O

Oxygen

15.9994

The chemical properties of oxygen are shown in the excerpt above, from the periodic table.

1. *What is the atomic number?*
2. *What is the atomic mass?*
3. *How many protons does oxygen have?*
4. *How many neutrons does oxygen have?*

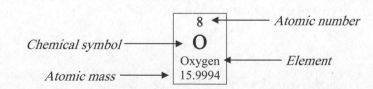

1. *The atomic number is 8.*
2. *The atomic mass is 15.9994 atomic mass units (AMU).*
3. *The number of protons is the atomic number, which is 8.*
4. *The number of neutrons + the number of protons = the mass number*
   The number of neutrons + 8 = 15.9994 rounded
   The number of neutrons = 15.9994 – 8 (by subtracting 8 from both sides)
   The number of neutrons is 8.

ⓟ *Practice problems*

Solutions to the practice problems are located in the back of this book.

1. Describe the construction of an atom.

Use the following excerpt from the periodic table to answer the following four questions.

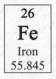

26
Fe
Iron
55.845

2. What is the atomic number of iron?

3. What is the atomic mass of iron?

4. How many protons does iron have?

5. How many neutrons does iron have?

Protons, Neutrons, and Electrons

The protons, neutrons, and electrons found within an atom each contribute to the atom's mass and charge in unique ways. (An atom's **charge** refers to the positive or negative distribution within it.) An atom's charge is dominated by the total number of protons or electrons. Since neutrons are neutral subatomic particles found in the nucleus of an atom, they do not possess any charge. Each proton's positive (+1) charge is exactly counterbalanced by each electron's negative (–1) charge. An electrically neutral atom will possess the same number of electrons and protons. However, as seen in Example 3.11, an electrically charged atom will have an excess (or imbalance) of protons or electrons.

 Example 3.11:   *Neutral carbon is known to have six protons and six electrons. However, if an electron is released to the environment (by a collisional or absorptive process), the carbon atom will have only five electrons. The atom will have an excess of positive charge (in this case, a +1 amount).*

An atom's mass is dominated by the total number of protons and neutrons (since the electron's mass is small by comparison). The protons and neutrons found within the nucleus of an atom have approximately the same mass as each other. The mass number is a defining characteristic of each atom of a given element, as well as the **isotopes** (atoms with the same number of protons, but different numbers of neutrons) of each element (see Example 3.12). Every element is found to have multiple isotopes.

 Example 3.12:   *Carbon is known to have three isotopes that contain 6, 7, and 8 neutrons (all with the same 6 protons). The mass number then distinguishes each isotope as C-12, C-13, and C-14, respectively.*

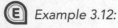 *Practice problems*

Solutions to the practice problems are located in the back of this book.

Use Figure 3.16 to answer the following two questions.

1.   How many protons would a positively charged isotope ion of O-18 have?

2.   How many protons would a negatively charged isotope ion of C-14 have?

Purpose of Catalysts

Catalysts control the rate of chemical reactions, or reactions in which atoms react to come to a stable state. Reaction rates may be increased by the use of promoters or reduced by the use of inhibitors. The reaction rates depend largely on the frequency of contact of reactants with the catalysts. This may be artificially accomplished by increasing the **substrate** (i.e., the molecular surface acted upon by an enzyme) surface area. Catalysts are generally not consumed in a primary reaction. However, they may be destroyed or regenerated in secondary steps.

Catalysts increase reaction rates by lowering **activation energy**. The potential barrier of products compared to reactants is reduced, resulting in a reaction path requiring less energy. The general reaction may be symbolically represented as the following four-step process:

1) $X + C \rightarrow XC$
2) $XC + Y \rightarrow XYC$
3) $XYC \rightarrow CZ$
4) $CZ \rightarrow C + Z$

In this process, the catalyst (C) generates a product (Z) from the reactants (X and Y). Notice that the catalyst is present with the product, and is thus available to continue the reaction anew.

Important examples of catalysts occur in nature, ranging from biological processes to fusion within a star's core. Catalytic reactions are also responsible for the production of about 90% of all commercial chemical products. Examples 3.13 through 3.15 use catalysts:

(E) *Example 3.13:*   *The breakdown of hydrogen peroxide (H_2O_2) using a manganese dioxide catalyst:*

$$2H_2O_2 \rightarrow 2H_2O + O_2$$

(E) *Example 3.14:*   *The breakdown of carbon monoxide (CO) using platinum and rhodium in catalytic converters:*

$$2CO + 2NO \rightarrow 2CO_2 + N_2$$

(E) *Example 3.15:*   *The breakdown of ozone (O_3) by chlorine ions donated by chlorofluorocarbons (CFCs) in the upper atmosphere (a harmful example):*

$$Cl + O_3 \rightarrow ClO + O_2$$

(P) *Practice problems*

Solutions to the practice problems are located in the back of this book.

1. Given reactants (X and Y), a catalyst (C), and a product (Z), order the following steps in the general catalytic reaction process.

    - $XYC \rightarrow CZ$
    - $CZ \rightarrow C + Z$
    - $X + C \rightarrow XC$
    - $Y + XC \rightarrow XYC$

2. How does a catalyst increase the rate of a chemical reaction?

Physical and Chemical Patterns Within the Periodic Table

The periodic table is arranged into a series of rows and columns that obey specific chemical patterns. The original design of the periodic table of the elements is credited to Gregor Mendeleev in the 1800s. By studying the known elements of his day, Mendeleev noted that these elements could be arranged by atomic mass according to specific patterns. The discovery of other elements could be inferred from the numerous gaps within his periodic table. However, it was subsequently noted that some of the element masses did not quite fit according to pattern, due to isotope mass variation. In the early 1900s, Henry Moseley proposed that the periodic table be modified such that elements would be arranged by atomic number rather than atomic mass. Moseley's format is recognized as the correct format for the modern periodic table.

As seen in the periodic table (see Figure 3.16), each row (or period) displays elements according to an increasing number of systematic **orbital shells** (the arrangement of electrons within orbits around the nucleus). The naming of the shells is reflected within the electronic configuration for each element (see Example 3.16). As a result, the elements become populated by an increasing number of electrons from left to right on the periodic table. In addition, several chemical properties exhibit dramatic change from left to right within each row, as outlined in the following paragraphs.

(E) *Example 3.16:*   *The electron configuration of certain noble gas elements includes the following: helium = $1s^2$; neon = $1s^2 2s^2 2p^6$; argon = $1s^2 2s^2 2p^6 3s^2 3p^6$*

The coefficients 1, 2, and 3 refer to the first 3 rows of the periodic table and are the primary shell numbers for each row.

The s and p refer to subshells of electrons within each shell. The s subshell may have 2 electrons, while the p subshell may have 6 electrons (note the raised numbers to the right of each s and p symbol).

The sum of all the raised numbers equals the number of electrons found within the neutral atom for that element.

Further discussion of other subshells (d and f) requires a much fuller explanation.

From left to right across a period, electrons are added to the outer energy shell, one at a time. Within a shell, electrons cannot shield each other from the attraction to protons. The number of protons is also increasing, thus the effective nuclear charge increases. This causes the atomic radii to decrease. For instance, argon is found to have a smaller atomic radius than aluminum, even though they are both found in the same period.

Moving down a group (or column), the number of electrons and filled electron shells increase, but the number of **valence electrons**, electrons in the outermost shell of an atom, remain the same. The outermost electrons in a group are exposed to the same effective nuclear charge; however, electrons are found farther from the nucleus as the number of filled energy shells increases. Therefore, the atomic radii increase. For instance, bromine is found to have a larger atomic radius that fluorine, even though they both belong to the halogen family.

The ionization energy, or ionization potential, is the energy required to completely remove an electron from a gaseous atom or ion. Ionization energies increase moving from left to right across a period (decreasing atomic radii). Argon would have a larger ionization energy than aluminum, due to argon's smaller atomic radius. However, ionization energy decreases moving down a group (increasing atomic radii). Bromine has a smaller ionization energy than flourine, due to bromine's larger atomic radius.

Electronegativity is a measure of an atom's attraction on electrons in a chemical bond. The greater the electronegativity of an atom, the greater its attraction for bonding electrons. Elements that have low ionization energies have low electronegativity because their nuclei do not exert strong attractive forces on electrons. Elements that have high ionization energies have high electronegativity due to the strong pull exerted on electrons by the nuclei. For instance, the electronegativity of argon is greater than that of aluminum. Within a group, electronegativity decreases as atomic number increases. This is a result of increased distance between the valence electrond and the nuclei (greater atomic radius). For instance, the electronegativity of bromine is smaller than that of fluorine.

Specifically, the rules of **chemical bonding** (the chemical merging of atoms due to their electron arrangements) are determined by an element's location within a given row. Due to bonding rules, a transition between **metals** (elements that donate highly conductive electrons to their environment) and nonmetals is also found to exist from left to right within each row. As each shell becomes filled (or row becomes completed), a new shell (or new row) becomes necessary to accommodate elements of higher periods. Metalloids, which are found next to the stairstep line on the periodic table, are considered to have transitional properties between metals and nonmetals.

Each column (or family) displays elements that are similar in their chemical properties due to having a similar arrangement of outer shell electrons. For example, the alkali family (first column) may donate one electron that is available for chemical bonding, whereas the alkali Earth family (second column) may donate two electrons that are available for bonding. By contrast, the halogens (seventh column) may accept one electron for bonding, whereas the noble gases (eighth column) are electronically stable (resistant to bonding) due to their full outer shells.

Regarding physical patterns at standard temperature and pressure, the elements in the periodic table are dominated by the solid state as their natural forms. Only 10 elements on the right-hand side of the periodic table are identified as gases, whereas only two (mercury and bromine) are recognized as liquids.

 Practice problems

Solutions to the practice problems are located in the back of this book.

1. Complete the following sentence.

    Within a given family on the periodic table, atomic radii _____ while electronegativity _____.

2. Which groups on the periodic table contain the most metalloids?

3. A student has two material samples. One is a metal (A), and the other is a nonmetal (B). The student is trying to determine which one is the metal. Which of the following could the student observe? (Select all that apply.)

    A) Samples A and B both conduct an electric current.
    B) Sample A cools rapidly when refrigerated, but Sample B does not.
    C) Sample B heats very slowly when heat is applied, but Sample A heats very quickly.

Enzymes

Enzymes act as the catalysts for special chemical reactions within the human body. These enzymes are found as protein molecules (organic compounds composed of amino acids) within body tissue. **Globular proteins** (proteins that are water soluble) are built from amino acids that form chains ranging from a few dozen to thousands of members. Each amino-acid sequence produces a specific 3-D structure.

Cell processes require the use of enzymes for rapid reactions (often millions of reactions per second). The activity is driven by external factors such as temperature, pH, and substrate concentration. The **pH** value is a measure of hydrogen ion concentration within a solution, and a substrate is a molecular surface acted upon by an enzyme. Enzymes are highly selective. Only a few **metabolic pathways** (chemical reactions with a cell) are preferred, and they depend on the needs of the cell. Even so, enzymes participate in thousands of chemical reactions throughout the human body.

The biomolecules recognized as enzymes perform their functions by attaching to substrate molecules and subsequently convert these molecules into products. The flexibility of an enzyme allows its active site surface to reshape when placed in contact with a substrate. A typical chemical reaction involving an enzyme (E), substrate (S), and product (P) may be identified symbolically by as follows:

$E + S \rightarrow ES \rightarrow E + P$

Here, the second step represents the catalytic process. The enzymes act to lower the activation energy. As a result, the potential barrier between the products and reactants is lessened, allowing a greater reaction rate to occur. However, inhibitors (e.g., drugs and poisons) can compete with the substrate by blocking its active sites, causing greatly reduced activity.

Enzymes can also catalyze forward and reverse reactions equally so that equilibrium is maintained. For instance, in the following equation, H_2CO_3 produces H_2O and CO_2 in the lungs using an enzyme called carbonic anhydrase:

$H_2CO_3 \rightarrow H_2O + CO_2,$

In the reverse equation, H_2O and CO_2 produce H_2CO_3 in tissues using the same enzyme:

$H_2O + CO_2 \rightarrow H_2CO_3,$

Applications of enzyme reactions include food processing (e.g., baby food and dairy products), brewing (e.g., making sugar from starches), and manufacturing (e.g., biofuels and detergents).

(P) *Practice problems*

Solutions to the practice problems are located in the back of this book.

Identify whether the following statements are TRUE or FALSE.

1. Enzymes participate in a limited number of chemical reactions throughout the human body.

2. Enzymes act to lower the activation energy of chemical reactions.

3. An enzyme can reshape itself when placed in contact with a substrate.

4. The amino-acid structure of an enzyme is important to its function.

Acid and Base Solutions

The pH scale is used to measure the strength of **acidic solutions** (solutions with a pH value less than 7) and the strength of **basic solutions** (solutions with a pH value greater than 7). Pure H_2O at 25° Celcius is recognized as the standard of neutrality between acids and bases because it has a pH value of 7.0. Stronger acids will have smaller numerical values on the pH scale than weaker acids, and stronger bases will have greater numerical values than weaker bases. Some sample values are illustrated in Table 3.7.

Table 3.7 Substances With Approximate pH Scale Values

Substance	pH scale value
Battery acid	pH below 1
Gastric juice	pH about 2
Orange juice	pH between 3 and 4
Milk	pH about 6.5
Blood	pH between 7.34 and 7.45
Hand soap	pH between 9 and 10
Bleach	pH about 12.5

The calculation of pH is based on the activity (a_H) of hydrogen ions (H+) dissolved in solution. Specifically, the pH range of numbers is based on a logarithmic scale:

$$pH = -\log(a_H)$$

Log functions are used to rescale very large numbers (or very small numbers) into values much closer to 1. This is often done to deal with more reasonable numbers (for pH, 1 to 14). Mathematically, the negative sign in the formula means that a_H must be less than 1, as seen in Examples 3.17 and 3.18.

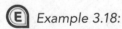 *Example 3.17:* *Suppose the activity of hydrogen ions in solution is 1 part per thousand (i.e., 1/1,000 or 0.001). In scientific notation, this number equals 1×10^{-3}. To calculate the pH value, do the following:*

$$pH = -\log(a_H)$$
$$pH = -\log(1 \times 10^{-3})$$
$$pH = -(-3)$$
$$pH = 3$$

This value would then be considered to represent an acid of similar strength to orange juice, as seen from the previous table.

Example 3.18: *Suppose the activity of hydrogen ions in solution is 1 part per billion (i.e., 1/1,000,000,000 or 0.000000001). In scientific notation, this number equals 1×10^{-9}. To calculate the pH value, do the following:*

$$pH = -\log(a_H)$$
$$pH = -\log(1 \times 10^{-9})$$
$$pH = -(-9)$$
$$pH = 9$$

This value would then be considered to represent a weak base. Hand soap has a similar pH value.

Since activity (a_H) measures concentrations of hydrogen ions, the numerical value is typically found to be much less than 1. In addition, since a larger number of hydrogen ions is associated with an acid than a base, the activity value for acids will be larger for acids than bases. If activity values are not readily known, a **pH indicator** is used to qualitatively determine the pH. A known weak acid or base (such as litmus paper) changes color when introduced to an unknown acid or base. Litmus paper will indicate red for acidic solutions and blue for basic solutions. Even though pH indicators will not give precise measurements of pH, they are usually sufficient when only an approximate value is needed.

(P) *Practice problems*

Solutions to the practice problems are located in the back of this book.

1. Suppose the activity of hydrogen ions in a solution is 1 part per ten thousand. Find the pH value of the solution. Is this a basic or acidic solution?

2. Complete the following sentence.

   Regarding bases, a ____ number of hydrogen ions is associated with a basic solution (as opposed to an acidic solution), and red litmus paper will turn _____ in the presence of a base.

3. What does a difference of one unit on the pH scale below represent?

$[H^+]$	pH	$[OH^-]$
10^{-1}	1.0	10^{-13}
10^{-2}	2.0	10^{-12}
10^{-3}	3.0	10^{-11}
10^{-4}	4.0	10^{-10}
10^{-5}	5.0	10^{-9}
10^{-6}	6.0	10^{-8}
10^{-7}	7.0	10^{-7}
10^{-8}	8.0	10^{-6}
10^{-9}	9.0	10^{-5}
10^{-10}	10.0	10^{-4}
10^{-11}	11.0	10^{-3}
10^{-12}	12.0	10^{-2}
10^{-13}	13.0	10^{-1}
10^{-14}	14.0	10^{-0}

Chemical Bonds Between Atoms in Common Molecules

Chemical bonding primarily occurs through **ionic** (the electrical attraction between ions of opposite charges) and **covalent** (sharing of electrons between atoms) methods. Common molecules use both bonding methods. For example, **hydrocarbons** like methane, propane, and butane bond to hydrogen and carbon atoms. Carbon possesses four valence electrons, as shown in Figure 3.17, which are available for bonding with other carbon and hydrogen atoms within the hydrocarbon structure. This is readily seen from the periodic table, where carbon resides in group IVA. The addition of four electrons will provide the carbon with the maximum electron stability possible, since the outer valence shell will then become complete.

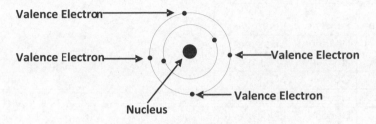

Figure 3.17 Carbon atom.

Hydrocarbons are generally subdivided into saturated and unsaturated categories. Saturated hydrocarbons (also known as **alkanes**) are the most basic structure of the hydrocarbons. These compounds are composed entirely of single bonds and are **saturated** (carbon is completely connected) with hydrogen. The general formula for saturated hydrocarbons is C_nH_{2n+2}, where n is a whole number greater than or equal to 1 (see Example 3.19). Saturated hydrocarbons are the basis of petroleum fuels.

(E) Example 3.19: *Let n=2. The chemical composition may be found using the formula C_nH_{2n+2}.*

The hydrocarbon is ethane, with the formula C_2H_6 (substitute 2 in for the n in the formula C_nH_{2n+2}).

Unsaturated hydrocarbons have one or more double or triple bonds between carbon atoms. Those with one double bond are called **alkenes**, with the general formula C_nH_{2n}. Those containing triple bonds are called **alkynes**, with the general formula C_nH_{2n-2}. In both of these formulas, n is again a whole number greater than or equal to 1 (see Example 3.20). Unsaturated hydrocarbons permit the attachment of other atoms to the unbonded carbon atoms within the molecule.

(E) Example 3.20: *Let n=3. The chemical composition may be found using the formula C_nH_{2n}.*

The hydrocarbon is propene, with the formula C_3H_6.

Each hydrocarbon and its molecular formula have a special geometry associated with them. However, a given formula may possess two or more molecular structures known as isomers. Although the bonding is identical, a different geometric structure can lead to widely differing properties (e.g., explosive versus poisonous).

Hydrocarbons are abundant within living things, foods, fuels, and plastics (to name a few). The basis of **organic chemistry** is connected with the study of hydrocarbon structure. Some hydrocarbons are even found in the solar system. Lakes of liquid methane and ethane have been discovered on Saturn's largest moon.

The names of simple hydrocarbons with up to 10 carbon atoms and their variations are shown in Table 3.8.

Table 3.8 Simple Hydrocarbons and Their Variations

Number of carbon atoms	Alkane	Alkene	Alkyne
1	Methane	—	—
2	Ethane	Ethene	Ethyne
3	Propane	Propene	Propyne
4	Butane Isobutane	Butene	Butyne
5	Pentane Isopentane	Pentene	Pentyne
6	Hexane	Hexene	Hexyne
7	Heptane	Heptene	Heptyne
8	Octane	Octene	Octyne
9	Nonane	Nonene	Nonyne
10	Decane	Decene	Decyne

(P) *Practice problems*

Solutions to the practice problems are located in the back of this book.

1. Identify the name and formula of the common saturated hydrocarbon that has four carbon atoms.

2. Identify the name and formula of a common unsaturated hydrocarbon that has five carbon atoms.

Chemical Bonds Resulting From Sharing or Transferring Electrons

The electrons found within various orbits around the nucleus interact with other atoms. These interactions represent forces that are electrical in nature, involving complicated patterns of attraction and repulsion. Chemical bonds may be established through such electron interaction, resulting in the formation of new molecules. This chemical bonding is generally categorized by covalent, ionic, or metallic bonds. Even though one of these three forms is treated as the dominant type for each particular molecule, all bonds possess some degree of each.

The periodic table (see Figure 3.16) is artificially separated by the zigzag, stairstep line between boron and aluminum and between polonium and astatine. Metals are to the left, nonmetals are to the right, and metalloids are in contact with the stairstep line. **Metalloids** are elements that may accept or donate electrons readily, and possess a mixture of metallic and nonmetallic properties.

The identical atoms within a metal share electrons so readily that metallic bonding results in the treatment of that metal as one large molecule. However, a metallic ion (which tends to be a **cation**, or positive ion) and a nonmetallic ion (which tends to be an **anion**, or negative ion) may also form chemical bonds due to their electrical attraction. These ionic bonds complete one another by the donation and acceptance of electrons to form stable outer electron shells. For instance, common table salt (NaCl) forms from the positive Na+ ion and the negative Cl- ion.

A covalent bond is a form of chemical bonding that involves electron sharing between atoms. The valence electrons of both atoms are being shared cooperatively to form a stable outer shell for both atoms. Covalent bonding is greatest between atoms of similar **electronegativities**, or similar attractions for electrons. Electronegativity tends to increase from left to right on the periodic table, so covalent bonding often results between atoms on the same side of the table. While such bonding does occur for like atoms, the two atoms do not have to be identical, as long as they are of comparable electronegativity.

Lewis structures (or Lewis dot diagrams) provide visual representations of covalent bonding between atoms of a molecule. The atoms are symbolically shown and surrounded by dots that represent each of the valence shell electrons. The dots are arranged such that the molecule is shown to have the atoms in the most completely filled shell configuration of paired electrons (see Examples 3.21 and 3.22).

(E) *Example 3.21:*   *Draw the Lewis structure to display the ionic bonding between sodium (Na⁺) and chlorine (Cl⁻) to form table salt.*

The metallic ion Na⁺ and the nonmetallic ion Cl⁻ form an ionic bond due to their electrical attractions (i.e., sodium has one positive ion and chlorine has one negative ion). The ionic bond completes the outer electron shells of both ions. The Lewis structure should be drawn as follows:

$$Na\cdot + \cdot \ddot{\underset{\cdot\cdot}{Cl}} : \; = \; Na : \ddot{\underset{\cdot\cdot}{Cl}} :$$

(E) *Example 3.22:*   *Draw the Lewis structure to display the covalent bonding between hydrogen and oxygen to form water.*

Hydrogen (H) has 1 valence electron and oxygen (O) has 6 valence electrons. These electrons combine to complete the outer shells, which forms water ($H_2 + O \rightarrow H_2O$).

$$\begin{matrix} H\cdot \\ H\cdot \end{matrix} + \cdot \ddot{O} : \; = \; H : \underset{\underset{H}{\cdot\cdot}}{\overset{\cdot\cdot}{O}} :$$

(P) *Practice problems*

Solutions to the practice problems are located in the back of this book.

1. Why does hydrogen gas exist as H_2 and never just H? (That is, why do two hydrogren atoms need to be connected together in the natural state?)

2. Regarding the Lewis structure for sulfur (S), how many unshared pairs of electrons will sulfur have (refer to Figure 3.16)?

Important Chemical Reactions: Balancing and Identifying

Chemical reactions occur throughout nature and are critical for sustaining life. Every reaction undergoes a dynamic interplay of reactants that combine in special ways to manufacture products through well-defined rules. For instance, reactions must be balanced according to atomic number and charge. The first part of this discussion focuses on balancing a chemical equation. The second part discusses the most important types of chemical interactions, which include certain oxidation-reduction and acid-base reactions.

Balancing Chemical Equations

A chemical equation represents an actual chemical reaction and includes formulas for elements and compounds. Formulas on the left side of the reaction sign ($\rightarrow$) are substances consumed or altered in the chemical reaction. These are called the **reactants**. The substances formed as the results of a chemical reaction are called the **products** and are located to the right of the reaction sign. The goal of balancing an equation is to make certain that there are equal numbers of each atom on the reactant side and the product side.

Most equations contain formulas with small numbers called subscripts, which are at a lower level than the element that they follow. This subscript indicates how many atoms of that element are in the formula. Only one atom is present if it has no subscript. For example, consider the following reaction:

$$NI_3 \rightarrow N_2 + I_2$$

The reactant, NI_3, has 1 atom of nitrogen (N) and 3 atoms of iodine (I). On the product side, there are 2 atoms of nitrogen and 2 atoms of iodine. This reaction it is not yet balanced (i.e., numbers of each kind of atom are not equal on each side of the reaction sign). The only way to balance this reaction is to place a number, called a coefficient, in front of one or more of the formulas. If no coefficient is in front of a formula, then only one of that formula is in the reaction. Example 3.23 balances this reaction.

An important rule to remember is that a subscript cannot change, because that would change the chemical.

(E) *Example 3.23:*   *Balance the following equation: ___ $NI_3 \rightarrow$ ___$N_2 +$ ___I_2*

Start with the easiest fix first, which would be nitrogen. Two N are on the right side, and only one N is on the left. Place the coefficient 2 in front of NI_3:

$$2NI_3 \rightarrow \text{___}N_2 + \text{___}I_2$$

Nitrogen is now balanced on both sides of the reaction, but the coefficient 2 also applies to another element in the formula — the iodine. In fact, the coefficient multiplies iodine's subscript, 3, by 2 so that there are now 6 atoms of iodine on the left. The only way to have 6 atoms of iodine on the right is to place the coefficient 3 in front of I_2 on the product side (the coefficient 3 multiplies the subscript 2):

$$2NI_3 \rightarrow N_2 + 3I_2 \text{ balanced}$$

Sometimes there is a group of atoms with parentheses and a subscript outside the parentheses, as in $Ca(OH)_2$. In this formula, the subscript 2 indicates that there are 2 of each atom inside the parentheses: 2 hydrogen and 2 oxygen atoms. It is important to remember this point when balancing equations.

Oxidation-Reduction and Acid-Base Reactions

Oxidation-reduction reactions involve the donation and acceptance of electrons (see Example 3.24). **Oxidation** involves electron donation to produce a more positive ion. **Reduction** involves electron acceptance to produce a more negative ion. Oxidation-reduction reactions have many applications in our lives. Some of these applications are common, while others are not obvious. A few examples of oxidation-reduction reactions include combustion (see Example 3.25), photosynthesis (see Example 3.26), and **metabolism** (see Example 3.27), which refers to the chemical reactions in living organisms that are necessary to maintain life.

(E) **Example 3.24:** *As a general example, the overall reaction between the* diatomic molecules *(molecules consisting of two atoms) of hydrogen and fluorine involves two half-reactions that must be balanced according to charge and atomic number. The oxidation reaction and the reduction reaction yield the sum of the reactants and products.*

Oxidation reaction: $H_2 \rightarrow 2H^+ + 2e^-$
Reduction reaction: $F_2 + 2e^- \rightarrow 2F^-$
Reactants and products: $H_2 + F_2 + 2e^- \rightarrow 2H^+ + 2e^- + 2F^-$.
Canceling the electrons along with ionic bonding then yields:

$$H_2 + F_2 \rightarrow 2\ HF$$

(E) **Example 3.25:** *An example of combustion involves the burning of propane (C_3H_8). The carbon atoms are oxidized by combining with oxygen to form carbon dioxide. The oxygen is reduced by combining with hydrogen to form water. The excess heat could then be used for cooking or to drive heat engines, according to the reaction:*

$$C_3H_8 + 5\ O_2 \rightarrow 3H_2O + CO_2 + Heat$$

(E) **Example 3.26:** *An example of photosynthesis is carried out by green plants. The plants harness sunlight energy using a series of oxidation-reduction reactions that produce oxygen and sugar, such as glucose ($C_6H_{12}O_6$). The overall equation may be expressed as:*

$$6CO_2 + 6H_2O \rightarrow C_6H_{12}O_6 + 6O_2$$

(E) **Example 3.27:** *An example of metabolism in cellular respiration is the oxidation of glucose ($C_6H_{12}O_6$) to carbon dioxide (CO_2) and the reduction of oxygen (O_2) to water (H_2O). The half-equations (not shown) may be combined to yield the overall reaction for this metabolic process as:*

$$C_6H_{12}O_6 + 6O_2 \rightarrow 6CO_2 + 6H_2O$$

An **acid** is any compound with a hydrogen ion activity greater than water (pH < 7). A **base** is any compound with a hydrogen ion activity less than water (pH > 7). Although acids and bases do not generally undergo oxidation and reduction, their reaction will produce water and **salts**, which act to neutralize the pH. Generally,

$$acid^+ + base^- \rightarrow salt + water$$

As shown in Examples 3.28 and 3.29, the positive ion from a base forms a salt with the negative ion from an acid.

(E) **Example 3.28:** *A sodium hydroxide base (NaOH) can combine with sulfuric acid (H_2SO_4) to form water and a sodium sulfate salt (Na_2SO_4) according to the balanced equation:*

$$2NaOH + H_2SO_4 \rightarrow 2H_2O + Na_2SO_4$$

(E) **Example 3.29:** *Sodium hydroxide can combine with hydrochloric acid (HCl) to form water and table salt according to the balanced equation:*

$$HCl + NaOH \rightarrow H_2O + NaCl$$

(P) *Practice problems*

Solutions to the practice problems are located in the back of this book.

1. Balance the following chemical reaction:

    ___Ca(OH)$_2$ + ___HCl → ___H$_2$O + ___CaCl$_2$

Identify whether the following statements are TRUE or FALSE.

2. pH neutralization is an important oxidation-reduction reaction.

3. Metabolism is an important oxidation-reduction reaction.

4. Combustion is an important acid-base reaction.

5. Photosynthesis is an important acid-base reaction.

Chemical Properties of Water

Water possesses several unique chemical properties that distinguish it from other molecules. It is these chemical properties that give water its physical properties and allow it to serve as the essential basis for life on Earth.

Water is considered a polar molecule of hydrogen (H) and oxygen (O), with oxygen possessing the higher electronegativity. (A **polar molecule** is a molecule that possesses both positive and negative atomic structure.) Electrons gravitate toward the oxygen within the molecule. The resulting H_2O molecule is a stable substance due to the sharing of electrons between the hydrogen and oxygen by covalent bonding. Despite this stability, the energetic input from **electrolysis** can chemically split the liquid water molecule into gaseous components, according to the balanced equation $2H_2O \rightarrow 2H_2 + O_2$.

Pure H_2O serves as a pH standard, which is central to acid-base neutrality and enzyme function. Pure water also possesses a low electrical conductivity. However, small concentrations of impurities (e.g., NaCl) can significantly increase conduction.

Due to its chemical structure, water is characterized by a maximum density at 4° Celcius (C), where **density** is the ratio of mass per volume for a substance, and **Celsius** is a metric temperature scale that is defined (at standard pressure) by the melting point of ice (0° C) and the boiling point of liquid water (100° C). At this temperature of 4° C, water is considered a standard value of 1 gram/milliliter. This unique property means that ice is less dense than liquid water; therefore, it floats. That is why aquatic animals can survive under an ice covered lake.

The boiling point of water depends on pressure. For instance, at 29,000 feet above sea level water boils at 68° C, while at sea level the boiling point is at 100° C. In the metric system, the **Kelvin** scale is alternately used to express temperature. Kelvin is a metric temperature scale defined by an absolute zero reference point (0 K = -273° C). Kelvin temperatures are standardized by the **triple-point** of water (the temperature and pressure at which water will coexist as a solid, liquid, and gas [273.16 K = 0.01° C]).

Water chemically possesses the second highest specific heat (after ammonia). (**Specific heat** is the energy required to raise one unit of mass of a substance by 1° C.) This large specific heat enables water to undergo minor temperature changes compared to the environment. Also, water has a high **heat of vaporization**, which is the amount of heat necessary to cause a phase transition between a liquid and a gas. Since a large amount of heat is needed to vaporize liquid, water acts to moderate Earth's climate.

This tasteless, odorless, and transparent substance acts as a universal solvent. Water dissolves many solids, liquids, and gases into aqueous solutions. In addition, water's polarity results in high surface tension and adhesion. Water is also essential and central to metabolic processes – anabolic (creation of larger molecules) and catabolic (creation of smaller molecules) – within living things. Water is abundant throughout the universe as a byproduct of star formation. Water is known to be heavily concentrated on comets as well as other planets. The presence of water is considered a necessity for the formation of life.

(P) Practice problems

Solutions to the practice problems are located in the back of this book.

Identify whether the following statements are TRUE or FALSE.

1. Water serves as the standard for pH and has a value of 6.

2. Water is used as the standard density at 4° C.

3. Water has the standard electronegative value on the periodic table.

4. The Kelvin temperature scale is based on water's triple-point.

Atoms or Molecules in Liquids, Gases, and Solids

Kinetic theory states that atoms (or molecules) are always in motion. Depending on intermolecular forces, these atoms may undergo a range of motions from highly ordered to entirely random. In addition, atomic motion may involve atoms in very close proximity to one another or highly separated from each other. The atomic order and separation are strongly dependent on macroscopic factors such as temperature and pressure, since temperature is directly related to the speed of the particles and pressure is the force of particle interaction over a certain area. As one (or both) of these quantities changes, the physical state (or phase) of the atoms may transition between a solid, liquid, or gas.

The solid state is considered to have a fixed shape and volume. A solid's fixed shape may range from possessing a **crystalline order**, in which the atoms are arranged in a highly ordered state, to a state in which the atoms lack true order. Solids are often considered to exist at relatively high pressures and low temperatures. By contrast, the liquid state of the same atom generally has a fixed volume of greater size, in addition to a changing shape. While the atoms within the liquid still maintain intermolecular forces with one another, the **physical bonding**, or the physical connection between atoms (or molecules) that does not alter the chemical nature of the atoms (or molecules), is of a weaker attractive nature. As a result, the liquid will spread out over a greater volume. Relative to the solid state, a liquid exists typically at a much higher temperature (the pressure is still high).

While most liquids are considered amorphous, some have a crystalline form. To contrast further, the gaseous state of an atom has a changing volume as well as a changing shape. The difference in volume between the gaseous state and the liquid state is much more pronounced than the volume difference between the liquid state and the solid state. For neutral gases, the forces between atoms are of the weakest nature, such that movement is nearly random. Relative to the liquid state, gases are found to exist at much higher temperatures (or much lower pressures).

The transitions between solid, liquid, and gas phases are achieved by adding or subtracting energy from the system. The amount of energy necessary for a phase transition depends on the value of the latent heat of the atom. **Latent heat** is related to the energy needed to cause a phase transition at a fixed temperature. Generally, more energy is needed to transition from a liquid to a gas (as opposed to a liquid from a solid). The greater energy results in a much more pronounced atomic separation within gases.

(P) *Practice problems*

Solutions to the practice problems are located in the back of this book.

1. Suppose a phase transition occurs between a liquid and gas at –196° C. What is the Kelvin temperature?

Identify whether the statements associated with the following situation are TRUE or FALSE.

A certain amount of a substance is in a solid state, but it is then melted to form a liquid, and finally vaporized to form a gas. The solid had a volume of 1 cubic centimeter, the liquid occupied 0.75 cubic centimeters, and the gas expanded to 10 cubic meters.

2. The liquid is more dense than the gas.
3. The liquid is less dense than the solid.
4. The solid is more dense than the gas.
5. The liquid has the highest density of the three forms.

Evaporation, Vaporization, and Condensation

The transition between the liquid and gas phases of an atom (or molecule) is achieved by adding or removing heat from a system. **Heat** is the flow of energy due to a difference in temperature. The liquid to gas transition, through evaporation or vaporization, requires an addition of heat, and the gas to liquid transition, through condensation, requires a subtraction of heat. Although evaporation and vaporization are related, it is important to contrast them carefully.

Evaporation of a liquid is often achieved due to the high heat, low humidity, and fast movement of the surrounding air mass. Evaporation occurs by physical collisions at the surface layer of a liquid, and it acts to remove the faster-moving liquid molecules, thereby removing the more energetic atoms from the liquid. This results in a cooler system (e.g., a person's skin after air drying).

By contrast, vaporization occurs through a phase transition from a liquid to a gas. A **phase transition** is an alteration of the physical state between a solid, liquid, and gas. This transition from a liquid to a gas takes place by breaking the physical bonds within the liquid. The amount of heat of vaporization (H) necessary for this phase transition depends on the mass (M) and the latent heat (L), or heat per mass needed for a phase change at a constant temperature, of the atom (see Example 3.30). As long as this amount of heat (H) is continually added to the liquid at the boiling point, a hybrid state of liquid and gas will exist until only the gas state remains.

 Example 3.30: *Suppose a 100-gram (g) mass of water is at the boiling point. Given that the latent heat of water is 540 calories/gram (cal/g), the amount of heat added to fully vaporize the liquid can be calculated by:*

$$H = M \times L$$
$$= 100 \text{ g} \times 540 \text{ cal/g}$$
$$= 54,000 \text{ cal}$$
$$= 54 \text{ kilocalories (Note: 1,000 cal = 1 kcal)}$$

Condensation occurs through a phase transition from a gas to a liquid. This transition takes place by creating physical bonds within the gas. As demonstrated in Example 3.31, the amount of heat of vaporization (H) necessary for this phase transition requires a removal of heat. As long as this amount of heat H is continually removed from the gas at the boiling point, a hybrid state of liquid and gas will exist until only the liquid state remains.

 Example 3.31: *Suppose a 100-g mass of water is at the boiling point. Given that the latent heat of water is 540 cal/g, the amount of heat removed to fully condense the gas can be calculated by:*

$$H = - M \times L$$
$$= - 100 \text{ g} \times 540 \text{ cal/g}$$
$$= -54,000 \text{ cal}$$
$$= - 54 \text{ kcal}$$

Note: The negative sign indicates a removal of heat from the system. However, the total amount of heat compared to Example 3.30 remains the same (the reverse process).

P *Practice problems*

Solutions to the practice problems are located in the back of this book.

1. Complete the sentence below.

    The heat of vaporization refers to the energy necessary (at constant temperature) to cause a complete phase change from a _____ to a _____.

2. Suppose a substance A has a mass of M grams and a latent heat of L cal/g. If substance B has a mass three times that of substance A and a latent heat 1/6 of that of substance A, what will be the ratio of the heat of vaporization of A compared to B?

SECTION 4: ENGLISH AND LANGUAGE USAGE

The English and Language Usage section of the TEAS® covers material related to grammar, word meaning, spelling, punctuation, and sentence structure.

GRAMMAR AND WORD MEANINGS IN CONTEXT

Parts of Speech

It is important to be able to identify elements of a sentence, not only to eliminate errors, but also to communicate effectively. If someone cannot separate a verb from a preposition, for example, that person will have a hard time making sure that no subject-verb agreement error exists in his or her essay. Table 4.1 provides short definitions of the different parts of speech.

Table 4.1 Definitions of the Parts of Speech

Parts of speech	Definition
Adjective	a descriptive word that modifies a noun or pronoun
Adverb	a word that modifies a verb, adjective, or another adverb and indicates *when*, *how*, *where*, *why*, or *how much*
Article	a word that is used to limit a noun, either indefinite (*a* and *an*) or definite (*the*)
Clause	a group of words that are related and contain both a subject and a verb
Direct object	the noun or pronoun that receives the action of the verb and answers the question *whom*, or *what*
Noun	a word for a person, place, or thing
Object of the preposition	the noun, pronoun, phrase, or clause to which the preposition refers
Phrase	a group of words that are related but do not contain a verb and a subject together
Possessive pronoun	a pronoun used to indicate ownership
Preposition	a word such as *by*, *at*, *to*, or *from* that gives additional information, usually in relationship to something else in the sentence
Pronoun	a word that replaces and refers to a noun
Subject	a noun or pronoun that performs the action of the verb. If a sentence contains a verb of being or a linking verb such as *be*, *feel*, *become*, or *look*, the subject of the sentence is the noun or pronoun being described.
Verb	a word that shows an action or a state of being

The following sentence exemplifies some of the different parts of speech:

The	young	boys	enjoy	soccer	practice.
(definite article)	(adjective)	(subject-noun)	(verb)	(adjective)	(direct object)

This straightforward sentence can be parsed or diagrammed easily. In this sentence, both adjectives clearly modify the nouns they precede (boys and practice), the subject of the sentence (boys) performs the action, which is the verb (enjoy), and the direct object (practice), answers the question *what* after the verb (i.e., "What do the boys enjoy?" practice). However, not all sentences are so easily described.

One area that often poses problems for students is the prepositional phrase. A prepositional phrase is usually composed of a preposition, an article, and an object of the preposition, with modifiers added sometimes as well. Here is a sentence with the prepositional phrases underlined:

Bryan headed <u>to the mall</u> <u>for the latest release</u> <u>by the band</u> <u>from his home state</u> <u>of Oregon</u>.

One way to identify some prepositions is by remembering this mnemonic about a box: The boy can sit <u>on</u> the box, <u>by</u> the box, <u>above</u> the box, <u>below</u> the box, <u>around</u> the box, or <u>near</u> the box. However, this does not allow for <u>to</u> and <u>from</u>, which are two of the most common prepositions.

Possessives also give writers problems. A possessive pronoun shows possession automatically; that is its purpose. As an example, consider the following sentences: That green Volvo is <u>mine</u>. Did you drive <u>your</u> Explorer? <u>Their</u> new Lexus is larger than <u>our</u> older model. In these sentences, there are no apostrophes added as there are with proper nouns.

Table 4.2 provides the most common possessive pronouns:

Table 4.2 Common Possessive Pronouns

	Singular	Plural
First person	mine, my	our, ours
Second person	your, yours	your, yours
Third person	her, hers, his, its	their, theirs

Notice that the possessive pronoun *its* has no apostrophe. Compare this with the contraction *it's,* which always means *it is.* Similarly, adding an apostrophe to *theirs* is always incorrect. Since *their* is a possessive pronoun, *their's* is not a word.

Adverbs are words that usually modify verbs, though they can modify adjectives or other adverbs. When thinking of adverbs, the *–ly* ending is commonly remembered. Consider the following sentence:

> That student performs <u>poorly</u> in a test environment, but he performs <u>well</u> in a relaxed setting.

In this sentence, the adverb *poorly* clearly shows *how* the student performs. In the second clause, *well* is also an adverb, though an irregular one, telling *how* the student performs in different conditions.

 Practice problems

Solutions to the practice problems are located in the back of this book.

1. Underline the verb(s) in the paragraph below.

   I go to concerts frequently, and I went to my favorite singer's concert yesterday. I had already been to her concert when I was in the seventh grade. I had not planned to go to this one, but my younger sister wanted me to take her. I hope that in the future my brother will take her to these concerts.

2. Underline the adjective(s) in the sentence below.

   The thick, brown molasses slides rapidly down the sides of the warm, fragrant pancakes.

3. Underline the adverb(s) in the sentence below.

   The multicolored snake inches smoothly forward despite the rocky terrain blocking its path.

4. Underline the direct object(s) in the sentence below.

   Tim Cratchit offers a prayer of gratitude at the end of Dickens's story. His utterance exemplifies the simplicity and generosity Dickens wanted to illustrate. Through this character, the author accentuates the social ills then prevalent in London.

5. Underline the prepositional phrase(s) in the sentence below.

   The man in the company of the noisy partygoers attempts to extricate himself from the rabble.

Subject-Verb Agreement

A native speaker of English understands basic subject-verb agreement as a result of learning the language as a child. A child may claim that a scraped knee feels fine now, but it "feeled bad" the day before. As the child grows, he or she will gradually learn that *feel* is an irregular verb and the regular rule for making a verb past tense–adding *–ed* to the ending–will not work in this case. In the same way, most difficulties with verbs fade with childhood, but problems with subject-verb agreement, which means making the subject of the sentence agree (or match) in number with the verb, may still arise.

A subject and verb agree in number when they are both either plural or singular. Consider the child again. A child may say, "I feels bad," when he or she means, "I feel bad." The child has used a singular subject, *I*, with a plural verb, *feels*. To think about this more clearly, consider the conjugation of the verb *run* shown in Table 4.3.

Table 4.3 Conjugation of the Verb *Run*

	Singular	Plural
First person	I run	We run
Second person	You run	You run
Third person	He runs	They run

Demonstrated in this table, the third person singular form of regular verbs in English has an *–s* at the end. The other forms of the verb are alike. Usually, this rule is very clear, and a native speaker can easily move from first person to second person while making subjects and verbs agree. Consider the following sentence:

> The two women work well together in their group assignment.

In this sentence, the plural subject *women* agrees with the plural verb *work*. However, not all sentences are this straightforward. When subjects and verbs are separated by other words, agreement can become more difficult. Take a look at this example:

> A physician, constantly surrounded by many patients who need help with their ailments and illnesses, easily become overwhelmed.

In this case, the descriptors or modifiers set off in commas make the subject-verb agreement error obvious. The sentence should state that "A physician... easily *becomes* overwhelmed." Now try this one:

> Sometimes the conference planner, holding the nametags and information packets for the newly arrived participants, many of whom have already introduced themselves, seem unneeded.

Though not quite so obvious, after omitting the descriptive information between the subject and the verb, it is easy to see the error. The sentence should state that "The... planner... *seems* unneeded."

Another issue regarding subject-verb agreement involves the use of *or, nor,* and *and.* When *or* or *nor* is used to connect multiple subjects that are singular, a singular verb is required; when *and* is used, a plural verb is necessary:

> Neither Mark nor Ann <u>enjoys</u> studying obstetrics, but both Mark and Ann <u>enjoy</u> studying geriatrics.

> The main argument or dispute between the couple who is in the process of divorcing <u>is</u> the welfare of the children, but both the topic and debate <u>are</u> well known in the judge's courtroom.

In this latter example, *or* requires the singular verb *is,* while *and* requires the plural verb *are.*

Finally, be careful when using nouns that seem plural but are actually conjugated with singular verbs; many of these end in *one*:

> Everyone *hopes* to score well on the exam.
> Any of us *has* the opportunity to score well.
> None of the students *uses* the break period to study English.
> Anyone *is* welcome to study in the library.

(P) Practice problems

Solutions to the practice problems are located in the back of this book.

The following sentences may or may not be correct. If the sentence is incorrect, write the correct sentence in the space provided. If the sentence is correct, write "no change" in the space provided.

1.	The planes was flying overhead.
Corrected sentence:	

2.	Everyone have a favorite dessert.
Corrected sentence:	

3.	Several of the members chooses not to vote.
Corrected sentence:	

4.	They say a woman's home is her castle.
Corrected sentence:	

5.	The man and woman eats at 3:00 p.m.
Corrected sentence:	

Pronoun-Antecedent Agreement

A pronoun replaces a noun so that the noun does not have to be repeated. Table 4.4 provides a list of pronouns:

Table 4.4 Pronouns

	Singular	Plural
First person	I, me, mine, my	we, us, our, ours
Second person	you, your, yours	you, your, yours
Third person	he, she, him, her, it, hers, his, its	they, them, their, theirs

The noun that a pronoun refers back to is called its **antecedent**. For example, consider the following sentence:

> Mom went to the store before I could remind her to buy ingredients for my favorite dish, her special spicy spaghetti.

In this sentence, the first pronoun *her* refers back to *Mom*, a noun. The antecedent for the pronoun *her* is thus *Mom*. The second pronoun *her* is a possessive pronoun, but it still refers back to Mom. *I* and *my* are pronouns as well, replacing the proper name of the speaker, which is not given in this sentence. Notice how funny the same sentence without pronouns would be:

> Mom went to the store before Michael could remind Mom to buy ingredients for Michael's favorite dish, Mom's special spicy spaghetti.

A pronoun and its antecedent must agree in number, meaning that whether the antecedent is singular or plural, the pronoun must be the same. A singular antecedent must have a singular pronoun, and a plural antecedent must have a plural pronoun. According to Table 4.4, if the noun *apples* is replaced with a pronoun, the plural pronoun *they* (or one of the other pronouns from the third person plural category) must be used, since the word *apples* is plural.

Frequently, people will use *they* or *them* as a singular pronoun to avoid using **gendered language** (language that specifies male or female gender using words such as *he or she*). This practice is increasingly common and will likely be acceptable at some point in the future. However, at this time, it is still considered incorrect in most writing guides. It is correct to replace words with the possessive pronouns *his* and *her* or a combination of the two (e.g., *his or her*):

> The senator stated that the responsibility of each <u>citizen</u> is to become involved in <u>his or her</u> local political organization.

The antecedent (*citizen*) is singular, so the pronouns (*his or her*) must be singular as well. If the senator had stated that the responsibility of each citizen is to become involved in *their* local political organization, the possessive pronoun *their* (plural) would not agree in number with the antecedent noun *citizen* (singular).

Opt for a plural noun when possible so that the plural pronouns *they* or *them* can be used. Rather than writing about a *person* who dreams of *his or her* ideal occupation in *his or her* future, for example, write about *people* who dream of *their* ideal occupations in *their* various futures.

Additionally, agreement between a pronoun and its antecedent can be technically correct, yet still problematic if it is unclear which noun is the antecedent. If a friend said, "My dad often goes with my brother to soccer practice, but he gets tired quickly," it is unclear whether the friend's brother becomes tired from playing soccer or the father grows tired of watching it. For that reason, it's important to use pronouns only when the antecedent is clear; if the antecedent is not clear, either replace the pronoun with the noun or recast the sentence entirely. As an example, consider the following sentence:

> The nurse saw his former patient in the mall and wished that he had greeted him more cordially.

The pronoun and antecedent in this sentence agree in number, but the relationship is unclear, which makes the meaning unclear as well. In this sentence, both *nurse* and *patient* are singular, as are the pronouns *he* and *him*. However, the reader cannot tell if the nurse wished that the patient had greeted the nurse more cordially, or if the nurse wished that he himself had greeted the patient more cordially.

Ⓟ Practice problems

Solutions to the practice problems are located in the back of this book.

The following sentences may or may not be correct. If the sentence is incorrect, write the correct sentence in the space provided. If the sentence is correct, write "no change" in the space provided.

1.	Each girl was presented with their varsity letter.
Corrected sentence:	

2.	The guide reiterated the possibility of danger to each person as they entered the bus.
Corrected sentence:	

3.	The boy's childish behavior is reminiscent of days gone by when he would throw temper tantrums daily at his nursery.
Corrected sentence:	

Use of Dialogue

Using dialogue is effective in a variety of situations: it can create immediacy and specificity in a college essay, it can provide a specific example in a presentation, or it can be a vivid example to spice up a letter or e-mail. This contrasts to indirectly communicating what a speaker says. Notice the difference between **indirect dialogue** (or indirect discourse) and **direct dialogue** (or direct discourse). Indirect dialogue tells *about* what someone said:

A'ishah says that he hasn't finished studying for the exam and it begins in 1 hour.

Direct dialogue tells exactly what someone said rather than telling about it:

A'ishah said, "I haven't finished studying for the exam and it begins in 1 hour."

Direct dialogue offers a more specific perspective than indirect dialogue, because the reader can see the exact words the speaker used, rather than hearing about them through another person.

It is important to punctuate dialogue properly. Quotation marks are always used to indicate exactly what someone says. If one quote exists inside another quote, then single quotation marks are used to designate the inside quote. Otherwise, the quotation marks should be double pairs. In the following example, the **attributive tag**, which is the part of the sentence that indicates who said a direct quote, is followed by a comma, and the quotation marks open and close the direct dialogue:

Alex said, "After babysitting my sister all afternoon, I hope that I never have to sing 'The Wheels on the Bus' again."

In this example, a song title is within the dialogue. Because song titles should also be enclosed in quotation marks, the double quotation marks that would have been used for the song title are replaced with single quotation marks, made with the apostrophe key on the keyboard.

Quotation marks open the quotation, occurring immediately to the left of the first quoted word (with no space in between), and a second set of quotation marks closes the quotation. If the quoted material occurs at the end of a sentence, a period should be placed within the quotation marks; if the quoted material is in the middle of a sentence, a comma should be placed inside the closing quotation marks; if the quotation marks enclose a question or an exclamation, then a question mark or exclamation point should be included within the quotation marks; and if the question mark or exclamation point applies to the whole sentence, then it should be placed outside of the quotation marks. Consider the following two examples:

(1) After Alejandro forgot to pick me up for the ballgame, I asked him, "Don't you ever think about anyone other than yourself?"

(2) How is it possible that I can say to my daughter, "Pick up your room before going out to play," but she hears, "Pick up your room at some point in the not-too-distant future"?

In sentence (1), the quotation marks surround the direct dialogue and also the question mark because the question mark is part of the dialogue. In other words, the direct dialogue is a question, so the question mark goes inside the quotation marks. Though periods and commas always go inside closing quotation marks, other punctuation marks can go inside or outside, depending on context. In sentence (2), the quoted dialogue is not a question in either case, but the sentence as a whole is. Therefore, the question mark occurs after the quotation marks.

Note, too, that a comma follows or precedes an attributive tag (depending on where the quote is placed) like *John said* or *According to the professor*. Also, the first word of direct dialogue is capitalized if the quote contains a complete sentence.

(P) *Practice problems*

Solutions to the practice problems are located in the back of this book.

The following sentences may or may not be correct. If the sentence is incorrect, write the correct sentence in the space provided. If the sentence is correct, write "no change" in the space provided.

1.	"Apparently, there is a monotone among us," chided the choir director.
Corrected sentence:	

2.	I should have chosen the red sports car, said Fahari regretfully.
Corrected sentence:	

First, Second, and Third Person

Point of view is often studied in literature classes to explore how a writer tells his or her story. As a writer, consider the most effective way to convey information to readers. The perspective from which an author writes is called the **point of view**.

When writing from a **first-person** point of view, the narrator is a character within the story. In nonfiction writing, that character is the author, and in fiction writing, the narrator may be any of the characters in the story. When using a first-person point of view, a writer should use the pronouns *I* and *my* or possibly *we* and *our*. As shown in the following sentence, information conveyed via a first-person point of view stresses the personal account of the speaker or writer (or the narrator, when writing fiction):

> I appreciate the opportunities I have had to visit the campuses of many fine universities over the last few years, and I look forward to visiting many more in the future.

Using the first-person point of view is an effective way to communicate a story about oneself or one's personal feelings and attitudes toward a subject. While at one time it was considered inappropriate to use first person in a formal setting, that opinion is gradually changing and first person can be found in a wide range of writings. A student might, for example, find a first-person point of view in a current issue of an academic journal–a collection of articles by professionals for professionals–though that same journal might have prohibited the use of first person in years past. When writing in an academic setting such as a classroom, it is important to ask the instructor whether or not the use of first-person point of view is permitted.

Frequently, students will add first-person statements like *I think, I feel,* or *I believe* that do not convey any information and that actually serve to weaken writing. In the sentence, *I truly believe that science has the power to transform our culture*, for example, it is unnecessary to say *I truly believe* because the reader knows a writer believes what he or she is writing; such phrasing also suggests that the author's personal attitude to this and other subjects must continually be expressed. This style can become monotonous. Additionally, students sometimes use this type of phrasing in an almost apologetic way, as if to say, "It's just my opinion and you may not agree." Again, this is unnecessary and deflates the writing.

Third-person point of view is generally considered the most formal writing style. The narrator of a story that is written from a third-person point of view will reference the thoughts or actions of other characters. This viewpoint can offer a more generalized perspective through the use of pronouns such as *everyone* or indirect nouns like *people*. The following sentence, for example, shows that information conveyed via a third-person point of view is more formal and creates a distance between the writer (or narrator) and the reader that is common to formal writing:

> Ikuto appreciates the opportunities he has had to visit the campuses of many fine universities over the last few years, and he looks forward to visiting many more in the future.

Compare a third-person approach with a first-person comment:

> People sometimes fail to realize the significance of obtaining a driver's license as a rite of passage in our culture. (third person)

> I did not realize the significance of obtaining a driver's license as a rite of passage in our culture. (first person)

The third-person passage is broader in scope and suggests an issue of larger significance, while the first-person passage makes the same issue more a matter of personal reflection. Either approach is equally correct; just consider the approach that is desired and the message that is to be conveyed.

A **second-person** point of view is another option. Text that is written from a second-person point of view specifically refers to the reader using the pronoun *you*. Though a second-person viewpoint is often considered too informal for academic writing, it has many other uses. Textbooks and study guides, for example, may employ a second-person viewpoint, and a letter or e-mail is usually written from this point of view. The use of a second-person point of view is like speaking directly to another person, so it's important to consider whether or not such directness will be appropriate.

If we change our earlier example to second person, it becomes quite different:

> You have failed to realize the significance of obtaining a driver's license as a rite of passage in our culture.

When this second-person sentence is read, it could seem accusatorial, depending on the context. Therefore, it is very important to consider the subtle changes in meaning that various points of view create.

(P) *Practice problems*

Solutions to the practice problems are located in the back of this book.

1. Identify whether the following sentence is written from a first-, second-, or third-person point of view:

    You should appreciate the opportunities you have had to visit the campuses of so many fine universities over the last few years, and you should be looking forward to visiting many more in the future.

2. Decide the most appropriate narrative voice to use in each of the following situations:

    A)   A formal writing about the history of the American Revolution
    B)   A diary entry
    C)   A letter

Grammar for Style and Clarity

Studying writing often begins in middle school, where issues of correctness are confronted. Does a comma go before or after the coordinating conjunction? Is this a regular or an irregular verb conjugation? Does that sentence require a period or a question mark? As mastery over these issues develops and moves beyond thinking only about whether or not a sentence is punctuated correctly or a capital letter is used as it should be, writing style begins to develop. Writers will start to think about which writing style is preferable based upon the purpose of the writing.

Some options might initially seem to make little difference. For example, there are several ways to combine sentences with coordinating conjunctions. **Coordinating conjunctions** are words that join two or more words, phrases, or clauses so that each conjoined element is equal. The coordinating conjunctions are *for, and, nor, but, or, yet,* and *so* (FANBOYS). Here are some possible sentences:

> My mom went shopping yesterday. She forgot to stop by Fabulous Foods, her favorite grocery store.

> My mom went shopping yesterday; she forgot to stop by Fabulous Foods, her favorite grocery store.

> My mom went shopping yesterday, but she forgot to stop by Fabulous Foods, her favorite grocery store.

All three of these sentences convey the same information, and all three are grammatically correct. The only decision to be made is a matter of style. Which might better provide sentence variety? Which might be better for a third-grade audience? Which might make a smoother transition from a previous idea? These are the sorts of stylistic questions that should become a part of a writer's revising process. Thus, revising or rethinking a paper becomes more than proofreading for grammar or mechanical errors. It involves making the best choice for the particular writing task at hand.

With the above examples, a writer might want to stress the mom's forgotten stop. To show that stress, a subordinating conjunction could be used. A **subordinating conjunction** is a word that joins two or more clauses and makes the clause that contains it dependent on another clause; therefore, the clause that contains the subordinating conjunction is of less importance. Some common subordinating conjunctions are *because, though, although, as, as if, when,* and *while*.

> Although my mom went shopping yesterday, she forgot to stop by Fabulous Foods, her favorite grocery store.

Though the difference is slight, the meaning of this sentence is altered from the same sentence using a coordinating conjunction. In the current version, the fact that the mom went shopping is a supporting statement, while the focus is on the mom forgetting to go to Fabulous Foods. In the previous examples, both facts are treated with equal weight.

Nominalization refers to the making of a noun from a verb, adverb, or adjective. Writers sometimes use this method because they think it sounds more sophisticated, but repeated use of vague, abstract nouns can become boring. To cure the problem, opt for active verbs. **Active verbs** are verbs that show an action performed by the subject of the sentence. For example, the first sentence in each of the following pairs of sentences uses nominalization, while the second sentence uses an active verb.

(1) He had a negative <u>reaction</u> to the nutritionist's presentation.

      The better version without nominalization:

(2) He <u>reacted</u> negatively to the nutritionist's presentation.

(1) My aunt made a <u>statement</u> about the red vehicle hitting the black one.

      The better version without nominalization:

(2) My aunt <u>stated</u> that the red vehicle hit the black one.

The question of which to use is again a stylistic choice dependent on purpose and **audience** (i.e., the person or people who will be reading the piece of writing). However, using active verbs whenever possible is a good rule of thumb to follow.

Passive verbs are comprised of *be* plus a past participle that shifts the action of a sentence from the subject to the object of the sentence. Consider this example:

> The dog chewed the bone.
>   →   →   →

To make this sentence passive, the action should be moved from the subject of the sentence, *the dog*, to the direct object of the sentence, *the bone*. The subject of the original sentence now performs the verb on the object, in other words. Now notice a passive construction:

> The bone was chewed by the dog.
>   ←   ←   ←

In this example, the bone is not doing the chewing; the noun performing the action has been relegated to the position of object of the preposition. A passive construction can also eliminate the "doer" altogether:

> The bone was chewed.

This type of construction is frequently used in formal settings or in situations for which no subject or actor is known:

> I was told that there would be refreshments at this meeting.

In this situation, the speaker or writer either does not know who made the remark, does not remember who made the remark, or does not want to divulge who made the remark about the refreshments. In any case, the passive construction is clearly less informative in this example. As with the other stylistic choices shown, the use of passive verbs is not wrong. However, a writer should be aware of the choice being made and should choose passive voice for the right reason. Often, the **passive voice** is useful in situations for which the writer does not wish to assign blame, which may be the case in the example above. However, most teachers will encourage the use of active verbs and discourage passive verbs.

There are many choices that a writer makes when constructing a sentence: active or passive verb, syntax (word order), modifiers, word choice (diction), and punctuation. It is important when writing and especially when revising that the writer be aware of the possibilities and make choices with an eye toward purpose and audience.

Ⓟ *Practice problems*

Solutions to the practice problems are located in the back of this book.

1. Underline the conjunctions in the sentence below.

    My eyes glazed over as I reviewed the math problems, but I forged ahead with renewed vigor when I remembered the upcoming exam and the necessity of scoring well to pass the course.

2. Underline the words that are nominalizations of verbs in the sentences below.

    I made an estimation of the number of possible scenarios. I had a transformation when I saw the moon shining brightly overhead. I had a realization that there was plenty of available light on the night of the crime.

3. Underline the active and passive verbs in the sentences below. Identify whether each verb is active or passive.

    Malcolm raced past the hall monitor, burst into the English class, slid into his seat, and then calmly glanced at the teacher as if nothing had happened. He was seen by everyone in the class, but he was effective in appearing nonchalant.

Context Clues

Context clues are words surrounding an unfamiliar word that can help in discerning the meaning of the unfamiliar word. Context clues may not appear in the same sentence as the unfamiliar word, but may be located in nearby sentences.

Table 4.5 contains eight types of context clues. An example follows each type of context clue as clarification.

Table 4.5 Context Clues

Context clue	Explanation	Example
Definition	The definition of the unfamiliar word is given in the sentence.	In his woodworking, he used a type of file known as a <u>rasp</u>.
Description	A description of the unfamiliar word is given in the sentence.	Allen is a <u>malcontent</u>; he is constantly changing jobs, moving to different apartments, and trading in cars. He complains and expresses his dissatisfaction with every aspect of life.
Example	Examples of the unfamiliar word are given in the sentence.	The menu listed such <u>delicacies</u> as frog legs, octopi, and chocolate-flavored worms.
Synonym	A synonym of the unfamiliar word is given in the sentence.	The <u>ophthalmologist</u>, or eye doctor, prescribed eyedrops.
Antonym	An antonym of the unfamiliar word is given in the sentence.	Unlike the sophisticated life in the city, life in Scottsville was a <u>quaint</u> existence.
Comparison	A comparison is used in the sentence that helps give meaning to the unfamiliar word.	Elliott is wealthy and generous as is his father, who is a <u>philanthropist</u>.
Contrast	The unfamiliar word is contrasted to known words or phrases.	The instructor would often <u>deviate</u> from the topic, rather than remain focused on the subject he introduced at the beginning of the lecture.
Explanation	The unfamiliar word is defined in the sentence through an explanation of a situation.	He was awarded a degree <u>posthumously</u>; he died a month before graduation.

ⓟ *Practice problems*

Solutions to the practice problems are located in the back of this book.

In each of the following sentences, decipher the meaning of the underlined word based on clues provided in the sentence. Then, identify the context clues.

1.	Scrubbing floors, washing dishes, and sifting garbage are just a few of the <u>menial</u> jobs he worked.
Definition:	
Context clue(s):	

2.	The man is <u>cantankerous</u>. He quarrels and starts arguments with everyone.
Definition:	
Context clue(s):	

3.	The guide <u>reiterated</u> the possibility of danger by repeating the warnings again and again.
Definition:	
Context clue(s):	

4.	Much to our surprise, Don was not <u>hostile</u>, but warm and friendly.
Definition:	
Context clue(s):	

5.	Many movie stars attend the <u>premiere</u>, or first showing, of a movie.
Definition:	
Context clue(s):	

6.	She had <u>surmounted</u> many challenges, but she would not overcome this one.
Definition:	
Context clue(s):	

Word Structure

The English language contains a wide variety of words. Etymology, root words, prefixes, and suffixes are all parts of **word structure** (the way in which the parts of a word are arranged together) used to determine a word's meaning. **Etymology** refers to the history of a given word or its origin. A **root word** is a word in its simplest form, before any affixes are attached. The **prefix** of a word is a group of letters added to the beginning of a word that modifies or extends the word's meaning. Finally, the **suffix** of a word is a group of letters added to the end of a word that modifies or extends the word's meaning.

Many readers will seek out a dictionary to assist with defining words. Yet, there is another way to determine the meaning of words that does not require a dictionary. The reader can determine how to pronounce and identify a word, as well as unlock its meaning, by considering the word parts used in the structure of the word. By knowing some common prefixes, suffixes, and root words, the reader can determine the meanings of many words, even when the reader did not previously have an understanding of the word as a whole.

There are four common prefixes found in the English language that are helpful in providing clues to a word's meaning. These are shown in Table 4.6.

Table 4.6 Common Prefixes

Prefix	Possible definition	Example
un	not	unavailable, unarmed, unattractive
re	again	reacquaint, readjust
in	not	invisible, inaccurate
dis	not	disorganized, disagreeable

Suffixes can be more difficult to determine because they often have more abstract meanings. Table 4.7 lists some common English suffixes.

Table 4.7 Common Suffixes

Suffix	Possible definition	Example
ia, y	state or condition	amnesia, democracy
ic, ical, ac	having to do with	endoscopic, physical, cardiac
ism	belief in	nationalism, activism
ology	the study of	archeology, bacteriology
or, er	one who takes part in	conductor, reporter, fighter

The majority of English words have Latin or Greek origins. Table 4.8 lists some root words that can be found in the English language.

Table 4.8 Common Root Words

Root	Possible definition	Example
arch	ruler	archenemy, tetrarch, hierarchical
audio	sound	audiovisual, audiocassette
bio	life	biochemistry, biodegradable
chrom	color	monochrome
geo	earth	geometry, geode, geologic
graph	written	biographic, calligraphy, mimeograph
morph	form	endomorph, isomorphic, morphine
ortho	correct	orthodontia, unorthodox
ped	foot	backpedal, millipede
terra	earth	terrace, terrarium, extraterrestrial
therm	heat	exothermal, endothermic, geothermal

Ⓟ *Practice problems*

Solutions to the practice problems are located in the back of this book.

1. What is the prefix in the word *invisible*? What does the prefix mean?

2. What is the suffix in the word *socialism*? What does the suffix mean?

3. What is the root of the word *audible*? What does the root mean?

STRUCTURE

Simple Sentences

A **simple sentence** is a sentence that contains only one clause that has a complete meaning (a clause that has a complete meaning is called an **independent clause**). Simple sentences, such as those in Example 4.1, are the easiest type of sentences to identify. They must not contain any dependent clauses. A **dependent clause** is a clause that is made dependent or incomplete because of the addition of a subordinating conjunction. Because a simple sentence cannot contain a dependent clause, it need only have a subject and verb to be complete:

 Example 4.1:   *Simple sentences: I am going. Don't cry. Never fear. I'll return.*

A simple sentence may also have additional parts of speech: prepositions, adjectives, and adverbs. As seen in Example 4.2, these develop sentences into more meaningful ways of communicating:

 Example 4.2:   *Simple sentences: I am going away from this noisy, crowded cafeteria. Don't cry over that exam last period. Never fear defeat while learning. I'll return to help you study after lunch period.*

The additional modifiers change the meaning of these sentences. However, they are still simple sentences. They do not contain one or more dependent clauses, which would make them **complex sentences**. A complex sentence appears in Example 4.3.

 Example 4.3:   *Complex sentence: When this happens, I don't try to pull my thoughts back to the present.*

The only difficulty in writing a simple sentence is in conjugating the verb. Students occasionally confuse a **verbal**, a word that is sometimes a verb but not acting as a verb in a particular sentence, with a conjugated verb. First look at this sentence:

> The sixteen members of the newly formed Friendship Club traveled to Quebec's famous hotel, Le Chateau Frontenac, for a spring break field trip.

In this sentence, the subject, *members*, and the verb, *traveled*, convey the meaning of the sentence. The other words give additional information about the members or the traveling. Together, the parts form a cohesive whole. Compare the simple sentence above with the following:

> The sixteen members of the newly formed Friendship Club traveling to Quebec's famous hotel, Le Chateau Frontenac, for a spring break field trip.

This sentence fragment cannot be called a simple sentence because the verb is not properly conjugated. Though *traveling* looks like a verb, it is a participle and must have an auxiliary verb like *are* to make it complete. Without that helper, *traveling* becomes a modifier; it is not a conjugated verb, so this sentence is not correct.

In addition to simple sentences and complex sentences, there are also compound sentences. As seen in Example 4.4, a **compound sentence** differs from a simple sentence because it contains two (or more) independent clauses joined together with a coordinating conjunction or a semicolon.

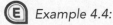 *Example 4.4:*   *Compound sentence: I enjoy watching golf matches on television, especially on Sundays near the end of the tournaments, but I also like to play golf with friends at our local nine-hole course.*

> *This compound sentence is just two simple sentences joined together with the coordinating conjunction* but. *Notice that the subjects and verbs of both sentences,* I enjoy *and* I like, *are conjugated properly.*

Ⓟ *Practice problems*

Solutions to the practice problems are located in the back of this book.

1. Read the following sentence. Then, answer the question.

    Of the three volunteers at the annual cheerleader car wash, only Jeff was washing cars.

    Is the sentence above a simple sentence? Explain why or why not.

2. Read the following sentence. Then, answer the question.

    Mark imagines a successful future for himself that includes a large family with at least eight children, a large number of dogs, cats, hamsters, and guinea pigs, a job that he looks forward to performing each day, and plenty of money in the bank for extra security.

    Is the sentence above a simple sentence? Explain why or why not.

Organized and Logical Paragraphs

When we read, we are accustomed to seeing our text divided into different sections or paragraphs. A **paragraph** is a group of sentences that forms a cohesive whole due to its similar topic or theme. One of the reasons we use paragraphs is to help us absorb smaller units of information; if we had a three-page paragraph, for example, we would have a difficult time trying to hold all points of that paragraph in our heads until we finished reading it and were ready to make some assessment of it.

Another reason for breaking writing into paragraphs is to group similar ideas together. A paragraph should be a cohesive unit sharing a particular topic. Dividing writing into clearly identifiable, separate points will prevent paragraphs from being collections of illogical, random ideas with no clear focus. The topic is usually given at or near the beginning of the paragraph in a **topic sentence**. The function of the topic sentence, in addition to giving the topic of the paragraph, is to tie the topic of the paragraph to the overall theme of the piece of writing, and often to provide a clear **transition** (i.e., a smooth movement from one point to the next). Example 4.5 provides an example of a topic sentence.

 Example 4.5:   *Topic sentence*

In addition to grading papers, a teacher's day is spent preparing the next day's lesson.

In this example, the topic sentence gives the topic of the paragraph (preparing the next day's lesson), ties that topic to the main theme (how a teacher spends his or her day), and transitions from the previous point (grading papers).

After the topic sentence, a paragraph should contain sentences that support the topic. This **support** may come in the form of details and examples that clearly explain the topic of the paragraph. Continuing Example 4.5, Example 4.6 adds specific details about how a lesson is prepared:

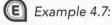 *Example 4.6:*   *Support*

A literature teacher might have to dedicate some time to rereading the assigned portion of Beowulf *and creating relevant discussion points. A history teacher might have to supplement his or her knowledge of the Civil War with current scholarship about the subject. An algebra teacher might have to create some new word problems to test the students' understanding of quadratic equations. A biology teacher might need to create a slide show presentation about the alimentary canal.*

This support further explains the main topic of the paragraph through specific, detailed examples.

After providing support, a writer might want to assess or analyze the information given. This will help to defend the supporting sentences and provide a conclusion. An analysis of Example 4.6 might look like Example 4.7:

 Example 4.7:   *Analysis*

Though these tasks might seem unnecessary for a teacher who has been in the classroom for twenty or thirty years, a good instructor can never fall back on previously learned material. Each lesson is not only a result of the accumulation of knowledge, but also a continued engagement with the subject matter.

This paragraph has concluding remarks for the continued example.

After an assessment or concluding remark, the writer is then ready to move to the next topic. As you can see from this example, a well supported paragraph will be of some length. Though there is no hard-and-fast rule about how long a paragraph must be, you should avoid writing short paragraphs of three or four sentences (or even less). As shown in Example 4.8, good writers have paragraphs that are at least five sentences long, though they are often considerably longer.

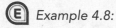 *Example 4.8:*   *Paragraph*

> *My father, after considering what my punishment should be for staying out past curfew, decided to adopt a new tactic. First, he sent me to my room to "consider the profound consequences" that might have resulted from my behavior. Then, after I spent 2 hours trying to imagine what on earth he meant by "profound consequences," he came into my room and quizzed me on the thoroughness of my consideration: "Do you know what might have happened to you wandering around town past midnight? Did you consider how worried your mother and I would be? Can you imagine all of the frightening possibilities we were imagining? Do you want to have your driving privileges taken away completely?" After an hour of these unanswerable questions, the punishment became even worse. I had to write a letter to my future children explaining to them why I had stayed out so late and why I was so unspeakably wrong for doing so. As I sat at my computer for the next 2 hours, I at least had the pleasure of knowing that my punishment was coming to an end; I could hear Dad snoring in the family room as I signed my letter, "Your older, wiser, and not-too-soon-to-be father."*

The topic sentence of the paragraph, here the first sentence, gives the topic of the paragraph, the father's new tactic.

The support for that topic sentence is in three parts: thinking about the mistake, talking with the father about it, and writing the letter about it to the future children.

To conclude the paragraph, the writer shows that the new tactic is at an end since the father has fallen asleep and the letter is finished.

In addition to transitioning between paragraphs, it is important to clearly transition between ideas and sentences. Abrupt changes in direction within a piece of writing will leave the reader confused, making it necessary for the reader to re-read your writing. For example, use transition words, such as *first*, *then*, and *next*, when writing a chronology, and use contrasting words like *but* or *however* to signal to your reader that what you are about to write contrasts with the previous statements. Words that show a continuation of ideas, such as *similarly*, *in addition to*, or *moreover*, can also be helpful, as can words that show a judgment or conclusion, such as *therefore* or *in conclusion*.

Practice problems

Solutions to the practice problems are located in the back of this book.

Read the following paragraph. Then, identify each of the statements as TRUE or FALSE.

> At that point I wasn't sure what to do. Should I continue as planned or come up with a new idea? Either way seemed fraught with difficulty. I weighed my options: If I called Mom and asked her to bring my science project, then I wouldn't fail the assignment in biology class, but by calling her, I was telling her what happened before I'd had the chance to see if I had left the bag in Madison's car. I imagined the disappointed look on Dr. Conrad's face as I sat in Biology I, my favorite class. Then I imagined Mom's glare as she realized I had lost yet another book bag, and my answer was clear. Dr. Conrad's wrath was not nearly as lethal as Mom's angry stare and long sigh, so I took a deep breath and headed for biology class. It wasn't the easiest decision I had ever made, but I felt confident in the choice I had selected.

1. The paragraph above includes a topic sentence.

2. The paragraph above includes support.

3. The paragraph above includes a concluding remark.

Sentence Fluency

An awareness of writing style is important to prevent monotony and to keep a reader engaged with the subject matter. Beginning readers' books use simple sentences, but the repeated use of simple sentences in adult writing is not appropriate.

One way to enliven writing is through sentence variety. William Faulkner, the acclaimed fiction writer of the early twentieth century, is famous for his use of very long sentences, sometimes a whole paragraph long, followed by a very short sentence. This juxtaposition of long sentences and short sentences captures the reader's attention and enables the writer to focus that attention toward a particular point. When writing, you should also work to vary sentence lengths. Follow long sentences with short ones, or even use a couple of short sentences together for an abrupt focus on a particular point. Challenging the reader in this way will ensure that he or she stays engaged and alert.

In addition to sentence length, sentence variety is important. Rather than using a long string of simple sentences, follow a simple sentence with a complex sentence, and a complex with a compound sentence.

A good writer can also opt for more complicated sentence structures, such as a **periodic sentence**, in which the meaning or point of the sentence is delayed until the end, usually in the form of an independent clause, or a **cumulative sentence** (also known as a **loose sentence**), in which the independent clause of the sentence comes first and is followed by modifiers that further develop the initial idea. See Examples 4.9 and 4.10. Varying sentence structures should be a part of the editing process after the rough draft is completed.

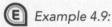 Example 4.9:   *Periodic sentence*

Propelled by my jet-propulsion backpack, speeding past my astonished parents, blasting through the limits of the atmosphere, and careening into the blackness of outer space, I imagined myself as the first astronaut to orbit the earth without a space ship.

A periodic sentence often contains a string of parallel modifiers followed by the main clause. In this case, parallel means that the string contains all of the same elements, whether they be prepositional phrases, single adjectives, or as in the example here, participial phrases.

Example 4.10:   *Cumulative sentence*

I still dream of traveling in space, floating through feathery clouds, slipping past lone-flying birds, soaring towards the heavens, all the while pitying the ground-dwellers below.

A cumulative sentence is like a periodic sentence, but reversed. In a cumulative sentence the main clause comes first and is followed by a parallel string of modifiers. Parallel means that the string contains all of the same elements, whether they be prepositional phrases, single adjectives, or as in the example here, participial phrases.

Practice problems

Solutions to the practice problems are located in the back of this book.

Identify each of the following sentences as a simple sentence, compound sentence, complex sentence, periodic sentence, or cumulative sentence.

1. I dream of being an astronaut.

2. When I was younger, I asked for a space suit every year for Christmas.

3. I dream of being an astronaut, but I also imagine myself as a great trapeze artist.

SPELLING AND PUNCTUATION

Spelling

There are many spelling rules in the English language. There are also many exceptions. The information provided in Table 4.9 includes common English language rules and exceptions.

Table 4.9 Common English Language Rules and Exceptions

Type of word	Rule	Example		Exception	
ie and *ei* words	*i* before *e*, except after *c*– or when sounded like *a* as in the words *neighbor* and *weigh*	**"ie"** believe friend grievous niece siege	**"ei"** ceiling conceit conceive neighbor receipt receive reign sleigh veil weigh	**"ie"** ancient conscience efficient policies species science society sufficient	**"ei"** either foreign height leisure neither protein seize weird
Suffixes for words ending in *e*	If a word ends in a silent *e* and the added suffix begins with a consonant, then keep the letter *e* when adding the suffix.	awe + some = awesome hate + ful = hateful		—	
	If a word ends in a silent *e* and the added suffix begins with a vowel, then drop the letter *e* when adding the suffix.	age + ing = aging enforce + ing = enforcing true + ism = truism		If a word ends in *-ce* or *-ge* and the added suffix is *-able* or *-ous*, then keep the letter *e*: change + able = changeable courage + ous = courageous enforce + able = enforceable notice + able = noticeable outrage + ous = outrageous trace + able = traceable If a word ends in a silent *e* and the added suffix is *–ing*, then keep the silent *e* when adding *ing* only if dropping the *e* would create ambiguity: singe + ing = singeing (not to be confused with singing)	
Suffixes for words ending in *y*	If a word ends with a *y* preceded by a vowel, keep the *y* when adding a suffix.	annoy + ance = annoyance buy + er = buyer convey + ance = conveyance delay + ed = delayed employ + er = employer enjoy + able = enjoyable journey + ed = journeyed pay + able = payable survey + or = surveyor		—	
	If a word ends with a *y* preceded by a consonant, change the *y* to an *i* before adding a suffix.	carry + ed = carried glory + ous = glorious hurry + ed = hurried magnify + cent = magnificent necessary + ly = necessarily satisfy + ed = satisfied silly + est = silliest victory + ous = victorious charity + able = charitable		If a word ends with a *y* preceded by a consonant and the suffix being added is *-ing*, then keep the *y*. carry + ing = carrying hurry + ing = hurrying ready + ing = readying bury + ing = burying	

Type of word	Rule	Example	Exception
Suffixes for words ending in a consonant-vowel-consonant pattern	In general, if a word has one syllable and ends with a consonant-vowel-consonant pattern, then double the final consonant before adding a suffix that begins with a vowel.	bag + age = baggage bar + ed = barred bed + ing = bedding get + ing = getting rub + ed = rubbed run + ing = running sag + ing = sagging shut + ing = shutting sit + ing = sitting	—
	In general, if a word has more than one syllable, but the accent is on the last syllable, then double the final consonant before adding a suffix that begins with a vowel.	compel + ing = compelling control + ing = controlling corral + ed = corralled excel + ence = excellence forget + able = forgettable occur + ence = occurrence omit + ed = omitted prefer + ed = preferred refer + ed = referred allot + ed = allotted	—
Suffixes for words ending in c	In general, if a word ends in a c and a suffix beginning with e, i, or y is added, then the letter k should be inserted following the letter c.	colic + y = colicky frolic + ed = frolicked mimic + ed = mimicked panic + y = panicky shellac + ed = shellacked	—

Words ending in -ceed, -sede, and -cede	In English there are four words that end in -ceed, and one word that ends in -sede. Other words with the same sound end in -cede.	<u>-ceed</u> <u>-sede</u> <u>-cede</u>
		emceed supersede accede
		exceed antecede
		proceed concede
		succeed intercede
		                    recede
		                    retrocede
			—

Words ending in -able or -ible	In general, if the root word is a complete word, then add -able. (If the root ends in e, drop the e before adding -able.)	accept + able = acceptable avail + able = available depend + able = dependable profit + able = profitable enjoy + able = enjoyable retrieve + able = retrievable believe + able = believable love + able = lovable desire + able = desirable	—

	In general, if the root word is not a complete word, then add -ible.	aud + ible = ible
		divis + ible = divisible
		ed + ible = edible
		feas + ible = feasible
		invis + ible = invisible
		horr + ible = horrible
		terr + ible = terrible
			There are many exceptions, these are just a few:
			   digestible
			   flexible
			   responsible
			   irritable
			   accessible
			   inevitable
			   collectible/collectable
			   discernible/discernable

Words ending in -ance, -ancy, -ant or -ence, -ency, -ent	In general, if the suffix is preceded by a hard c or g sound, then the suffix is -ance, -ancy, or -ant.	elegance elegant extravagance extravagant significance significant vacancy vacant	—

Type of word	Rule	Example		Exception
	In general, if the suffix is preceded by a soft *c* or *g* sound, then the suffix is *-ence*, *-ency*, or *-ent*.	absence absent agency agent beneficence emergency emergent indigence innocent innocence negligence negligent		—
Words ending in -*tion*, -*sion*, or -*cian*	In general, if the root word ends in -*t*, then the suffix -*tion* can be added. If the root word ends in -*s*, the suffix -*sion* can be added.	**-*tion*** abduction addiction deduction distraction exception	**-*sion*** procession profession regression succession depression	—
	In general, if a word names a person, then it should end in -*cian*.	**-*cian*** magician musician physician politician technician		—

Homophones are words that sound alike but are spelled differently. Before writing a word, determine its context to make sure that the word being spelled is not a homophone for the intended word. Table 4.10 lists some common homophones and their definitions.

Table 4.10 Homophones

Homophone	Part of speech	Definition
affect effect	verb noun	to have an effect on something that is brought about by a cause
ascent assent	noun noun	a slope that angles upward agreement
all ready already	adjective adverb	everyone or everything is ready by this time
all together altogether	adjective adverb	everyone in a group entirely, completely
altar alter	noun verb	a structure used in worship to change
bear bare	verb verb	to carry or support to expose
capital capitol	noun noun	a leading or governing city a building that houses a state's lawmakers
cite site	verb noun	to use as an example; to quote a location
complement compliment	noun noun	an element that completes a remark of appreciation
council counsel	noun noun	a body of people assembled for advice advice
descent dissent	noun noun	a slope that angles downward disagreement
dying dyeing	verb verb	ceasing to live coloring a fabric
forth fourth	adverb noun	forward in place or time the element in a series that is next after the third element
principal principle	noun noun	chief or leader a belief or a rule of conduct
stationary stationery	adjective noun	not moving paper for writing letters
their they're there	adjective adjective	belonging to them contraction of they are in that place
to too two	preposition adverb adjective	indicates movement or intent also something that has two units
whose who's	adjective	belonging to whom contraction of who is
your you're	adjective	belonging to you contraction of you are

(P) *Practice problems*

Solutions to the practice problems are located in the back of this book.

1. For words ending in *–able* or *–ible*, which is the correct suffix for the word if the root is a complete word?

Identify each of the following four words as spelled CORRECTLY or INCORRECTLY.

2. conceive

3. receive

4. wierd

5. seize

6. In which of the following words is the ending *y* changed to an *i* prior to adding a suffix?'

    A) destroy
    B) victory
    C) delay
    D) journey

7. Which of the following root words remains unchanged when adding the suffix *–able*?

    A) desire
    B) love
    C) enforce
    D) believe

8. Which of the following words is an exception to the rules of *–able* and *–ible*?

    A) enjoyable
    B) credible
    C) feasible
    D) inevitable

Identify the correct word in the following sentences.

9. The judge ended the debate on a matter of (principal/principle).

10. The race was conducted on a course that wound around (their/they're/there) home.

Commonly Misspelled Words

Words that are commonly misspelled may be misspelled for a variety of reasons, such as the word being an exception to a spelling rule or the word being a homophone. To identify if a word is incorrectly spelled, it is important to know common spelling rules and exceptions to spelling rules (see the previous section titled "Spelling"). It is also helpful to know which words are commonly misspelled. Table 4.11 provides nearly 350 commonly misspelled words.

Table 4.11 Commonly Misspelled Words

accidentally	cemetery	deferred	exercise	influential	ninth
accept	changeable	definite	exhaust	innocence	noticeable
accommodate	changing	descent	exhilaration	instance	notoriety
accompanied	characteristic	describe	existence	instant	nucleus
achieved	chauffeur	description	explain	intellectual	obedience
across	colonel	desirable	explanation	intelligence	obligation
address	column	desperate	extraordinary	intelligent	oblige
aggravate	commit	device	familiar	intelligible	obliged
aisle	committed	devise	fascinate	intentionally	obstacle
allot	committee	dictionary	February	intercede	occasion
allotted	comparative	diphtheria	fiery	interest	occur
alright	comparatively	disappear	finally	irresistible	occurred
all right	comparison	disappoint	financial	legitimate	occurrence
amateur	compel	disastrous	forehead	leisure	omission
annual	compelled	discipline	foreign	liable	omit
anxiety	competent	discuss	foremost	library	omitted
apparent	competition	discussion	forfeit	lightning	operate
appearance	completely	disease	fraternity	likely	opinion
appropriate	compulsion	dissatisfied	furniture	literature	optimistic
arctic	conceivable	dissatisfy	ghost	livelihood	organization
argument	conceive	dissipate	government	loneliness	outrageous
arrangement	conception	distribute	grammar	magazine	pageant
association	confident	dormitories	grandeur	maintain	pamphlet
attendance	conqueror	drudgery	grief	maintenance	parallel
auxiliary	conscience	ecstasy	grievous	manual	parliament
awkward	conscientious	efficiency	guidance	marriage	pastime
bachelor	conscious	eighth	handkerchief	material	permissible
barbarian	contemptible	eligible	height	mathematics	perseverance
barbarous	convenient	eliminate	hesitancy	mattress	persistent
barren	coolly	eminent	hesitate	medicine	persuade
beggar	course	emphasize	hindrance	messenger	physically
believe	courteous	enemy	hoping	miniature	physician
beneficial	courtesy	environment	hurriedly	minute	picnic
benefited	cruelty	equip	hygiene	mischievous	picnicking
biscuit	curiosity	equipment	hypocrisy	misspell	piece
brilliant	cylinder	equipped	imaginary	momentous	pleasant
business	deceit	equivalent	imitation	mortgage	politician
cafeteria	deceive	especially	imminent	muscle	possess
calendar	deception	exaggerate	incidentally	naturally	possession
candidate	decide	exceed	incredible	nickel	possible
career	decision	excel	indigestible	niece	practically
carriage	defer	excellent	indispensable	ninetieth	prairie
ceiling	deference	except	inevitable	ninety	precede

precedence	quantity	repetition	secretary	surprise	tyranny
preceding	rally	representative	seize	syllable	unanimous
prefer	realize	reservoir	sentinel	symmetry	unusual
preference	recede	resistance	separate	temperament	usage
preferred	receive	restaurant	severely	temperature	valuable
prejudice	recognize	rhetoric	shriek	tendency	vengeance
presence	recommend	rhythm	siege	tournament	vigilance
prevalent	refer	ridiculous	similar	tragedy	villain
procedure	reference	sacrifice	soliloquy	transfer	Wednesday
proceed	referred	sacrilegious	sophomore	transferred	wholly
processor	region	safety	strenuous	tried	writing
pronunciation	reign	salary	studying	tries	written
propeller	relieve	scarcely	suffrage	truly	yoke
psychiatrist	religious	schedule	supersede	try	yolk
psychology	repeat	science	suppress	twelfth	

 Practice problems

Solutions to the practice problems are located in the back of this book.

Identify each of the following words as spelled CORRECTLY or INCORRECTLY.

1. accommodate

2. disipate

3. hypocrisy

4. temperament

5. diptheria

Capitalization

Capital letters are to be used according to rules established by custom or standard usage. Several capitalization rules are listed in Table 4.12. Knowledge of basic capitalization rules, such as capitalizing the first word at the beginning of a sentence, is assumed.

Table 4.12 Capitalization Rules

Rule	Example	Exception
Capitalize geographical locations such as cities, continents, counties, countries, islands, peninsulas, beaches, bodies of water, mountains, streets, parks, forests, canyons, dams, sections of the country or world, city streets, parks, and buildings.	Kansas City United States North America Hawaii Jackson County Venice Beach Atlantic Ocean Italian Peninsula Grand Canyon the Far East Park Avenue Lincoln Park Chapman Building	Do not capitalize any geographical labels that are not used as or with proper nouns. Example: They ride their bikes down the *street* to the park by the *beach*.
Capitalize the cardinal directions and their compounds when they refer to particular regions.	West Canada the South	Do not capitalize a cardinal direction when it refers to a point of the compass or when it refers to a part of a state. Example: drive east western Kansas
Capitalize names of specific organizations, companies, institutions and government bodies.	Spanish Club (organization) Ford Foundation (company) University of New Mexico (institution) Department of Defense (government body)	—
Capitalize the names of historical events or documents, months, days of the week, special events, and calendar items.	French Revolution (historical event) Atlantic Pact (historical document) August (month) Sunday (day of the week) World Series (special event) Junior Prom (special event) Christmas Eve (calendar item) Labor Day (calendar item)	—
Capitalize the names of nationalities, races, and religions.	Turkish (nationality) African-American (race) Muslim (religion)	—
Capitalize the names of monuments, ships, planes, and awards.	Longfellow Monument (monument) Mayflower (ship) Purple Heart (award)	Do not capitalize the names of general school subjects. Only capitalize the languages and specific course names, including those followed by a number; the words senior, junior, sophomore, and freshman are not capitalized when used to refer to a student.
Capitalize proper names and titles of rank or honor.	Dr. Larry Smith General Marcus Clark President Lincoln J. Weston Walsch Reverend John Thompson Queen Elizabeth	Do not capitalize a title or rank of honor when it follows a name. Example: George Washington was the first president of the United States.

Rule	Example	Exception
Capitalize words showing family relationship when they are parts of titles or when they can be substituted for proper nouns.	Uncle Elson Cousin Li Aunt Margaret	Do not capitalize words showing family relationship when preceded by a possessive. Examples: my cousin Rob your mother Mohammed's brother
Capitalize the main words in the titles of books and poems, plays, articles, musical compositions, chapters of books, etc.	the New York Times (newspaper) A Tale of Two Cities (play) Computers for Dummies (book) Moonlight Sonata (musical composition)	—
Capitalize words referring to specific deities.	Lord Savior Messiah Shiva Yahweh Shango Osiris Allah	The word "god" should not be capitalized when speaking of gods in general. Example: The Greek gods are portrayed as being fickle.
Capitalize the first word in every line of poetry and the first word of a complete quotation.	Twinkle, twinkle little star, How I wonder what you are. Mr. Jackson said, "You will always remember your high school days with fond recollection."	—
Capitalize the names of seasons only if they are personified or are part of a specific event. Otherwise, they are not capitalized.	(1) "Heralded in trumpet blare, comes Spring across the threshold in scented frock and maiden hair." (2) My favorite season is summer. (3) I can't wait for the Winter Olympics. Sentence (1) personifies the word *Spring* (i.e., spring is given the features of a person). Sentence (2) does not personify the word *summer* or refer to an event. Sentence (3) refers to a specific event.	—

(P) *Practice problems*

Solutions to the practice problems are located in the back of this book.

For each of the following three sentences, determine if the capitalization is correct or incorrect. If the capitalization is incorrect, rewrite the sentence with the correct capitalization.

1. My aunt lives in Louisiana.

2. He lives in eastern Mississippi.

3. Drive East to the lake.

4. Which of the following categories of words always requires the first letter of the word to be capitalized? (Select all that apply.)

   ☐ Geographical names

   ☐ Historical events

   ☐ Special events

   ☐ Cardinal directions

   ☐ Government bodies

   ☐ Nationalities

   ☐ Subjects in school

   ☐ Names of awards

   ☐ The relationship name of a family member

   ☐ Names of deities

   ☐ Seasons

Ellipses, Commas, Semicolons, Colons, Hyphens, and Parentheses

Table 4.13 addresses the correct use of punctuation, specifically, the use of ellipses, commas, semicolons, colons, hyphens, and paranetheses. Learning and reviewing these rules of punctuation will help make errors in punctuation more readily noticeable.

Table 4.13 Rules for Ellipses, Commas, Semicolons, Colons, Hyphens, and Parentheses

Punctuation	Use	Example	Exception
Ellipses [...]	<u>General use</u>: Ellipses are used to suggest hesitation, attempt to conceal something, signal a trailing or unfinished thought, indicate difficulty in directly expressing oneself, or denote the omission of part of an original material within a quotation. Different style guides have different rules regarding the use of ellipses. A style guide should be consulted when writing documents that must be consistent with a specific style. However, it is helpful for writers to be aware of how these rules may vary. <u>Points</u>: An ellipsis always contains three points. <u>Spacing</u>: Guidelines may also vary on the use of spacing within an ellipsis and surrounding one. The amount of space that should be placed between points of an ellipsis should be determined, although many word processing programs will automatically adjust this spacing during writing. The writer should also ascertain whether or not spaces are required before or after an ellipsis, because some styles require spaces whereas others do not. <u>Appropriate Use</u>: Style guides also differ regarding rules of appropriate usage. Some may require an ellipsis to be inserted at the beginning of a quotation, whereas others will find this unnecessary. Some may instruct writers to use an ellipsis to mark indecipherable text, whereas others will prefer a dash for this purpose. Some may require an ellipsis to be inserted on a blank line when a paragraph is omitted, whereas others will find it sufficient to include the ellipsis at the end of the line of text.		Some styles require that an ellipsis be followed by a period when it is used at the end of a complete sentence (for a total of four points). For other styles, a three-point ellipsis, without a consequent period, will suffice at the end of a sentence.
Commas [,]	Any two words or phrases in a series of three or more should be separated by a comma.	Red, green, and yellow balloons were chosen for decorations.	The last comma in a series (the one placed before the *and* in the example) is optional.

Punctuation	Use	Example	Exception
	When a dependent clause precedes an independent clause in a complex sentence, a comma should separate the two.	If time were gold, some of us could not spend it more foolishly.	—
	The introductory words *yes* and *no* should be set apart by commas.	"Yes, sir!"	—
	Nonrestrictive phrases and **nonrestrictive clauses** (groups of words that do not contain information that is necessary to interpreting the meaning of the sentence) should be offset by commas.	Jack Smith, who studied drama in New York City, is a fine actor.	—
	Parenthetical expressions, words of direct address, and appositives should be offset by commas.	The weather, a key factor in scheduling the tour, was ideal.	—
	Use commas to separate a quotation from interrupting text.	"The time to leave," she shouted sternly, "is right now!"	—
	A comma should be used to separate a city from a state. In text, a comma should also follow the state.	We visited Madison, Wisconsin, last summer.	No comma is necessary after the state if it is abbreviated.
	Commas should be used within dates to separate two textual elements or two numerical elements that appear next to each other.	We will be getting married on Saturday, January 14, 2008.	—
	A comma should follow the salutation of an informal letter.	Dear Mom,	—
Semicolons [;]	A semicolon may be placed between two related, independent clauses.	Adelaide sings beautifully; she plays the piano well, too.	—
	Use a semicolon to precede conjunctive adverbs, such as *however* or *therefore*, that connect sentence elements of equal rank.		—
	When a sentence contains a series of elements that contain one or more commas, the division between the elements should be marked with a semicolon.	He is annoying; he has a bold, obdurate personality; and he delights in the displeasure of others.	—
Colons [:]	A colon should be used to herald something that is to immediately follow an independent clause. Often, this information comes in the form of a list.	I would like to perform the following activities during my vacation: hiking, snorkling, and canoeing.	—
	The colon should be used to separate the hour from the minute when expressing standard time.	3:23 p.m.	—
	A colon should follow the salutation of a formal letter.	To whom it may concern:	—
	A colon should be used between the title and subtitle of a book.		
	A colon can be used between two independent clauses if the second explains, expands upon, or illustrates a point made in the first.	When dealing with people, keep this in mind: always be master of the situation.	—
Hyphens [–]	Although a style guide should be consulted for specific rules and exceptions, the following guidelines provide a general overview of common hyphenation practices.		
	Use a hyphen to divide a word at the end of a line when it is necesssary for stylistic purposes and the entire word will not fit on one line. If this must be done, words should be divided between syllables and writers should avoid leaving fewer than three letters on either line. If possible, hyphenated words should be divided at the hyphen.		Words of one syllable should not be divided, nor should names.

Punctuation	Use	Example	Exception
	Use hyphens with spelled-out compound numbers from twenty-one to ninety-nine if they function as adjectives.	thirty-three-year-old man	—

	Use hyphens with fractions that are spelled out and used as adjectives.	a two-thirds majority	If the fraction serves as a noun in the sentence, do not use a hyphen.
			
			Example:
			    There was only one half left.
			
			If one of the numbers in the fraction already contains a hyphen, do not add another one.
			
			Example:
			    thirteen thirty-fifths

	A hyphen should be used to join any prefix to a proper adjective or noun.	mid-August pre-Renaissance	—
	Although many prefixes do not require the use of hyphens, there are some prefixes that should always be hyphenated. Consult style guides for individualized, complete lists.	self-sufficient self-esteem	—
	Hyphenate a compound adjective when it precedes the word it modifies and when doing so helps to clarify.	a well-known artist	Do not use a hyphen if one of the modifiers is an adverb ending in –ly Example: an easily remedied situation
	Use a hyphen to prevent confusion or awkwardness.	Although the prefix *re-* doesn't usually require a hyphen, including one in a phrase like, "*re-form the band*" prevents the reader from confusing the word with *reform*.	—
Parentheses [( )]	Parantheses are used to enclose supplementary or explanatory material that interrupts the main sentence. If the material inside of a pair of parentheses is a question, then a question mark should be inserted within the parentheses. If the material is an exclamation, an exclamation point should be inserted inside within the parentheses. This applies regardless of where the parentheses are located within the sentence.	Your employer called me on the telephone (did you know?) and inquired why you were not at work.	—
	If the material within a pair of parentheses is a complete sentence that is not located within another sentence, a period should be added before the closing parenthesis.	I haven't been to the movies in a year. (It's too expensive.)	If the parentheses occur within a sentence, a period before the closing parenthesis is unncessary. Example: I don't want anything to eat right now (I had a bad day).

(P) *Practice problems*

Solutions to the practice problems are located in the back of this book.

For each of the following sentences, determine if the sentence is correct or incorrect. If the sentence is incorrect, rewrite the sentence with the correct punctuation.

1.   He insisted on introducing the contractor of course.

2.   The weather was hot and dry there was no sign of rain.

3.   The equipment needed is as follows sleeping bag, flashlight, boots, fishing gear, and hunting knife.

4.   There were thirty-five people on the guest list.

5.   The speaker hesitated after receiving a question that he did not know how to answer, "That is a very interesting question. I believe well to be honest, I do not know!"

Quotation Marks and Apostrophes

Table 4.14 addresses the correct use of punctuation, specifically, the use of question marks and apostrophes. Learning and reviewing these rules of punctuation will help make errors in punctuation more readily noticeable.

Table 4.14 Rules for Quotation Marks and Apostrophes

Punctuation	Use	Example	Exception
Quotation Marks [" "]	Use quotation marks to enclose the exact words of a speaker or anything taken from a text or other copyrighted source.	"I won't do it," Chris said.	If the quotation is over a certain length, quotation marks may be omitted. Consult a style guide for specific guidelines.
	Use quotation marks to enclose titles of chapters, articles, short poems, short stories, songs, plays, and essays.	Before I read the next chapter, "Ten ways to be more active," I decided to take a nap.	Long works such as magazines, long poems, newspapers, books, etc. should be italicized or underlined rather than enclosed in quotation marks.
	Quotation marks may be used to enclose technical terms and slang words; however, some style manuals discourage this latter use.	Admiring his new "wheels," he performed a complete circuit of the driveway.	—
	Use single quotation marks when making a quotation within a quotation.	"'The curfew tolls the knell of parting day,' is the line I want," said Mr. Song.	
Apostrophes [']	To form the possessive case of a noun or indefinite pronoun that doesn't end in an *s*, add an apostrophe and an *s*.	The boy's cat was stuck in a tree.	Some style manuals will allow that when a word ends in an *s* sound, the singular possessive may be formed by adding the apostrophe only (i.e., *the witness' testimony* or *for her conscience' sake*). However, other manuals require that the word have more than one syllable if the *s* after the apostrophe is to be omitted, and some demand an *s* after the apostrophe anytime that the noun is singular.
	To form the possessive case of a plural noun that ends in an *s*, it is generally considered appropriate to add only the apostrophe. Plural nouns that do not end in an *s* form the possessive by adding an apostrophe and an *s*, just as singular nouns do.	The trees' leaves looked beautiful.	—
	Use an apostrophe in certain expressions of time.	a week's vacation	—
	Use an apostrophe to pluralize letters, numbers, and words that normally do not have plurals.	*dot your i's, grouped by 4's, and no if's or and's about it*	—
	Use an apostrophe to show omission of letters or numbers as in contractions or dates.	*can't* or *class of '05*	—

(P) *Practice problems*

Solutions to the practice problems are located in the back of this book.

For each of the following sentences, determine if the sentence is correct or incorrect. If the sentence is incorrect, rewrite the sentence with the correct punctuation.

1. I should have chosen the red sports car, said Sharon regretfully.

2. They won't be here until 10 o'clock.

3. The cars motor needed repair.

SECTION 5: SOLUTIONS TO PRACTICE PROBLEMS

The solution section is divided into four categories: reading, mathematics, science, and English and language usage.

READING

Paragraph and Passage Comprehension
Primary Sources

1. Answers may vary.   Possible responses:
   - letters
   - diaries/memoirs/autobiographies
   - interviews
   - audio/video recordings
   - works of art
   - films
   - literature
   - photography
   - statistical data
   - publication of research results
   - census or demographic records

2. Answers may vary.   Possible responses:
   - A) farming tools
   - B) sketches
   - C) The Declaration of Independence
   - D) audio recording of an interview
   - E) courtroom hearing
   - F) novel
   - G) composer's original score
   - H) polls
   - I) speeches
   - J) voting records.

Facts, Opinions, Biases, and Stereotypes

1. This bit of text from a local newspaper blends facts and opinions, biases, and stereotypes, despite the convention that a news article should only report facts. The first four sentences are strictly factual, reporting indisputable events: a crash occurred, one driver was seriously injured and taken to a hospital, the occupants of the other vehicle escaped serious injury, slippery roads contributed to the accident. The final sentence suggests that another contributing factor of the crash was that the driver was only 17 years old. Although it is a fact that the driver was 17 years old, it is a matter of opinion as to whether or not age was a contributing factor to the accident.

   The final sentence not only contains opinions, but also hints at the writer's biases and stereotypes. While the age of the pickup truck driver (17) is an easily verifiable fact, the article states that the driver's age contributed to the accident. This is pure opinion, not fact; it suggests that the writer has a bias against younger drivers. Possibly the writer believes in the stereotype that all young drivers are reckless and accident prone, while older drivers are cautious and prudent.

   The last two sentences turned what started as a purely fact-based report into one colored with the writer's opinions. A passive reader would not notice this, while a critical reader would correctly pick out the article's facts from its opinions.

2. Only Option A has no trace of the author's opinions. The statement cites a report from *Pharmaceutical Insider* magazine, which anyone can look up and verify. It also states when the medication was approved and when it appeared in stores; both of these are also easily verifiable facts.

   Options B, C, and D mix facts with opinions.
   Option B states that the 20-mg pill is "best for most people," while the 30-mg pill is "too strong": both statements are author opinions.
   Option C characterizes the other allergy medications on the market as "excellent" (an opinion) and speculates that Allergone will have trouble finding buyers. Speculation is opinion.
   Option D makes an opinionated statement about Allergone's manufacturer, telling us that it is "reputable" and "*high-quality.*" Descriptive phrases that make blanket judgments about people or things (e.g., *excellent, trustworthy, poor-quality, dishonest,* and *cheaply made*) tend to be opinions, not facts.

3. The correct answer is option B. Options A, C, and D all cite concrete, reasonably logical reasons for picking this team. Option A cites the excellent quarterback, option C cites expert opinions, and option D cites the return of a player.

   Opinion B, on the other hand, is based on a personal bias about sportswriters. This fan is very critical of sportswriters' opinions. He is so critical, in fact, that he doesn't just ignore them – he believes they are more likely to be wrong than right. Therefore, he automatically picks the team the sportswriters do not favor. His reasoning process does not even take the most important factor – the relative quality of the two teams – into consideration.

Characteristics of Different Passage Types

1. This is narrative: in other words, a piece of text that tells a story.

    This narrative contains a good deal of information. Technical writing, persuasive writing, and expository writing also contain information. What, then, classifies this text as narrative?

    Technical writing is generally writing that explains how to perform a specific procedure. Although there are facts in this text, they are not really teaching the reader how to do anything.

    Expository writing typically introduces a topic or provides background information so that a topic can be understood. That is not what is happening here.

    Narrative is storytelling. In narrative, one thing leads to another in a chain of causal events. That is how this text is organized: it tells a story. First the ship gets stuck in the ice, then the men wait several weeks, then they set out across the ice in hopes of surviving. Telling the facts out of sequence, or leaving some of them out, would make the text impossible to understand. That is a common feature of narrative.

2. This is expository writing.

    Notice that this text covers the same incident as the text in Practice Problem 1. However, it does so in a different way.

    This text steps back and discusses the incident in abstract terms. It briefly relates the story of the ship getting stuck – but that is just one paragraph, not the focus of the entire text. Paragraphs two, three, and four do not relate any sort of story whatsoever. Therefore, this is not narrative writing.

    Though the text does provide several ideas for avoiding future disasters, it is not a step-by-step set of instructions that the reader is meant to follow. This makes it hard to classify as technical writing.

    Though the text states opinions on how the expedition could have been managed better, it does not seem particularly concerned with selling these ideas or viewpoints to the reader. It is just listing the ideas, not trying to argue a case for them. That makes it hard to classify as persuasive writing.

    The text is providing information and analyzing it objectively so the reader can understand a concept – possibly so that the author can then go on to explain more concepts. That is a hallmark of expository writing.

3. This is persuasive writing.

    While this text touches on the same subject (arctic expeditions) as the previous problems, it deals with the subject in a very different manner.

    No story is told here, so this is not narrative writing. The text does not provide detailed information on how to accomplish a task or learn a new skill, so this is not technical writing.

    The text does present a number of facts, so it could be expository writing. But take a closer look, and it becomes clear that the facts are not there for their own sake. They are presented in order to make a persuasive argument: specifically, that arctic expeditions are not worthwhile and should be abandoned until the danger can be completely removed.

    Since this argument is the central purpose of the article, it can safely be considered persuasive writing.

Topic, Main Ideas, Supporting Details, and Themes

1. The article's main idea, or specific point, is that microchip production is increasingly happening in a few giant Asian factories instead of in dozens of smaller factories.

2. The article deals with the concept of a few giant factories doing the same work as many small factories. This qualifies as a theme.

3. The overall topic of the article is technology and industry. (If this article was being categorized in a library, these are headings under which it would likely appear.)

4. The fact that the new Asian factories can be entrusted with major brands' trade secrets is a supporting detail. It supports the main idea and helps to explain why the shift from small factories to modern megafactories is occurring.

Topic and Summary Sentences

1. "Recent years have shown a trend toward microchip consolidation, with manufacturing centered on a few giant, modern Asian factories, many in Taiwan."

    This is a difficult topic sentence to locate, mainly because it does not appear in the first paragraph. Instead, this article follows an unconventional format. The entire first paragraph serves as a brief history lesson, explaining to the reader the fragmented state of microchip production in the 1990s. It is only after that first paragraph that the article launches into its real topic.

    How can the topic sentence be identified? The best method is to read the text, decide what it is trying to say, and then find an early sentence that states that message. In this case, the article can be summarized like this: "Microchip manufacturing used to be done in lots of little factories, but now it's done in just a few Asian megafactories." That's exactly what the topic sentence says, although it uses slightly different words. For example, it uses the word *consolidation* to describe the process of many small factories being absorbed into a few larger ones.

2. "The future looks bright indeed for the largest chip manufacturers."

    This sentence appears at the end of the passage, draws a conclusion, and briefly summarizes the paragraph.

Logical Conclusions of a Reading Selection

1. The logical conclusion of this quote is, "Bikes are unsafe, especially in this city." One could also come up with slightly different ways of phrasing the conclusion: for example, "It is inadvisable to ride bikes around here; take your car instead."

    Note that this conclusion is not necessarily factual or correct, and the reader does not need to agree with it. Some of the information cited in the quote may be untrue, and different statistics may suggest that bikes are actually safer than cars. However, a text's logical conclusion is drawn from the ideas in the text, and every point in this text (the accident numbers and statistics, the criticism of the narrow bike lanes, the comparison of bikes' and cars' safety measures) suggests one conclusion: that biking in the city is unsafe.

2. The city of Moville should consider building additional parking lots in the downtown area to increase business revenue. Even though many of the claims or premises in the text may not be true or accurate, the logical conclusion is based on the assumption that the claims are facts. There may be other ways to increase revenue in this situation, but the text does not address solutions other than the addition of new parking lots.

Predictions, Inferences, and Conclusions

1. The reader should disregard this piece of literature as a gimmick (i.e., a way to catch the reader's attention and business). It is an attempt to appeal to the reader's personal desire to become smarter, but it does not appear to have any functional value or evidence for its effectiveness. Based on prior knowledge about intelligence and business tactics, the reader should draw the conclusion that the author is only interested in making a sale and does not actually have a product worth any value.

2. There are several inferences that the reader can make from the excerpt. For instance, it can be inferred that the author of the blog has a bias against the current president. Similarly, it may be inferred that the author is affiliated with a different political party from the president, or that he most likely did not vote for the current president. The reader should conclude that while some of the author's statements may be true, they are based on a distinct point of view and should only be interpreted with this bias in mind.

Position and Purpose

1. This is a recruiting letter: its purpose is to persuade a young athlete to join a university. The author's position is that Eastern Reserve University is the best fit for the young athlete.

    At first this may seem like a letter of congratulations, not a recruiting letter. This is not uncommon; many times, text does not reveal its main intention right away. This is not always because the text's author wishes to be deceitful. For example, a letter from a job seeker might begin with small talk, and only after a paragraph or two get down to the business of asking for the job. The employer is not expected to be misled by the small talk; it is just a way of breaking the ice.

    Similarly, an e-mail asking a friend for a favor might begin with a few paragraphs unrelated to the favor. Again, this is not necessarily because the author wants to trick his friend. Rather, he may think if he gets right to the point he will seem overly demanding.

2. The purpose of this text is strictly to entertain. The reader is supposed to be amused by Mr. Grundle's incompetence, and by the comical results of the tasks he tries to perform.

    Of course, not every reader will find a given piece of text entertaining. Some readers, for example, will simply be bored by this description of Mr. Grundle's incompetence. However, since the text is not trying to pass along any particular information, is not evoking a strong emotional reaction, and is not persuading the reader to adopt a particular viewpoint, it is a good bet that its purpose is simply to entertain.

Persuasive, Informative, Entertaining, or Expressive Passages

1. This author's intent is to inform.

    This passage appears to be taken from the business section of a newspaper. People read the newspaper's business page in hopes of gleaning information that will help them make money. Therefore, most business page articles are purely informative.

    There are exceptions to this rule. For example, a business page might feature a persuasive editorial about tax policy. On rare occasions, a humorous article with a financial angle might be printed, in hopes of entertaining the readers. But the text in this example, like most business articles, provides pure, straightforward information.

2. This text fragment is expressing emotions: specifically, it expresses Steven's fear as something emerges from the mausoleum, and then his relief as it turns out to only be the groundskeeper.

    One could also argue that the text is meant to entertain. It probably is; any literature that expresses emotions is likely written for entertainment as well. Think of a tear-jerking romantic novel in which the main character dies at the end: even though the subject matter is sad, many people enjoy experiencing the sad emotions. They buy the book for entertainment, and also to experience the same emotions that the characters experience.

Historical Context

1. Medieval people believed that personality traits could be affected by physical traits.

   The second paragraph explains that humour imbalances (physical problems) can lead to different temperaments (personality traits). This connection can only be drawn if one believes that the body can affect the personality.

   If the concept of body affecting personality was radical – if the typical medieval person disbelieved it – the author would have provided arguments and explanations to defend the idea. Since the author provides neither of those in this text, he probably assumed that the book's medieval readers were already comfortable with the concept.

2. In medieval times, people still believed in the concept of the four elements. (The concept of the four elements comes from ancient Greek times. It states that everything in the world is comprised of some mixture of four basic elements: earth, fire, air, and water.)

   In the third paragraph, the author states that each humour correlates to both an organ of the body, and to one of the four elements. If the "four elements" theory was no longer popular in medieval times, the author would probably not have mentioned it – and if he had, he would have been obliged to defend it. Since the author did not defend the theory, it is safe to assume that the four-elements theory still shaped how medieval people viewed the world.

3. At the time the text was written, people believed that foreigners' bodies were very different from their own.

   This is the only answer directly suggested by the fifth paragraph. This paragraph suggests that treating foreigners is completely different from treating locals, because foreigners' humours tend to be completely out of balance – much more so, apparently, than those of nonforeigners.

   It also states that many foreigners are completely incurable – a statement that is not made about locals.

   These statements suggest that the author (and his audience) has made an assumption about foreigners: not only do they come from far lands, but their bodies are physically very different from those of locals.

Ways That Literature from Different Cultures Presents Similar Themes

1. Option A is the correct answer. The first paragraph explicitly states that family elders – not the eligible bride and groom – should decide who marries whom. Young people, according to the text, are too inexperienced to make such a major decision for themselves. Options B and D come close to being right, but they do not quite go far enough. The text does not say that elders should merely give advice to young people, or help them out: it says that elders are completely in charge of the decision. Option C is not correct. The text does not address this statement.

2. The author's culture takes honor very seriously. The importance of honor is demonstrated by the way the author discusses gifts. Instead of saying how much the bride and groom might appreciate a nice gift, or recommending that wedding gifts have a personal touch, the author describes gifts as potential hazardous to the gift-giver's personal honor. Specifically, failure to give an appropriate wedding gift may result in a loss of honor that can last an entire lifetime – so the author, quite logically, recommends spending a little more to ensure that the gift is adequate. This advice drives home the notion that in the author' culture, honor is a serious business.

3. The author's culture believes in both astrology and good-luck rituals. This information comes from two places in the text. First, the second paragraph recommends that astrological signs be consulted before two people marry. In other words, the author believes in astrology. Then, in the fourth paragraph, the author states that children should be encouraged to play on the newlyweds' bed, as this will enhance the newlyweds' fertility. This qualifies as a good-luck ritual. Since the author mentions both of these superstitions in a very matter-of-fact way, it can also be assumed that his intended readership shared these beliefs.

Text Structure

1. This is a sequence, or list, of ideas. It is formatted as a numbered list, which makes it easier for the reader to identify the text structure. Sequences lend themselves to lists, since in effect they are lists. However, a sequence is not always formatted as a list – especially in casual writing.

2. This text uses a problem-solution structure. The problem is that text is hard to read; the solution is to change the Web site's background color, as explained in the answer. Question and answer formatting usually indicates a problem-solution structure. The question portion gives the problem, and the answer portion provides the solution.

Informational Source Comprehension
Sets of Directions

1.

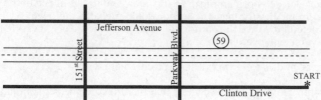

2.   Northwest

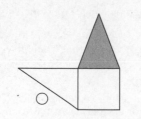

Labels' Ingredients and Directions
1.   No. The reader should note that 1 cup of this product contains 0 grams of dietary fiber, making it a poor food choice for a high-fiber diet.

2.   The woman should note in her log that she has consumed 400 calories. The reader can see that there are 2 servings per container. The 200 calories per serving should be multiplied by 2 to arrive at total calories consumed.

Definitions in Context
1.   capable of making errors

2.   dark; gloomy; obscure

3.   diminishing; fading

Printed Communications
1.   It is stated in the memo that the date for the annual fundraising event is Saturday, April 15.

2.   The advertisement states that the pups are currently 6 weeks old but will not be ready to go home for another 5 weeks, indicating that they need to be 11 weeks old before they are taken home or adopted out.

Indexes and Tables of Contents
1.   The information can be found on pages 554 and 556 to 559. Notice how the main index entry for Washington, DC does not have a page listing. Instead, it is followed by several subentries covering aspects of the topic; these entries do have page numbers. This is a common format for index entries about complex subjects.

2.   Since Chapter 3 includes a section on "Asking for Testimonials," the couple should start with this area of the book.

Product Information: One Product is the More Economical Buy
1.   Company D offers the best price. Since they offer free shipping on all orders over $50.00, and the textbook is $90.00, the instructor's total is $90.00. The price at Company A would be $95.00 total, the price at Company B would be $105.00 because the instructor is not located in California, and the price at Company C would be $100.00 total.

2.   Company B offers the best price. The reader should locate the stores in San Francisco and then identify the least expensive book without worrying about shipping since she will physically visit the store.

Information From a Telephone Book
1.   The best choice is Easy Rent Cars. Their yellow page advertisement states they will match the price of any other rental service.

2.   His best choice is Dale's Oil & Filter, because their advertisement states that no appointment is needed, and they are open until 10 p.m. on weekdays.

Sources for Locating Information Given a Topic
1.   Answers may vary. One possible answer is a road atlas or an electronic map. Either of these can provide the number of miles between her driving locations. With this information she can calculate approximately how long it will take her to reach her destination.

2. Answers may vary. One possible answer is a library catalog. Library catalogs are used to itemize the locations of all printed resources in a library. Each item corresponds to a book, is organized by topic and author, and is associated with a call number that directs the patron to the book's location within the library.

Sample Listings of Items and Costs

1. The cost of a Friday movie ticket for a student is $6.50. The movie ticket costs vary according to day of the week as well as age group.

2. The cost associated with playing 9 holes of golf without a cart on Wednesdays between 7:00 a.m. and 9:00 a.m. is $10.00. Golf rates vary according to the number of holes played, whether or not a golf cart is used, the day of the week, as well as the time of the day.

Graphic Representations of Information

1. Tuition was unchanged between 1999 and 2001. The reader should find the portion of the chart that contains two straight, horizontal lines side by side between the squares. A line that neither rises nor falls will show unchanged tuition costs. The two outer squares will show the time span when the reader consults the years along the bottom of the graph.

2. The reader should find the area marked $60.00 at the left side of the graph, then find where the line on the graph first rises above that mark. Follow that point down to the year area to determine that the answer is 2002.

Scale Readings

1. The correct answer is approximately 24° Centigrade (C). The reader should find the C that represents *Centigrade* at the top of the thermometer, and note where the temperature line stops along the numbers. In this case, it stops near 24.

2. The correct answer is 50° Fahrenheit (F). The reader should refer to the thermometer and note that each 10° span in Centigrade is equal to 18° F. Since the starting point on the thermometer is 32° F, 32 must be added to 18 to get to the correct answer of 50° F.

Legends and Keys of Maps

1. According to the map, there are two National Parks in the recreational area. The reader needs to refer to the key where they will find that National Parks are marked by a $ sign. In the map, there are two parks that have the $ sign in their designated areas.

2. The distance is approximately 4 miles. The reader can use the distance scale on the legend to determine the length on the map that is equivalent to 1 mile. Together, the two lines between the possible roadblock symbols are about four times as long as the mile designation.

Headings and Subheadings

1. Since all of the other subheadings are descriptions of the colors indicated in the headings, the "Painting with Yellows" subheading under the heading of "Yellow" breaks the set pattern and could cause a reader confusion.

2. Another color name, perhaps indigo. Since the chapter is titled "The Colors of the Spectrum" and all of the other headers are names of colors, the next logical header would be another color name.

Text Features

1. The superscript indicates a reference to a footnote (a small aside printed at the bottom of the page). By placing the number "1" in superscript, it is immediately clear that it refers to a footnote. This is a typical convention used in scholarly texts. Without the superscript, the 1 would look strange and out of place. The reader might even think it was a typographical error.

2. The use of bold text was used to show when the character Lori was speaking.

MATHEMATICS

Numbers and Operations
Order of Operations

1. 0 $\qquad$ $-2(3 - 5 + 2) = -2(-2 + 2) = -2(0) = 0$

2. 20 $\qquad$ $2 + 6 \times 3 = 2 + 18 = 20$

3. 45 $\qquad$ $(24 \div 3) \times 5 - 6 + 2 \times 7 - 3 = 8 \times 5 - 6 + 2 \times 7 - 3 = 40 - 6 + 14 - 3 = 45$

Subtraction of Whole Numbers with Regrouping

1. 901

```
  0  9  9  10
  X  8̷  8̷  0̷
-       9   9
  9  0  1
```

2. 158,378

$$\begin{array}{ccccccc} 1 & 14 & 16 & 10 & 13 & 13 \\ \cancel{2}\cancel{5} & \cancel{7} & \cancel{1} & \cancel{4} & \cancel{3} \\ - & 9 & 8 & 7 & 6 & 5 \\ \hline 1 & 5 & 8 & 3 & 7 & 8 \end{array}$$

3. 2,391

$$\begin{array}{ccccc} & 6 & 9 & 18 \\ \cancel{7} & \cancel{8} & \cancel{8} & 1 \\ - & 4 & 6 & 9 & 0 \\ \hline & 2 & 3 & 9 & 1 \end{array}$$

One- and Two-Step Word Problems with Whole Numbers

1. $389,147   Profit = $637,312 − $248,165

2. 20 inches   Since the distance between A and B is 30 inches, the distance between A and C is 30 ÷ 3 = 10. Therefore, the distance between C and B is 30 − 10 = 20 inches.

Addition and Subtraction of Fractions or Mixed Numbers With Unlike Denominators

1. $1\frac{1}{12}$ $\frac{2}{3} = \frac{8}{12}$, so $\frac{8}{12} + \frac{5}{12} = \frac{13}{12} = 1\frac{1}{12}$

2. $1\frac{5}{24}$ $\frac{3}{8} = \frac{9}{24}$ and $\frac{5}{6} = \frac{20}{24}$, so $= \frac{9}{24} + \frac{20}{24} = \frac{29}{24} = 1\frac{5}{24}$

3. $-2\frac{1}{3}$ $3 = \frac{9}{3}$ and $5\frac{1}{3} = \frac{16}{3}$, so $\frac{9}{3} - \frac{16}{3} = -\frac{7}{3} = -2\frac{1}{3}$

4. $\frac{3}{25}$ $\frac{3}{15} = \frac{1}{5} = \frac{5}{25}$, so $\frac{5}{25} - \frac{2}{25} = \frac{3}{25}$

Division and Multiplication of Fractions or Mixed Numbers

1. $1\frac{7}{12}$ $2\frac{3}{8} = \frac{19}{8}$, so $\frac{19}{8} \times \frac{2}{3} = \frac{19 \times 2}{8 \times 3} = \frac{19 \times 1}{4 \times 3} = \frac{19}{12} = 1\frac{7}{12}$

2. $6\frac{1}{4}$ $\frac{5}{3} \div \frac{4}{15} = \frac{5}{3} \times \frac{15}{4} = \frac{5 \times 15}{3 \times 4} = \frac{5 \times 5}{1 \times 4} = \frac{25}{4} = 6\frac{1}{4}$

3. $3\frac{3}{5}$ $3 + \frac{2}{3} \times \frac{9}{10} = 3 + \frac{2 \times 9}{3 \times 10} = 3 + \frac{1 \times 3}{1 \times 5} = 3 + \frac{3}{5} = 3\frac{3}{5}$

4. $\frac{7}{9}$ $4\frac{2}{3} = \frac{14}{3}$, so $\frac{14}{3} \div 6 = \frac{14}{3} \times \frac{1}{6} = \frac{14 \times 1}{3 \times 6} = \frac{7 \times 1}{3 \times 3} = \frac{7}{9}$

Decimal Placement in a Product or Quotient

1. 47.88   63 × 76 = 4788. In the problem, 6.3 × 7.6, there is one number to the right of the decimal point in 6.3 and one number to the right of the decimal point in 7.6. So, count back a total of two decimal places from the end of 4788 to get the solution of 47.88.

2. 14.2 $0.05\overline{)0.710} = 5\overline{)71.0}$ with quotient 14.2

3. 0.036   3 × 12 = 36. In the problem, 0.3 × 0.12, there is one number to the right of the decimal point in 0.3 and two numbers to the right of the decimal point in 0.12. So, count back a total of three decimal places from the end of 36 to get the solution of 0.036.

4. 20 $0.02\overline{)0.4} = 2\overline{)40.}$ with quotient 20.

Conversion Between Irrational Numbers and Approximate Decimal Form

1. A) R and Rat   B) R and Rat   C) R and Irr   D) R and Rat   E) R and Rat   F) R and Rat   G) R and Irr

2. 2.15   Since $\sqrt[3]{8} = 2$ and $\sqrt[3]{27} = 3$, the $\sqrt[3]{10}$ must be between 2 and 3. Therefore, 2.15 is a reasonable answer.

3. $\sqrt{11}$ 3.3166 is greater than $\sqrt{9} = 3$ and less than $\sqrt{16} = 4$. Since 3.3166 is about a third of the way between $\sqrt{9}$ and $\sqrt{16}$, the equivalent irrational number is likely to be a third of the way between 9 and 16 (temporarily ignoring the square root symbols). Therefore, 3.3166 is approximately $\sqrt{11}$.

Calculations of Percents

1. 8.5 $4\frac{1}{4}\% = 4.25\% = 0.0425$, so $0.0425 \times 200 = 8.5$

2. 20% $\square \times 25 = 5$, so $\square = 5 \div 25 = 0.20$ or 20%

3. 10%   Original amount = 50; new amount = 50 – 5 = 45; $\frac{50 - 45}{50} = \frac{5}{50} = 0.10$ or 10%

Conversions Between Percents, Fractions, and Decimals

1. A) $3\frac{19}{100}$ B) 3.19

2. A) 68.1%   B) $\frac{681}{1,000}$

3. A) 75%   B) 0.75

Comparisons of Rational Numbers

1. $\frac{4}{7} > \frac{5}{9}$ $\frac{4}{7} \times \frac{9}{9} = \frac{36}{63}$ and $\frac{5}{9} \times \frac{7}{7} = \frac{35}{63}$. Since $\frac{36}{63} > \frac{35}{63}$, it is true that $\frac{4}{7} > \frac{5}{9}$.

2. $\frac{11}{50}, 0.222, \frac{2}{9}$ Convert all fractions to decimals: $\frac{11}{50} = 0.22$, $\frac{2}{9} = 0.2\overline{2}$. Since $0.22 < 0.222$ and $0.222 < 0.2\overline{2}$, it is true that $\frac{11}{50} < 0.222$ and $0.222 < \frac{2}{9}$.

Estimation of the Solution to a Problem

1. Answers may vary.   One estimate is 67 gallons because $2,000 \div 30 = 66.67$, or about 67 gallons.

2. Answers may vary.   One estimate is 200,000 because $300,000 - 100,000 = 200,000$.

Reconciliation of a Checking or Savings Account

1. $440.96   The deposits (credits) total $1,543.42. The debits total $1,102.46. Therefore, the balance is $1,543.42 – $1,102.46 = $440.96.

2. $6,561.88   Previous balance + deposits – withdrawals – service charge. $9,369.23 + $1,472.65 – $4,270.00 – $10.00 = $6,561.88

Calculation of Take-Home Pay

1. $154.90   The monthly expenses total $1,125.60. The remaining money is $1,280.50 – $1,125.60 = $154.90.

2. $1,269.56   Gross pay – deductions = take-home pay
28.31×36 hours $\times 2$ weeks = $2,038.32
$2,038.32 – $768.76 = $1,269.56

Cost of a Given Set of Items

1. $242,017.45   Add all of the budgeted items together. Remember to line up the place values correctly.

2. $11.07   ($1.75 \times 2) + ($2.25 \times 1) + ($1.19 \times 2) + ($0.99 \times 1) + ($0.65 \times 3)$

Materials and Costs of Planning an Event

1. $102.38   (30 arrangements × $2.35) + (30 arrangements × $0.95) + (30 arrangements × 9 inches divided by 12 inches for each foot × $0.15) = $102.38

2. 60 square feet   To find the total area, find the area of the rectangle and the area of the two triangles. The area of the rectangle is 6 × 8 = 48 square feet. The area of each triangle is $\frac{1}{2}$ (4 × 3) = 6 square feet. The total area is 48 + 6 + 6 = 60 square feet.

One- and Two-Step Word Problems With Fractions or Decimals

1. $10\frac{7}{12}$ feet $3\frac{1}{2} + 5\frac{1}{3} + 1\frac{3}{4} = 3\frac{6}{12} + 5\frac{4}{12} + 1\frac{9}{12} = 9\frac{19}{12} = 10\frac{7}{12}$

2. $2.74   42.20 × 0.065 = 2.74300

Word Problems Involving Percents

1. 13.6% $\frac{710 - 625}{625} = \frac{85}{625} = 0.136$ or 13.6%

2. 12.5% $\frac{3}{24} = 0.125$ or 12.5%

3. 60 $\square$ × 30% = 18, so $\square = \frac{18}{0.30} = 60$

Word Problems Involving Ratios, Proportions, and Rates of Change

1. 325 miles $\frac{2 \text{ hours}}{130 \text{ miles}} = \frac{5 \text{ hours}}{? \text{ miles}}$. Solve the proportion: 2 × ? = 5 × 130, so ? $= \frac{650}{2}$.

2. 3 to 7   The ratio of male to female club members is 9 to 21, which simplifies to 3 to 7.

3. 30 gallons   4 + 3 + 2 = 9 gallons required to serve 72 people.

   $\frac{9 \text{ gallons}}{72 \text{ people}} = \frac{? \text{ gallons}}{240 \text{ people}}$. Solve the proportion: 9 × 240 = ? × 72.

   $\frac{3,780}{72} = ?$, so ? = 30 gallons.

Conversion Between Roman and Arabic Numerals

1. 554   D = 500, L = 50, IV = 5 −1 = 4

2. 1,445   M = 1,000, CD = 500 − 100 = 400, XL = 50 − 10 = 40, V = 5

3. CCCLXIX   300 = CCC, 60 = 50 + 10 = LX, 9 = 10 − 1 = IX

Measurement
Estimation of Metric Quantities

1. 5 miles   Since 1 kilometer = 0.62 miles and 1 mile = 1.6 kilometers, a mile is longer than a kilometer. Therefore, 5 miles is longer than 5 kilometers.

2. 5.02 inches   Since 1 centimeter = 0.394 inch, 12.75 centimeters = 0.394 inch × 12.75, or approximately 5.02 inches.

Conversion From One Measurement Scale to Another

1. 5,000 milligrams $\frac{1,000 \text{ milligrams}}{1 \text{ gram}} = \frac{x \text{ milligrams}}{5 \text{ grams}}$, so x = 5,000 milligrams

2. 13.2 pounds $\frac{1 \text{ kilogram}}{2.2 \text{ pounds}} = \frac{6 \text{ kilograms}}{x \text{ pounds}}$, so x = 6 × 2.2 = 13.2 pounds

3. 48 ounces $\frac{1 \text{ pound}}{16 \text{ ounces}} = \frac{3 \text{ pounds}}{x \text{ ounces}}$, so x = 3 × 16 = 48 ounces

4. 5 quarts $\frac{1 \text{ quart}}{4 \text{ cups}} = \frac{x \text{ quarts}}{20 \text{ cups}}$, so 4x = 20 and x = 5 quarts

Appropriate Units of Measure and Measurement Tools

1. Scale — A scale that is used to measure weights and grams is a weight measure. Therefore, a scale is the only choice. Beakers and measuring cups measure volumes and a ruler measures length.

2. Ruler; yard stick — A ruler should be used for the 11-inch section and a yard stick for the 13-inch section.

Measurements Based on Given Measurements

1. 16 feet — Since this is a 1:1 scale, with 1 inch equaling 1 foot, 16 inches on the blueprint equal 16 feet for the actual wall in the home.

2. 930 inches — Since this is a 1:100,000 scale with 1 inch equaling 100,000 miles, 93,000,000 miles would be 1×930 or 930 inches.

Data Interpretation
Dependent and Independent Variables

1. Score on the test — The score on the TEAS® depends on the amount of studying done for the test. Therefore, the score on the test is the dependent variable.

2. Treatment — The treatment is "put into" the experiment.

Interpretation of Data From Line, Bar, and Circle Graphs

1. From 11:00 a.m. to 2:00 p.m.

2. 2002 — The earnings for Stock A were $12,000 in the year 2002. This was the greatest amount of earnings for the four years shown.

3. $8,000 — Stock B earned $8,000 more than Stock A in the year 2000. Stock A earned $8,000 and Stock B earned $16,000. (Note that the graph indicates that the earnings are in the thousands.) $16,000 – $8,000 = $8,000

4. 2002 — The earnings of Stock A exceeded the earnings of Stock B in the year 2002.

5. 10% — 8,000 voters voted in 1999. Thus $\frac{8,000}{80,000} = \frac{1}{10} = 10\%$ of the eligible voters voted.

6. 6,000 — There were 24,000 voters in 2002 and 18,000 voters in 2003. 24,000 – 18,000 = 6,000

Organization of Data Using Tables, Charts, and Graphs

1. Answers may vary. — Possible responses:
   - The company's profit in 1995 was $2,000,000.
   - The company's profit increased from 1995 to 1997 and from 1998 to 1999, the company's profits decreased from 1997 to 1998 and from 2000 to 2001.
   - The company's profit remained constant from 1999 to 2000.

2. Answers may vary. — Possible responses:
   - The chemist has the highest salary ($80,000).
   - The secretary has the lowest salary ($25,000).
   - The difference between the highest and lowest salaries is $80,000 – $25,000 = $55,000.

3. $\frac{1}{6}$ — Five of the 30 students made grades of B. $\frac{5}{30} = \frac{1}{6}$

Algebraic Applications
Addition, Subtraction, Multiplication, and Division of Polynomial Terms

1. $5x^2 – 12x + 9$ — To subtract $(6x^2 – 5x + 8) – (x^2 + 7x – 1)$ distribute $–1$ to the second polynomial to get:
   $6x^2 – 5x + 8 – x^2 – 7x + 1$
   Then combine like terms: $6x^2 – x^2 – 5x – 7x + 8 + 1 = 5x^2 – 12x + 9$.

2. $25x^2 - 16$

The FOIL method can be used to multiply two binomials. So $(5x - 4)(5x + 4)$ simplifies to:

$25x^2 - 20x + 20x - 16$

$25x^2 - \cancel{20x} + \cancel{20x} - 16$

The middle terms sum to zero, leaving $25x^2 - 16$.

3. $2x - \dfrac{1}{2} + y - \dfrac{1}{3xy}$

Since the divisor $12xy$ is a monomial, this problem can be divided into 4 fractions. The terms in the dividend $(24x^2y - 6xy + 12xy^2 - 4)$ can each be divided by the divisor to get

$$\dfrac{24x^2y}{12xy} - \dfrac{6xy}{12xy} + \dfrac{12xy^2}{12xy} - \dfrac{4}{12xy}$$

Simplify each fraction.

$$\dfrac{\overset{2}{\cancel{24}}\ \overset{x}{\cancel{x^2}}\cancel{y}}{\underset{1}{\cancel{12}}\ \cancel{xy}} - \dfrac{\overset{1}{\cancel{6}}\ \cancel{xy}}{\underset{2}{\cancel{12}}\ \cancel{xy}} + \dfrac{\cancel{12}x\ \overset{y}{\cancel{y^2}}}{\underset{1}{\cancel{12}}x\ \cancel{y}} - \dfrac{\overset{1}{\cancel{4}}}{\underset{3}{\cancel{12}}\ xy}$$

This then simplifies to the final answer:

$$2x - \dfrac{1}{2} + y - \dfrac{1}{3xy}$$

Translation of Word Phrases and Sentences into Expressions, Equations, and Inequalities

1. $5 < \dfrac{1}{2}n$

The unknown is the number that can be defined as n. When "is less than" or "is greater than" is present, this usually means this is an inequality. The inequality $\overset{\text{Five}}{5} \overset{\text{is less than}}{<} \underset{\text{half a number}}{\dfrac{1}{2}n}$

is $5 < \dfrac{1}{2}n$.

2. Answers may vary.

The unknown is the number that can be defined as n. The equation is

$$\underset{\substack{\text{is greater than or equal to}\\ \text{(also "is at least")}}}{\overset{\text{the product of a number and 4}}{4n} \geq \overset{\text{the sum of the number and 10}}{n + 10}}$$

which translates to, "The product of a number and 4 is greater than or equal to the sum of the number and 10, or "The product of a number and 4 is at least the sum of the number and 10."

Equations With One Unknown

1. $y = -2$

Use the distributive property to get rid of the parentheses.

$12y - 3 = 16y + 5$

Use the addition principle to move the variable terms to one side and constants to the other.

$12y \underbrace{-16y} - 3 = 16y \underbrace{-16y} + 5$

$-4y - 3 \underbrace{+3} = 5 \underbrace{+3}$

$-4y = 8$

Use the multiplication principle to isolate y. Multiply both sides by the reciprocal of -4.

$\left(-\dfrac{1}{\cancel{4}}\right)(\cancel{-4}y) = \left(-\dfrac{1}{4}\right)(8)$

$y = -2$

Check the solution by substituting -2 back in for y into original equation.

$$3(4y-1)=16y+5$$
$$3(4(-2)-1)=16(-2)+5$$
$$3(-8-1)=-32+5$$
$$-27=-27$$

The above is a true statement, so the solution is correct.

2. $x = \dfrac{25}{6}$

Remove fractions by multiplying both sides of the equation by the LCD of 60.

$$\frac{x}{10} = \frac{5}{12}$$

$$60\left(\frac{x}{10}\right) = 60\left(\frac{5}{12}\right)$$

6x = 25

Use the multiplication principle to isolate x. Multiply both sides by the reciprocal of 12 (or divide both sides by 12).

$$\frac{6x}{6} = \frac{25}{6}$$

Check the solution by substituting $\dfrac{25}{6}$ back in for x into original equation.

$$\frac{x}{10} = \frac{5}{12}$$

$$\frac{25/6}{10} = \frac{5}{12}$$

Cross multiply to make sure the above statement is true.

$$\left(25/6\right)(12) - (10)(5)$$
$$50 = 50$$

The above is a true statement, so the solution is correct.

3. $x = -14$

Multiply all of the terms by the LCD of 12 to remove fractions.

$$12\left(\frac{x}{4} - \frac{1}{6}\right) = 12\left(\frac{x}{3} + 1\right)$$

$$\overset{3}{\cancel{12}}\left(\frac{x}{\cancel{4}}\right) - \overset{2}{\cancel{12}}\left(\frac{1}{\cancel{6}}\right) = \overset{4}{\cancel{12}}\left(\frac{x}{\cancel{3}}\right) + 12(1)$$

$$3x - 2 - 4x + 12$$

Use the addition principle to get the variable terms to one side and constants to the other side.

$$3x \underline{-4x} - 2 = 4x \underline{-4x} + 12$$

$$-x - 2 \underline{+2} = 12 \underline{+2}$$

$$-x = 14$$

Use the multiplication principle to isolate x. Multiply both sides of the equation by –1.

$$(-1)(-x) = (-1)(14)$$
$$x = -14$$

Check the solution by substituting –14 back in for x into original equation.

$$\frac{(-14)}{4} - \frac{1}{6} = \frac{(-14)}{3} + 1$$

Evaluate each side of the equation to make sure the above statement is true.

$$\frac{-42}{12} - \frac{2}{12} = \frac{-56}{12} + \frac{12}{12}$$

$$-\frac{44}{12} = -\frac{44}{12}$$

The above is a true statement, so the solution is correct.

Equations or Inequalities Involving Absolute Values

1. All real numbers   To solve $|8x – 3| + 4 > 2$, first isolate the absolute value by subtracting 4 from each side.

$$|8x-3| + 4 \underline{-4} > 2 \underline{-4}$$

$$|8x-3| > -2$$

Since $|8x – 3|$ will always result in a positive value regardless of the value of x, the solution is *all real numbers*. In other words, no matter what x is, $|8x – 3|$ *will always* be greater than a negative number like –2.

2. $-\dfrac{5}{3} < y < 3$ A compound inequality can be created to solve for y: $-7 < 3y – 2 < 7$

Solve the inequality by isolating y. Since this is a compound inequality, any operation that is performed on the center also must be done on the left and the right of the equation:

$$-7 \underline{+2} < 3y - 2 \underline{+2} < 7 \underline{+2}$$

$$-5 < 3y < 9$$

$$\frac{-5}{3} < \frac{3y}{3} < \frac{9}{3}$$

$$-\frac{5}{3} < y < 3$$

The solution includes all real numbers greater than $-\dfrac{5}{3}$, but less than 3.

Give both solutions as the answer. Also, verify that the solutions are correct by substituting the answer into the original inequality.

$$-7 = 3(-5/3) - 2 \quad \text{and} \quad 3(3) - 2 = 7$$
$$= -5 - 2 \qquad\qquad\qquad 9 - 2 = 7$$
$$= -7 \qquad\qquad\qquad\quad 7 = 7$$

SCIENCE

Scientific Reasoning
Reasons for Conducting Investigations
1. Answers may vary.   Possible responses:
   - Establishing procedures
   - Improving quality of life

2. Answers may vary.   Possible responses:
   - Prosthetics
   - Artificial organs

Questions and Concepts that Guide Scientific Investigations
1. This is not a good protocol to follow.

2. This is not a good protocol to follow.

3. This is a good protocol to follow. This protocol provides a decent number of patients per group, multiple groups, and different doses.

4. This is not a good protocol to follow.

Communication and Defense of Scientific Arguments
1. Identify a problem, ask questions, form a hypothesis, test the hypothesis, analyze the data, and form a conclusion.

2. Answers may vary.   Possible answers include that a bias may be shown or that results can not be repeated.

Reasons to Include Technology and Mathematics in Science Research
1. Answers may vary.   Possible responses:
   - Data is recorded in numbers.
   - Relationships are established by graphs and formulas.
   - Numerical models are used to describe mathematical relationships.

2. Answers may vary.   Possible response:
   - If mathematics were not used, scientific descriptions would be purely qualitative in nature.

Use of Technology and Mathematics to Improve Investigations and Communications
1. Answers may vary.   Possible responses:
   - Mathematical software like spreadsheets, intranet, and Internet have increased communication by providing ways to share information.
   - Fiber optics have increased communication speed and processing time.

2. Answers may vary.   Possible responses:
   - Forensics
   - Cosmology
   - Meteorology

Alternative Explanations and Models
1. Answers may vary.   Possible response:
   - New technology allows for new explanations, such as smaller increments of time and length so that more precise data can be collected.

2. Answers may vary.   Possible response:
   - Technology has allowed us to conclude that Earth revolves around the Sun, and we now know that there are millions of stars and more than just one solar system.

Formulation and Revision of Scientific Explanations and Models
1. Supported   There was a proportional rise in volume as the temperature was increased.

2. Deductive reasoning is when conclusions follow a general principle.
   Inductive reasoning is when conclusions are formed from specific facts.

Human Body Science
Anatomy and Physiology

1. A) i
   B) iv
   C) iii
   D) ii

2. A) xi
   B) i
   C) x
   D) vii
   E) ii
   F) v
   G) ix
   H) vi
   I) iv
   J) viii
   K) iii

Circulatory System

1. A   The mitral valve is on the left side of the heart, separating the ventricle and atrium. If it prolapsed, the blood would back up into the left atrium.

2. False   Blood that passes through the tricuspid valve enters the right ventricle.

3. False   Blood that passes through the mitral valve enters the left ventricle.

4. True

5. True

6. True

7. False   The pulmonary valve ensures that blood stays in the pulmonary artery.

Respiratory System

1. oxygen; carbon dioxide

2. alveoli

3. C   When the diaphragm contracts, the chest cavity enlarges, creating negative pressure in the chest cavity and pulling air into the lungs.

Nervous System

1. True

2. True

3. False   This is a function of the respiratory system.

4. False   This is a function of the integumentary system.

Digestive System

1. mouth

2. C   Peristalsis is the rhythmic contractions that occur in the stomach and intestines, which moves food from the stomach toward the anus.

3. B   Villi and microvilli are finger-like projections of tissue in the intestines that significantly increase the surface area from which nutrients are absorbed.

Immune System

1. D   Vaccines provide an artificial source (as compared to a natural source that comes from actually having a disease) of active immunity that stimulates antibody and memory cell production.

2. B   Damaged tissue releases cytokines, which attract white blood cells to the area of infection or injury.

3. D   The warm body temperature that occurs during a fever accelerates the destruction of pathogens and increases the activity of white blood cells.

Factors that Influence Birth and Fertility Rates

1. A   Fertility rates are higher in less-developed countries due to higher infant and child mortality rates.

2. A, B, C, E, G, H, I, J   Taxes and transportation do not have a direct relationship to birth rates.

Population Growth and Decline

1. T3   The curve labeled "T3" shows that most humans survive until the last part of the mean life span.

2. T1   The curve labeled "T1" shows high mortality among young individuals.

Life Science

Biological Classification System

1. A) iii   Each taxon becomes less specific. Therefore, the least inclusive listing is the species and the
    B) i   most inclusive is the kingdom.
    C) v
    D) ii
    E) iv
    F) vi
    G) vii

Natural Selection and Adaptation

1. Natural Selection

2. True

Nucleic Acids

1. True

2. Both DNA and RNA

3. Both DNA and RNA

4. Both DNA and RNA

5. DNA only   DNA contains adenine, cytosine, guanine, and thymine bases.

6. RNA only   RNA contains adenine, cytosine, guanine, and uracil bases.

Parts of a Cell

1. False   The mitochondria is the site of ATP production in cells.

2. False   Chloroplasts are involved in photosynthesis and the production of glucose for plants.

3. True

4. True

Cellular Organelles

1. D   Cytoplasm is contained in both types of cells.

2. nucleoid; nucleus   In bacteria, which lack nuclei, the large-massed nucleoids are found in the cytoplasm. In animals and plants, the nucleus separates the cytoplasm from the DNA.

Chromosomes, Genes, Proteins, RNA, and DNA

1. Chromosomes; genes   Each chromosome is a single molecule of DNA. Certain areas along this single molecule are transcribed into RNA. This makes them genes.

2. DNA   DNA, found in the cell nucleus, holds the code for protein production; however, it requires the messenger RNA to carry that code out of the nucleus to the ribosomes to complete protein production.

Cell Differentiation

1. True

2. An embryo is an animal or a plant in the early stages of development after fertilization.

RNA and DNA Involvement in Cell Replication

1. True

2. Enzymes initiate the process of unwinding DNA and releasing the two complementary strands of that DNA so DNA polymerase enzymes can duplicate them.

Mitosis and Meiosis

1. diploid; haploid   The original diploid cell will undergo two divisions to create four haploid cells.

2. False   Mitosis occurs to replace old cells in all cell types, while meiosis occurs in gametes to bring about genetic variation amongst offspring.

Photosynthesis and Respiration

1. A   Chloroplasts allow an autotroph to use sunlight to produce glucose. Mitochondria are found in heterotrophs, and glucose and ATP are products that are found in both autotrophs and heterotrophs.

2. Chloroplast; chlorophyll   Chlorophyll in the plant's chloroplasts gives the plant a green color and allows the energy from the Sun to be used by the plants chloroplasts to produce energy.

Storage of Hereditary Information

1. genes   These parts of the chromosome are comprised of DNA and contain information for particular traits.

2. True

Changes in DNA and Mutations in Germ Cells

1. DNA polymerase

2. True

Phenotypes and Genotypes

1. Genotypes; phenotypes   Genes comprise the genotype of an individual, and the phenotype is what can be seen or observed in an individual.

2. Phenotype   Coat color is what is seen or what is expressed by the cat, which is controlled by the genotype in the cat's DNA.

Mendel's Laws of Genetics and the Punnett Square

1.

	T	t
t	Tt	tt
t	Tt	tt

Two will be heterozygous for thorns and two will be homozygous and will not have thorns. The offspring will have a 50% chance of having thorns. Note that the only time an offspring will not have thorns is when it is homozygous for the recessive trait.

2. 50%

	A	a
A	AA	Aa
a	Aa	aa

The Punnett square shows that two of the four offspring are heterozygous (*Aa*) with one gene for the disease.

Earth and Physical Science
The Sun
1. x-ray, ultraviolet, infrared, radio

By knowing the order of wavelengths from long wavelength to short wavelength (radio, microwave, infrared, visible, ultraviolet, x-ray, and gamma) the reverse order can be determined.

2. Violet, indigo, blue, green, yellow, orange, red

Since the order of visible wavelengths from long to short is given by the mnemonic ROY G BIV, the reverse can be discerned.

Kinetic Energy, Potential Energy, and Other Energies
1. 300 Joules

Since potential energy is calculated by the expression PE = Mgh, it can be determined from the given information that PE = (5 kg)(10 meters/second^2)(6 meters) = 300 Joules. The appropriate units are Joules, which match kilograms and meters.

2. KE = 80 Joules
   PE = 20 Joules

Conservation of energy means that the sum of the KE plus the PE equals the total energy. Since the object has fallen $^1/_5$ of the way, the PE must be $^1/_5$ of the total energy. (There is no KE at the 10 meters height because it has no velocity there). If the PE equals 20 Joules, then the remaining energy of 80 Joules must be in the form of KE.

Measurable Properties of Atoms
1. An atom contains a nucleus in which protons and neutrons reside. Electrons circle the nucleus in varying energy levels.

2. Iron has an atomic number of 26, which is indicated by the *26* above the *Fe*.

3. 55.845 AMU

4. Iron has 26 protons, because the atomic number is 26.

5. Approximately 30, because 56 − 26 = 30.

Protons, Neutrons, and Electrons
1. 8

The number of protons depends only on the atomic number (from the periodic table) and is independent of the ionic charge and the isotope type. Since oxygen has an atomic number of 8, it has 8 protons.

2. 6

The number of protons depends only on the atomic number (from the periodic table) and is independent of the ionic charge and the isotope type. Since carbon has an atomic number of 6, it has 6 protons.

Purpose of Catalysts
1. (1) X + C → XC
   (2) Y + XC → XYC
   (3) XYC → CZ
   (4) CZ → C + Z

The catalyst acts on the raw reactants (X and Y) to create the four step product reaction chain, finally resulting in the product (Z) and catalyst (C). Notice that the catalyst is available to begin the reaction again.

2. By lowering the activation energy

Reaction rates are increased when activation energy decreases.

Physical and Chemical Patterns within the Periodic Table

1. increase; decreases   The number of filled shells increases from top to bottom within a family, so the size of the atoms increase. Also, the greater atomic radius decreases the electronegativity, because the attraction for an electron due to the nucleus is lessened.

2. 14, 15, 16   The metalloids are located next to the stairstep line on the periodic table. This line serves as a boundary that distinguishes metals from nonmetals.

3. A, B, C   Metals are excellent conductors of electricity; nonmetals are not. Metals also cool and heat faster than nonmetals. Although many nonmetals do not conduct electricity, there are some that do not conduct electricity, such as water.

Enzymes

1. False   Although enzymes are selective in their form and function, thousands of such reactions are known to occur throughout the body.

2. True

3. True

4. True

Acid and Base Solutions

1. pH = 4; acid $pH = -\log(a_H) = -\log(1 \times 10^{-4}) = -(-4) = 4$.

2. smaller; blue   The calculation of activity requires a smaller percentage of hydrogen ions to yield values larger than seven, and litmus paper turns blue for bases.

3. A concentration difference of 10   A difference of one unit on the pH scale represents a difference of 10 in strength of concentration, based on $\log_{10}[H^+]$ or $\log_{10}[OH^-]$.

Chemical Bonds Between Atoms in Common Molecules

1. Butane; C_4H_{10} Let n=4; The chemical composition may be found using the formula C_nH_{2n+2}. The hydrocarbon is butane, with a formula of C_4H_{10}.

2. Pentene; C_5H_{10} Pentyne; C_5H_8 Let n=5; The chemical composition may be found using the formula C_nH_{2n} for alkenes and C_nH_{2n-2} for alkynes. Pentene (C_5H_{10}) and pentyne (C_5H_8) are both examples of common unsaturated hydrocarbons with five carbon atoms.

Chemical Bonds Resulting From Sharing or Transferring Electrons

1. Hydrogren exists only in pairs because the atom is unstable on its own. A covalent bond is necessary to make the atom stable.

2. 2   Since sulfur belongs to the same family as oxygen, sulfur will have the same Lewis dot structure. Since there are six valence electrons (and since electrons form pairs), there will be two unshared pairs.

Important Chemical Reactions: Balancing and Identifying

1. The tally for the reactant (left) of the unbalanced reaction is: 1 Ca, 2 O, 3 H (both formulas), and 1 Cl. The product (right) side tally is 1 Ca, 1 O, 2 H, and 2 Cl. Only Ca is balanced, so begin with the easiest fix, which is Cl. Place a 2 in front of HCl:

   ___Ca(OH)$_2$ + 2HCl → ___H$_2$O + ___CaCl$_2$

   Because the right side has less H and O, a 2 needs to be placed in front of H$_2$O.

   Ca(OH)$_2$ + 2HCl → 2H$_2$O + CaCl$_2$

2. False   pH neutralization is an important acid-base reaction.

3. True

4. False   Combustion is an important oxidation-reduction reaction.

5. False   Photosynthesis is an important oxidation-reduction reaction.

Chemical Properties of Water

1. False   Water serves as the standard for pH and has a value of 7.

2. True

3. False   No standard for water exists with respect to electronegativity values.

4. True

Atoms or Molecules in Liquids, Gases, and Solids

1. 77   The Kelvin temperature is found by adding 273 to the Celsius value. So, –196 + 273 = 77.

2. A) True

    B) False   Density = mass/volume. Since the mass is constant in this problem, the phase with the smallest volume has the greatest density. The liquid has the highest density.

    C) True

    D) True

Evaporation, Vaporization, and Condensation.

1. liquid; gas   A phase transition between a liquid and a solid requires an amount of energy called the heat of vaporization.

2. 2:1   Recall that H = ML. For substance A, H_A = ML. For substance B, H_B = (3M)(1/6L) = 0.5 ML. Form the ratio by dividing: H_A / H_B = ML / (0.5 ML) = 1 / 0.5 = 2 / 1. So, the ratio must be 2:1.

ENGLISH AND LANGUAGE USAGE

Grammar and Word Meaning in Context

Parts of Speech

1. I go to concerts frequently, and I went to my favorite singer's concert yesterday. I had already been to her concert when I was in the seventh grade. I had not planned to go to this one, but my younger sister wanted me to take her. I hope that in the future my brother will take her to these concerts.

    - First sentence: *go* – simple present tense; *went* – simple past tense
    - Second sentence: *had been* – past perfect tense; *was* – simple past tense
    - Third sentence: *had planned* – past perfect tense; *to go* – infinitive; *wanted* – simple past tense; *to take* – infinitive
    - Fourth sentence: *hope* – simple present tense; *will take* – simple future tense

    Note: When using tenses in which an auxiliary, or helping, verb is required, be aware that the verb is more than just the auxiliary verb (e.g., *have* is the auxiliary verb in *have been*).

2. The thick, brown molasses slides rapidly down the sides of the warm, fragrant pancakes.

    Adjectives modify nouns or pronouns. When two (or more) adjectives are used to modify the same noun, the adjectives should be separated by a comma.

3. The multicolored snake inches smoothly forward despite the rocky terrain blocking its path.

    The underlined adverbs indicate how and where the snake inches.

4. Tim Cratchit offers a prayer of gratitude at the end of Dickens's story. His utterance exemplifies the simplicity and generosity Dickens wanted to illustrate. Through this character, the author accentuates the social ills then prevalent in London.

    The underlined direct objects all answer the question *what* after the verb:

    - Tim Cratchit offered what? A prayer
    - His utterance exemplifies what? The simplicity Dickens wanted to illustrate
    - His utterance exemplifies what? The generosity Dickens wanted to illustrate
    - The author accentuates what? The social ills (*Social* is an adjective that is modifying the direct object *ills*).

5. The man in the company of the noisy partygoers attempts to extricate himself from the rabble.

    The first two underlined prepositional phrases separate the subject from its verb. Be careful when checking for subject-verb agreement. *Partygoers* (plural) is not the subject; it is the object of the prepositional phrase. The verb *attempts* must be conjugated with *man*, not *partygoers*.

Subject-Verb Agreement

1. Answers may vary.   Possible solutions:
    - The planes *were* flying overhead.
    - The *plane* was flying overhead.

2. Everyone *has* a favorite dessert.

3. Several of the members *chose* not to vote.

4. No change

5. Answers may vary.   Possible solutions:
    - The man and woman *eat* at 3:00 p.m.
    - The *man* eats at 3:00 p.m.
    - The *woman* eats at 3:00 p.m.
    - The man *or* woman eats at 3:00 p.m.

Pronoun-Antecedent Agreement

1. Answers may vary. Possible solutions:
   - Each girl was presented with *her* varsity letter.
   - *The girls were* presented with their varsity letters.

2. Answers may vary. Possible solutions:
   - The guide reiterated the possibility of danger to each person as *he or she* entered the bus.
   - The guide reiterated the possibility of danger to each person as *he* entered the bus.
   - The guide reiterated the possibility of danger to each person as *she* entered the bus.
   - The guide reiterated the possibility of danger to *them* as they entered the bus.
   - The guide reiterated the possibility of danger to each person as *the bus was entered*.

3. No change

Use of Dialogue

1. No change

2. "I should have chosen the red sports car," said Fahari regretfully.

First, Second, and Third Person

1. This sentence is written from a second-person point of view.

2. A) Third person
   B) First person
   C) Second person or first person (or both)

Grammar for Style and Clarity

1. My eyes glazed over <u>as</u> I reviewed the math problems, <u>but</u> I forged ahead with renewed vigor <u>when</u> I remembered the upcoming exam <u>and</u> the necessity of scoring well to pass the course.

   Conjunctions connect two words, phrases, or clauses. In the sentence above, the subordinating conjunction *as* connects the first two clauses, the coordinating conjunction *but* connects the second clause with the third, and the subordinating conjunction *when* links the third clause to the fourth. The fourth conjunction, *and*, joins the compound direct objects, *exam* and *necessity*.

2. I made an <u>estimation</u> of the number of possible scenarios. I had a <u>transformation</u> when I saw the moon shining brightly overhead. I had a <u>realization</u> that there was plenty of available light on the night of the crime.

3. Malcolm <u>raced</u> past the hall monitor, <u>burst</u> into the English class, <u>slid</u> into his seat, and then calmly <u>glanced</u> at the teacher as if nothing had happened. He <u>was seen</u> by everyone in the class, but he <u>was effective</u> in appearing nonchalant.

   - Active verbs: *raced, burst, slid,* and *glanced*
   - Passive verbs: *was seen* and *was effective*

Context Clues

1. Definition: insignificant
   Context clues: *scrubbing floors, washing dishes,* and *sifting garbage* (examples)

2. Definition: argumentative
   Context clues: *quarrels* and *starts arguments* (description)

3. Definition: repeated
   Context clues: *repeating* and *again and again* (explanation of situation)

4. Definition: unfriendly
   Context clue: *warm and friendly* (antonym)

5. Definition: first
   Context clue: *first* (definition)

6. Definition: overcome
   Context clue: *overcome* (synonym)

Word Structure
1. Prefix: *in-*
    Meaning: not

2. Suffix: *-ism*
    Meaning: the belief in

3. Root: *audio*
    Meaning: sound

Structure
Simple Sentences
1. It is a simple sentence. Though this simple sentence is preceded by two long prepositional phrases, the subject, *Jeff*, and the verb, *was washing*, are conjugated correctly.

2. It is a simple sentence. The subject, *Mark*, and verb, *imagines*, are properly conjugated in this simple sentence. They are followed by a direct object, *future*, an indirect object, *himself*, and plenty of modifiers, but there are no additional clauses here.

Organized and Logical Paragraphs
1. False   The topic sentence is missing from the paragraph. The missing science project is not even mentioned until sentence four.

2. True

3. True

Sentence Fluency
1. Simple sentence: A simple sentence has a subject (*I*) with a properly conjugated verb (*dream*), and though it may have modifiers, such as a prepositional phrase (*of being an astronaut*), it does not have other clauses.

2. Complex sentence: A complex sentence contains one independent clause (*I asked for a space suit every year for Christmas*), which can stand alone, and one dependent clause (*When I was younger*), which contains a subordinating conjunction (*When*) that makes that part of the sentence dependent on the rest of the sentence for meaning.

3. Compound sentence: A compound sentence contains two simple sentences (*I dream of being an astronaut* and *I also imagine myself as a great trapeze artist*) joined by a coordinating conjunction (*but*).

Spelling and Punctuation
Rules of Spelling
1. *-able*   If the root word is *not* a complete word, then the suffix will be *-ible*.

2. Correct

3. Correct

4. Incorrect   The correct spelling is *weird*. This word is an exception to the "*i* before *e* except after *c*" rule.

5. Correct

6. B   The ending *y* is only changed to an *i* when the preceding letter in the root word is a consonant. Option B is the only word with a consonant preceding the ending *y*.

7. C   *Enforce* keeps the ending *e* when adding *-able*, whereas the other words all drop the *e* before adding the suffix.

8. D   In general, if the root word is not a complete word, the suffix is *-ible*. The root word in option D (*inevit*) is not a complete word, but the suffix is *-able*.

9. principle   A *principal* is a chief or leader, a *principle* is a belief or rule of conduct.

10. their   This word is referring to a home *belonging to them*.

Commonly Misspelled Words

1. Correct

2. Incorrect   dissipate

3. Correct

4. Correct

5. Incorrect   diphtheria

Rules of Capitalization

1. Correct

2. Correct

3. Incorrect   Problem: A cardinal direction should not be capitalized when it refers to a point of the compass.
Correct sentence: Drive east to the lake.

4. Geographical names, historical events, special events, government bodies, nationalities, names of awards, and names of deities always require the first letter of the word to be capitalized because they are proper names of people, places, or things. Cardinal directions, subjects in school, the relationship name of a family member, and seasons may or may not be capitalized. The use of these words must be analyzed to determine whether or not they should be capitalized.

Rules of Ellipses, Commas, Semicolons, Colons, Hyphens, and Parentheses

1. Incorrect   Problem: absence of parentheses or comma
Description of problem: of course (should be set off from the main idea using parentheses or a comma)
Possible correct sentences:
   - He insisted on introducing the contractor (of course).
   - He insisted on introducing the contractor, of course.

2. Incorrect   Problem: absence of semicolon
Description of problem: run-on sentence (punctuation should be added)
Correct sentence: The weather was hot and dry; there was no sign of rain.

3. Incorrect   Problem: absence of colon
Description of problem: as follows (a colon should precede a list)
Correct sentence: The equipment needed is as follows: sleeping bag, flashlight, boots, fishing gear, and hunting knife.

4. Correct

5. Incorrect   Problem: absence of ellipses
Description of problem: writer indicating hesitation (ellipses should be used when a writer wants to indicate hesitation)
Correct sentence: The speaker hesitated after receiving a question that he did not know how to answer, "That is a very interesting question. I believe...well...to be honest, I do not know!"

Rules of Quotation Marks and Apostrophes

1. Incorrect   "I should have chosen the red sports car," said Sharon regretfully.

2. Correct

3. Incorrect   The car's motor needed repair.

SECTION 6: COMPREHENSIVE PRACTICE TESTS

This section includes two comprehensive practice tests accompanied with solutions and rationales for the solutions. Keep in mind that the proctored TEAS® has a total of 170 items, 20 of which are unscored, pretest items. The total time allowed for the proctored TEAS® is 209 minutes.

Since these comprehensive practice tests do not include the 20 items used for pretest purposes, the time needed to complete each section is less than on the proctored test. Below is a recommended time allotment for taking these two practice tests:

Content areas	Number of items	Recommended time limit
Reading	42	51 minutes
Mathematics	30	45 minutes
Science	48	59 minutes
English and Language Usage	30	30 minutes
TOTAL	150	185 minutes

PRACTICE TEST 1

READING	MATHEMATICS	SCIENCE	ENGLISH AND LANGUAGE USAGE
1._____	1._____	1._____	1._____
2._____	2._____	2._____	2._____
3._____	3._____	3._____	3._____
4._____	4._____	4._____	4._____
5._____	5._____	5._____	5._____
6._____	6._____	6._____	6._____
7._____	7._____	7._____	7._____
8._____	8._____	8._____	8._____
9._____	9._____	9._____	9._____
10._____	10._____	10._____	10._____
11._____	11._____	11._____	11._____
12._____	12._____	12._____	12._____
13._____	13._____	13._____	13._____
14._____	14._____	14._____	14._____
15._____	15._____	15._____	15._____
16._____	16._____	16._____	16._____
17._____	17._____	17._____	17._____
18._____	18._____	18._____	18._____
19._____	19._____	19._____	19._____
20._____	20._____	20._____	20._____
21._____	21._____	21._____	21._____
22._____	22._____	22._____	22._____
23._____	23._____	23._____	23._____
24._____	24._____	24._____	24._____
25._____	25._____	25._____	25._____
26._____	26._____	26._____	26._____
27._____	27._____	27._____	27._____
28._____	28._____	28._____	28._____
29._____	29._____	29._____	29._____
30._____	30._____	30._____	30._____
31._____		31._____	
32._____		32._____	
33._____		33._____	
34._____		34._____	
35._____		35._____	
36._____		36._____	
37._____		37._____	
38._____		38._____	
39._____		39._____	
40._____		40._____	
41._____		41._____	
42._____		42._____	
		43._____	
		44._____	
		45._____	
		46._____	
		47._____	
		48._____	

Section 1. READING	Number of Scored Questions: 42
	Recommended Time Limit for Practice Test: 51 minutes*

*The proctored TEAS® has an additional six unscored questions for a total of 48 reading questions. The time limit on the proctored reading portion is 58 minutes.

Organic Landscaping

Keeping mature trees alive and healthy can be a challenge for any landscaper. The difficulties vary by tree species; this section will focus on caring for oak trees, which are quite common and also quite susceptible to a wide array of problems.

Oaks are beautiful shade trees. Many species of oak trees grow into true giants, and a single large tree can become the focal point of an entire yard or green space. But what happens when that tree becomes sick or dies? The cost and difficulty of replacing it – not to mention the trauma of losing such a majestic specimen – make it desirable to monitor your oaks and take aggressive action as needed.

Oak wilt is a common disease capable of affecting entire neighborhoods. Insects such as termites, weevils, and borers can seriously damage oaks. Also, when oaks grow old enough, a general condition known as "oak decline" may take effect.

Typical tree services and landscapers will attempt to use chemicals to solve all of the above problems. Typically, they use an injector to pump a commercial chemical product into the trunk; the chemical gradually spreads through the entire tree. A tree service or landscaper will use this same chemical regardless of the actual problems the oak faces, because chemical application is fast and relatively cheap. The chemical's effect is to slow down tree growth. Sometimes the chemical helps for a short while, because a slower-growing tree will focus more of its energy into maintaining existing foliage rather than creating new foliage. However, the chemical cannot mask serious problems indefinitely.

A good, environmentally conscious tree specialist will take a nonchemical approach. Dead and dying lower branches are pruned, because they absorb the tree's energy and provide an entry path for pests and tree diseases. Nutrients are applied to the soil. Nearby trees that have grown dangerously close are trimmed, because when trees are too close together, pests and diseases can easily pass from one tree to another.

In some cases, unfortunately, nothing can be done. Oak wilt is extremely fast acting once it gains a foothold in a tree, and oak decline is a mysterious process that is almost always irreversible. These are sad facts, but they are *not* limitations of the chemical-free approach. The standard tree-service chemicals provide no long-lasting solution to these problems, either.

Ultimately, a chemical-free approach to oak maintenance is the best approach. None of the chemicals on the market has been proven to give superior results to those of dedicated pruning and soil care. This is an important point for both the homeowner and the landscaper to consider.

The next five questions are based on this passage.

1. "Ultimately, a chemical-free approach to oak maintenance is the best approach."

   The sentence above appears as the first sentence in the last paragraph of the article. This sentence is best described as which of the following?

   A) Main idea
   B) Topic
   C) Theme
   D) Supporting detail

2. A homeowner has an oak tree infected with oak wilt. He happens to personally know the author of the above article, so he invites the author over to ask for advice. The homeowner tells the author that he respects his opinions on tree matters, but also that he is not prepared to spend a lot of money to save the tree.

    Based on the article, which of the following is a logical prediction of what the author will tell the homeowner to do?

    A) Use a chemical to prolong the tree's life, because even though chemicals are not a long-term solution, they might give the tree a few more years.
    B) Trim dead branches, and also trim any nearby trees that have grown too close to the infected tree.
    C) Begin a long-term program of adding nutrients to the soil around the tree.
    D) Do nothing; allow the tree to die a natural death.

3. The author of the article intends to do which of the following by using the words "the trauma of losing such a majestic specimen"?

    A) Persuade
    B) Inform
    C) Entertain
    D) Express feeling

4. Which of the following sentences is reflective of the author stating an opinion?

    A) Oak wilt is a common disease capable of affecting entire neighborhoods.
    B) Ultimately, a chemical-free approach to oak maintenance is the best approach.
    C) Insects such as termites, weevils, and borers can seriously damage oaks.
    D) Also, when oaks grow old enough, a general condition known as "oak decline" may take effect.

5. The author's description of chemical versus chemical-free interventions for mature tree maintenance is reflective of which of the following types of text structures?

    A) Sequence
    B) Problem-solution
    C) Comparison-contrast
    D) Cause-effect

Opinion on American Poetry (1930)

It is only in the last few decades that American literary contributions, particularly in the area of poetry, have attained any degree of maturity. There are exceptions, of course: Emily Dickinson and Henry Longfellow were noteworthy artists – but they were the lonely exceptions to the rule.

Indeed, the American poets have long tended to be loners and introverts, living in self-imposed exile from the bounds of ordinary society. Consider the bizarre, reclusive life of Emily Dickinson; the solitary wilderness sojourns of Henry David Thoreau; and, looking back a bit farther, the introverted, ghoulish visions of Edgar Allen Poe. Is it any wonder that the American literary tradition is fragmented, when each poet stands as an island unto himself?

By contrast, the English poets have traditionally been a social bunch. Consider the clannish pre-Raphaelites, the sometimes-incestuous Romantic poets, and, looking back across the centuries, the hundreds of literary collaborations (and feuds) that have played out across London's newspapers and literary journals. The British poets have always existed within the bounds of society, rather than lurking on its fringes. While not without drawbacks, that essential social interplay – that strong fraternity of writers – has, in the main, nurtured England's creative growth.

Even now, as the American literary scene finally matures, the cream of the American poets takes its inspiration from abroad. Longfellow spent several formative years in Europe; Ezra Pound and T. S. Eliot, two of the most celebrated, recent American poets, chose to move away from the United States. Indeed, it seems likely that the American literary tradition still needs time to grow. Perhaps another century, or even two, is required before American poetry can stand shoulder to shoulder with the heavyweights of world literature.

The next seven questions are based on this passage.

6. Which of the following sentences is the topic sentence for the entire passage?

   A) It is only in the last few decades that American literary contributions, particularly in the area of poetry, have attained any degree of maturity.
   B) Indeed, it seems likely that the American literary tradition still needs time to grow.
   C) Is it any wonder that the American literary tradition is fragmented, when each poet stands as an island unto himself?
   D) Even now, as the American literary scene finally matures, the cream of the American poets takes its inspiration from abroad.

7. Which of the following describes the word *isolation* as it relates to the passage?

   A) Theme
   B) Topic
   C) Main idea
   D) Supporting detail

8. Based on the passage, which of the following is the most likely inference?

   A) The author believes American poetry is superior to British poetry.
   B) The author believes British poetry is superior to American poetry.
   C) The author believes British and American poetry are of greater quality than other world literature.
   D) The author believes British and American poetry are of lesser quality than other world literature.

9. Which of the following conclusions may be drawn directly from the third paragraph of the passage?

   A) Some of America's best poets moved away and never returned.
   B) Social interaction leads to better, more mature literature.
   C) Emily Dickinson and Henry Longfellow were the greatest American poets.
   D) America's poets are not just loners – many of them are also a bit bizarre.

10. Which of the following is the author's main purpose for writing this passage?

    A) To state the lack of maturity of American poetry as compared to British poetry
    B) To pay tribute to noteworthy American poets
    C) To recognize that British poets are more social than American poets
    D) To inform the reader of the fact that many American poets move away from America

11. The passage is reflective of which of the following types of writing?

    A) Narrative
    B) Expository
    C) Technical
    D) Persuasive

12. Which of the following is an example of a summary sentence in the passage?

    A) It is only in the last few decades that American literary contributions, particularly in the area of poetry, have attained any degree of maturity.
    B) While not without drawbacks, that essential social interplay – that strong fraternity of writers – has, in the main, nurtured England's creative growth.
    C) Even now, as the American literary scene finally matures, the cream of the American poets takes its inspiration from abroad.
    D) Perhaps another century, or even two, is required before American poetry can stand shoulder-to-shoulder with the heavyweights of world literature.

Marley was a lean, quiet man who always seemed to blend into the background. When he entered a room for the first time, he had the peculiar habit of taking a long, hard look at every nook and cranny, as if carefully memorizing the location of the various pieces of furniture, the paintings, the knickknacks, the curios. He seemed quite a wealthy man, though no one knew his profession. He had moved into our neighborhood two years previously, during that summer when we had the record heat – the summer just before all the burglaries started.

The next three questions are based on this passage.

13. Which of the following is a logical conclusion that may be drawn from this description?

    A) It is likely that Marley is a private investigator.
    B) Marley prefers to be alone.
    C) Marley possibly committed the burglaries.
    D) The author does not care for Marley.

14. Based on a prior knowledge of literature, the reader can infer that this passage was taken from which of the following?

    A) A history textbook
    B) A science fiction novel
    C) An academic dissertation
    D) A mystery novel

15. What is the author's likely purpose for writing this description of Marley?

    A) To make the neighborhood seem more alive by describing some of its residents
    B) To give the reader a hint about whom committed the burglaries
    C) To provide historical background
    D) To describe a minor character's foibles in an entertaining way

Farmington Clinic Opens Monday

On Monday the twelfth, the new south-side Farmington Clinic opens its doors for the first time. It will be the area's largest full-service medical clinic and the largest of 14 Farmington Clinics throughout the Southeast.

The Farmington Clinic will have an entire wing devoted to Urgent Care. Urgent Care hours extend from 4 to 11 p.m., 7 days a week.

New patients can register starting at 8 a.m. Monday. The registration desk is located at the Pine Street entrance.

A number of secretarial and administrative positions at the new clinic remain unfilled. Prospective applicants may apply to the Farmington Clinic's main office for details.

The next two questions are based on this passage.

16. Which of the following is the author's intent in the passage above?

    A) To inform
    B) To persuade
    C) To entertain
    D) To express feelings

17. New patients can register starting at 8 a.m. Monday. The registration desk is located at the Pine Street entrance.

    In the context of the *entire document*, do the two sentences above provide a topic, a main idea, supporting details, or themes?

    A) Topic
    B) Main idea
    C) Themes
    D) Supporting details

The following e-mail was sent to a major company's director of human resources from another employee of the company.

Debra –

I just heard about the new executive opening. It seems a little unusual to add new people there, especially when some of the other departments need staff.

All that to the side, I think you should consider Alex Jones from Accounting. I think his skills are wasted at his current job; he would make an excellent manager. He's done everything we asked him to, and more. Everyone down here likes him, and I can't imagine him doing anything to disappoint you – or the company, for that matter. Just call him up for an interview, and I think you'll see what I mean.

Also – we're getting Chinese food delivered later, so give any menu requests to Andy.

Regards,

Hal

The next two questions are based on this passage.

18. Which of the following is the main purpose of the e-mail?

    A) The author wants to chat.
    B) The author wants to protest the company's hiring priorities.
    C) The author wants Alex Jones to be considered for the executive job.
    D) The author wants to tell Debra about the Chinese food being delivered later.

19. Which of the following statements best describes the e-mail author's biases?

    A) He has no bias about who should get the job.
    B) He has a secret bias in favor of Alex Jones.
    C) He is open about his bias in favor of Alex Jones.
    D) His biases are difficult to assess.

---

20. Read and follow the directions below.

    1. Imagine three colored marbles in a jar; one is red and two are blue.
    2. Remove a blue marble.
    3. Add a yellow marble.
    4. Add a red marble.
    5. Remove a blue marble.
    6. Add a yellow marble.

    Which of the following is the number of marbles of each color the jar now contains?

    A) 2 red, 2 yellow
    B) 2 blue, 2 yellow
    C) 2 red, 1 blue, 1 yellow
    D) 2 yellow, 1 red, 1 blue

21. Carbon, 254, 559-64, 670
    Cesium, 271, 655-6
    Chrome, 219
    Chromium, 220
    Chromium alloys, 221-2, 503
    Chromium oxidation, 223-4

    A chemistry student wants to learn about a chromium alloy. Using the excerpt above from a science textbook's index, on which of the following pages should the student begin to look?

    A) 219
    B) 220
    C) 221
    D) 223

22.

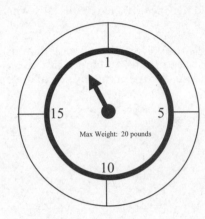

    A measurement of approximately how many pounds is represented on the above scale face?

    A) Less than 1 pound
    B) Between 1 and 20 pounds
    C) Exactly 20 pounds
    D) More than 20 pounds

23. Mrs. Crawford is a <u>gregarious</u> individual who can always be found laughing with friends.

    Which of the following is the definition of the word <u>gregarious</u>?

    A) High-spirited
    B) Energetic
    C) Sociable
    D) Inquisitive

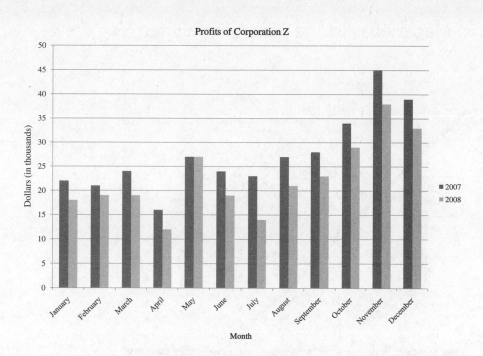

The next two questions are based on this chart.

24. Which of the following general statements may be made about Corporation Z's profits?

    A)   2008 was less profitable than 2007.
    B)   2008 was about as profitable as 2007.
    C)   2008 was more profitable than 2007.
    D)   It is impossible to tell from this data which year was more profitable.

25. Which of the following months is typically the *least* profitable for Corporation Z?

    A)   February
    B)   April
    C)   July
    D)   November

26.

Map of Blackstone Recreational Area

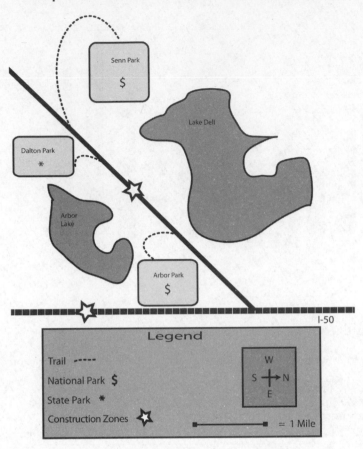

A family is driving via Interstate 50. They are traveling from south to north. If the family visits all three parks on the map above, and then turns around and drives back home using the same route, which of the following indicates the number of times their car will pass through a possible roadblock?

A) 1
B) 2
C) 3
D) 4

27.

Pricing Chart: Cases of Cleaning Fluid

Store	Shipping and handling
Janitor Depot	$30.00 total for any order
Hyperion Cleaning Supplies	$40.00 total for any order
Southern Cleaning and Maintenance	$30.00 for orders less than $100.00; free for orders $100.00 or more
Maid Central	$2.00 per case

A California company wants to buy 10 cases of cleaning fluid at $10.00 per case. Based on the pricing chart above, which of the following stores will provide the least expensive shipping and handling for this order?

A) Janitor Depot
B) Hyperion Cleaning Supplies
C) Southern Cleaning and Maintenance
D) Maid Central

28. The man in black was extremely clever. He pretended to bump into the elderly gentleman, and he used the ensuing distraction to <u>pick</u> the old man's pocket.

   Based on the context, which of the following is the definition of the underlined word in the sentence above?

   A) To provoke
   B) To steal the contents of
   C) To find fault with
   D) To choose or select

29. A voter is trying to decide whether or not to vote for Bill Williamson for political office. She plans to visit several Web sites to try to find unbiased information to help her make an informed decision. Based only on the following site names and tag lines, which of the following Web sites is most likely to provide this information?

   A) www.billwilliamson.org: "Vote Bill Williamson for Congress"
   B) www.candidateblender.org: "Devoted to Political Satire Since 1987"
   C) www.saynotobillwilliamson.org: "Why to Vote No for Bill Williamson"
   D) www.candidatestance.org: "Providing Comprehensive Facts on Candidate Views"

30. An individual is planning to drive from Nebraska to visit family members who live in Nevada. Which of the following is the most appropriate source of information to help the individual obtain the shortest route to her destination?

   A) Car owner's manual
   B) Road atlas
   C) Encyclopedia
   D) Nevada tourism brochure

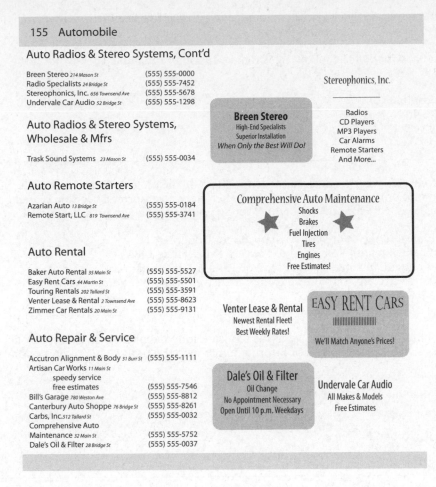

The next two questions are based on this sample yellow page.

31. A customer would like to have a CD player installed in her car. Which of the following businesses should she call?

A) Bill's Garage
B) Undervale Car Audio
C) Azarian Auto
D) Carbs Inc.

32. A car owner wants to take his car only to repair shops that state that they offer free estimates. Which of the following is an appropriate number for this person to call?

A) (555) 555-5752
B) (555) 555-1111
C) (555) 555-8812
D) (555) 555-0037

33. Each pain medicine has its own distinct benefits and drawbacks. Opiates, such as codeine, morphine, and a variety of derived products (such as hydrocodone and oxycodone) are extremely potent, but patients quickly build tolerance, and the potential for addiction is high. Another class of medications, which loosely encompasses both aspirin and ibuprofen, reduces pain, swelling, and inflammation. This makes these medications first-line treatments for many ailments, but caution must be used, as they can, to greater or lesser degrees, thin the blood. (Depending on the patient, the blood-thinning effect may be dangerous – but in some cases it may be desirable. Indeed, many older adults take aspirin precisely for its blood-thinning effect.) Acetaminophen stands by itself; it is not a narcotic and has no effect on swelling or inflammation. Its lack of a blood-thinning effect means that it is often prescribed in situations where ibuprofen is not. At unusually high doses it may cause stomach problems, though at recommended doses this is highly unusual.

A 72-year-old individual who has a history of addiction problems has been told by his doctor to avoid blood thinners. After reading the above information, which of the following pain medications is an appropriate choice?

A) Aspirin
B) Ibuprofen
C) Acetaminophen
D) Morphine

34. William Altucher was no fan of Scottish cooking; a long series of journal entries from his traveling days can attest to that fact:

> The meat was smelly and unrecognizable, and it was stuffed into a casing equally vile and of equally unknown origin. The vegetables, such that they were, had been boiled down to lifeless, colorless lumps. The sausages were accompanied by a soggy, beige pile that looked suspiciously like boiled oats – as if it were originally intended for the stable, not the dinner table.

Despite his culinary displeasure, the journals reveal that Altucher returned to Scotland on six separate occasions.

Which of the following signifies the use of the indentation in the passage above?

A) A piece of dialogue
B) A note from the author
C) A quotation from another work
D) A particularly important passage

35. The guide words at the top of a dictionary page are *dextral* and *diamond*. Which of the following words is an entry on this page?

A) Diamagnetic
B) Dexterity
C) Devilry
D) Dewdrop

36. Chapter 2: The Dinosaurs
    1. Where They Lived
       A. Africa
       B. Asia
       C. Australia
       D. _____
       E. North America
    2. When They Lived
    3. What They Ate

Examine the headings above. Based on the pattern, which of the following is a reasonable heading to insert in the blank spot?

A) China
B) Europe
C) Mexico
D) Ukraine

37.

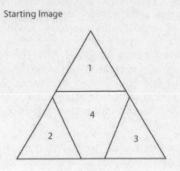

Starting Image

Start with the shape pictured above. Follow the directions to alter its appearance.

1. Draw a circle that completely encloses the shape.
2. Remove section 1 from the shape.
3. Remove section 3 from the shape.
4. Replace section 1 onto the shape, in its original spot.
5. Remove section 2 from the shape.

Which of the following does the shape now look like?

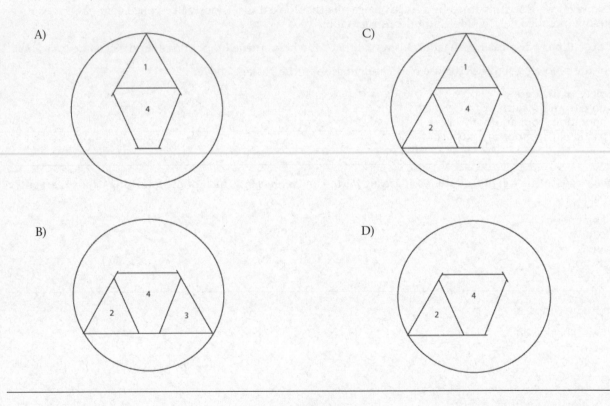

A)

C)

B)

D)

38. A traveler wants relevant, unbiased information about Rotuma, a little-known island in the Pacific Ocean, before deciding whether or not to visit. Which of the following information sources is most likely to be helpful?

A) *European Travel 2009*: A popular travel guidebook
B) *A Year in Rotuma*: A travel memoir, publication date 1975
C) "Visit Tropical Rotuma": A travel brochure printed by the Rotuma Department of Tourism
D) "A Guide to Pacific Island Destinations, 2009": An article covering all Pacific Islands

39.

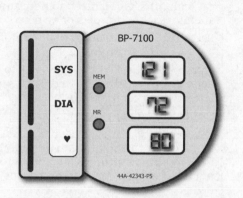

The diagram above represents a blood pressure monitor. Which of the following indicates the diastolic blood pressure reading?

A) 72
B) 80
C) 121
D) 152

Flea Control Products for Cats

Product name	Manufacturer	Cost	Rating from a cat magazine's product review (out of 10)	Description
Barton Flea Collar	Barton	$5.00	5	Standard 2-ounce flea collar lasts a cat 3 months.
Champion Deluxe Flea Collar	Champion	$15.00	7	Heavy-duty, 3-ounce flea collar lasts a cat 6 months. Guaranteed to not cause allergic reaction for pets or owners.
Super Flea Prevention Bath	Granville	$6.00	8	Bathe cat in this solution to prevent fleas for 4 months at a time.
Nordson Flea Inhibitor Spray	Nordson	$10.00	6	Spray on the back of the cat's neck to deter flea infestation. Enough sprays to last a typical cat 4 months.
Patton Flea Collar	Patton	$12.00	8	Standard 2-ounce flea collar lasts a cat 4 months.
Flea and Tick Control System	Redding	$7.00	7	Bathe cat in this solution to prevent fleas for 2 months at a time. Guaranteed to not cause allergic reaction for pets or owners.
ZenPet Flea Spray	ZenPet	$11.00	9	Spray on the back of the cat's neck to deter flea infestation. Enough sprays to last a typical cat 6 months.

The next two questions are based on this price listing.

40. A cat owner wants to buy enough of a flea control product to last for 1 year. The system must not cause an allergic reaction for her cat. Price is her secondary concern. Which of the following is the best product for the owner?

    A) Flea and Tick Control System
    B) Barton Flea Collar
    C) Champion Deluxe Flea Collar
    D) ZenPet Flea Spray

41. A pet owner needs a flea control product. It must be a collar, since his cat refuses to stand still for baths or sprays. He reads a popular cat magazine, and respects its reviews – but he is also on a budget. Therefore, he has decided to buy the highest-rated product that costs $30.00 or less for a year of protection. Based on the chart above, which of the following is the best product for this pet owner?

    A) Patton Flea Collar
    B) Barton Flea Collar
    C) Flea and Tick Control System
    D) Champion Deluxe Flea Collar

42. Jonathan was a debate champion *par excellence*. He never became flustered; he always had a ready response. His introductions and conclusions were both concise and precise. Indeed, he had a well-deserved reputation for spouting *mots justes*.

    The use of *italics* in the text above signifies which of the following?

    A) Foreign phrases
    B) Emphasized words
    C) References to footnotes
    D) Words used in unconventional ways

Section 2. MATHEMATICS	Number of Scored Questions: 30
	Recommended Time Limit for Practice Test: 45 minutes*

*The proctored TEAS® has an additional four unscored questions for a total of 34 mathematics questions. The time limit on the proctored mathematics portion is 51 minutes.

1. A man is putting a fence around his rectangular yard. His lot measures 13.5 feet (ft) long and 47.75 ft wide. The fencing comes in rolls that are 50 ft long. Which of the following is the number of rolls of fencing the man will need to buy?

    A)   1
    B)   2
    C)   3
    D)   4

2. $2\frac{1}{3} \times 4\frac{1}{2}$

    Simplify the expression above. Which of the following is correct?

    A) $6\frac{1}{6}$

    B) $8\frac{1}{6}$

    C) $10\frac{1}{2}$

    D) $20\frac{1}{2}$

3. Many buildings have a cornerstone that gives the date the building was completed. In Arabic numerals, which of the following dates is represented by MDCCCLIV?

    A)   1845
    B)   1846
    C)   1854
    D)   1855

4. A legal assistant works at a local law firm and earns $1,278.00 per pay period. The assistant's deductions each pay period are: federal tax $125.78, federal insurance $63.28, state tax $93.68, retirement plan $50.00, and health insurance $89.51. Which of the following is the assistant's take-home pay per pay period?

    A) $216.75
    B) $422.25
    C) $855.75
    D) $997.75

5. A fence is being built to enclose a backyard. The yard is 150 feet (ft) wide by 325 ft long. The back of the house (325 ft) will act as one side of the fence. Fencing sells for $13.00 per ft. Which of the following will be the cost of the fence?

    A) $6,175.00
    B) $8,125.00
    C) $10,400.00
    D) $12,350.00

6. A symphony has 125 musicians. Seventy-five of them are women. Which of the following is the ratio of the men to the total musicians in the symphony?

    A) $\frac{2}{5}$

    B) $\frac{3}{5}$

    C) $\frac{2}{3}$

    D) $\frac{5}{2}$

7. A student decides to have lunch at the school deli. The special for the day is a hamburger basket including fries for $6.95. The student adds a side salad for $2.45, a medium drink for $1.49, and a brownie for $1.19. Which of the following is the cost of this lunch?

    A) $10.89
    B) $11.99
    C) $12.08
    D) $12.20

8. Reconcile this checking account for the month of April 2009. The previous balance is $2,355.14. Deposits were made for $1,527.28. Checks were written for $1,203.97. Interest earned is $1.56 and there is a service charge of $5.00. Which of the following is the balance after reconciling this account?

    A) $2,675.01
    B) $2,671.89
    C) $2,678.45
    D) $2,685.01

9. $6 \times (5 + 7) \div 4 - 7 \times 2 + 3 \times 3$

    Simplify the expression above. Which of the following is correct?

    A) −72
    B) −5
    C) 13
    D) 75

10. Which of the following percents is equivalent to 0.003?

    A) 0.03%
    B) 0.3%
    C) 3%
    D) 30%

11. 215.4% of 55 = _____

Which of the following completes the equation above?

A) 11.847
B) 118.47
C) 1184.7
D) 11847

12. A school nurses' association is having its annual conference in September. Nurses' Elegant Events is catering the closing luncheon. Reservations have been received for 315 nurses and 53 guests. The luncheon cost for each nurse is $18.00 and for each guest it is $25.00. Which of the following is the cost of the luncheon?

A) $3,755.00
B) $6,545.00
C) $6,995.00
D) $8,829.00

13. A couple is buying living-room furniture. The sofa retails for $899.00, the chair with ottoman for $695.00, the coffee table for $379.00, end tables for $229.00, and a set of lamps for $149.00. Which of the following is an accurate estimate of the cost of the living room?

A) $2,200.00
B) $2,300.00
C) $2,600.00
D) $2,900.00

14. A father's age, y, is 4 less than three times his daughter's age, x.

Which of the following algebraic equations best represents the statement above?

A) $y = 3x - 4$
B) $y = 3x + 4$
C) $x = 3y - 4$
D) $x = 3y + 4$

15.

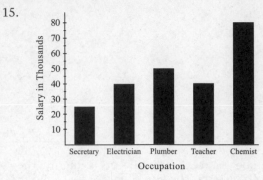

People in Certain Occupations

The graph above shows the average salaries of people in certain occupations in a given town. Which of the following is the difference between the lowest and highest salaries shown in the graph?

A) $25,000
B) $40,000
C) $55,000
D) $105,000

16. $\frac{x}{2} + 5 = 9$

Solve the equation above. Which of the following is correct?

A) $x = 4$
B) $x = 8$
C) $x = 13$
D) $x = 14$

17. $783 - 45$

Simplify the expression above. Which of the following is correct?

A)   732
B)   737
C)   738
D)   742

18. $|x+2| = 5$

Which of the following is the solution set for the equation above?

A)   {−7, 3}
B)   {−3, 7}
C)   {3, 7}
D)   {−7, −3}

19. A nurse is collecting categorical data on the different ethnicities of her clients. Which of the following graphs should the nurse use to present the data in terms of percents totaling 100?

A)   Pie chart
B)   Line graph
C)   Histogram
D)   Scatterplot

20. The enrollment at a college went up from 625 to 710 students over a period of 1 year. Which of the following is the percent of increase to the nearest tenth of a percent?

    A) 8.8%
    B) 11.4%
    C) 12.0%
    D) 13.6%

21. A chemist must measure exactly 2.3 milliliter of a chemical to add to his experiment. Which of the following measurement tools is appropriate for this task?

    A) Beaker
    B) Pipette
    C) Measuring cup
    D) Graduated cylinder

22. The scale on a map indicates that every 1 centimeter (cm) on the map equals 10 miles (mi) on the ground. The desired distance on the map measures 8 cm. Which of the following numbers represents the distance in miles?

    A) 0.8
    B) 8
    C) 80
    D) 800

23. Which of the following metric units of measurement is most reasonable to measure the amount of a liquid oral medication?

    A) milliliter (mL)
    B) liter (L)
    C) deciliter (dL)
    D) kiloliter (kL)

24. An average person grows taller with age.

    Which of the following is the independent variable in the event described above?

    A) Age
    B) Height
    C) Hair color
    D) Weight

25. Which of the following is the number of centimeters in 4 meters?

    A) 0.04
    B) 0.4
    C) 40
    D) 400

26. $(x^2 + 3x - 2) - (x^2 - 2x - 5)$

Simplify the expression above. Which of the following is correct?

A) $5x + 7$
B) $x^2 + 5x$
C) $x - 7$
D) $5x + 3$

27. Which of the following decimal numbers is approximately equal to $\sqrt{27}$?

A) 2.56
B) 3.14
C) 4.2
D) 5.2

28. Order the following list of numbers from least to greatest.

$-3, 4, \dfrac{11}{3}, 3.8$

A) $-3, 3.8, \dfrac{11}{3}, 4$

B) $4, 3.8, \dfrac{11}{3}, -3$

C) $-3, 3.8, 4, \dfrac{11}{3}$

D) $-3, \dfrac{11}{3}, 3.8, 4$

29. 5.13×0.02

Simplify the expression above. Which of the following is correct?

A) 0.1026
B) 1.026
C) 10.26
D) 1026

30. $\dfrac{7}{8} - \dfrac{5}{12}$

Simplify the expression above. Which of the following is correct?

A) $\dfrac{1}{12}$

B) $\dfrac{11}{24}$

C) $\dfrac{1}{2}$

D) $\dfrac{3}{5}$

| Section 3. SCIENCE | Number of Scored Questions: 48 |
| | Recommended Time Limit for Practice Test: 59 minutes* |

*The proctored TEAS® has an additional six unscored questions for a total of 54 science questions. The time limit on the proctored science portion is 66 minutes.

Periodic Table of the Elements

1 IA																	18 0
1 H	2 IIA											13 IIIA	14 IVA	15 VA	16 VIA	17 VIIA	2 He
3 Li	4 Be	3	4	5	6	7	8	9	10	11	12	5 B	6 C	7 N	8 O	9 F	10 Ne
11 Na	12 Mg	IIIB	IVB	VB	VIB	VIIB	[	- VIIIB -	]	IB	IIB	13 Al	14 Si	15 P	16 S	17 Cl	18 Ar
19 K	20 Ca	21 Sc	22 Ti	23 V	24 Cr	25 Mn	26 Fe	27 Co	28 Ni	29 Cu	30 Zn	31 Ga	32 Ge	33 As	34 Se	35 Br	36 Kr
37 Rb	38 Sr	39 Y	40 Zr	41 Nb	42 Mo	43 Tc	44 Ru	45 Rh	46 Pd	47 Ag	48 Cd	49 In	50 Sn	51 Sb	52 Te	53 I	54 Xe
55 Cs	56 Ba	71 Lu	72 Hf	73 Ta	74 W	75 Re	76 Os	77 Ir	78 Pt	79 Au	80 Hg	81 Tl	82 Pb	83 Bi	84 Po	85 At	86 Rn
87 Fr	88 Ra	103 Lr	104 Unq	105 Unp	106 Unh	107 Uns	108 Uno	109 Une									

Lanthanide Series	57 La	58 Ce	59 Pr	60 Nd	61 Pm	62 Sm	63 Eu	64 Gd	65 Tb	66 Dy	67 Ho	68 Er	69 Tm	70 Yb
Actinide Series	89 Ac	90 Th	91 Pa	92 U	93 Np	94 Pu	95 Am	96 Cm	97 Bk	98 Cf	99 Es	100 Fm	101 Md	102 No

1. Breakdown of which of the following begins in the small intestine?

A) Protein
B) Fats
C) Fiber
D) Carbohydrates

2. In geology, which of the following is considered a significant departure from previous ideas?

A) Ideology change
B) Theoretical refinement
C) A paradigm shift
D) Model adjustment

3. Which of the following terms describes the increase in alleles that permits a species to survive and reproduce better in an environment from generation to generation?

A) DNA
B) Genetic drift
C) Mutation
D) Adaptation

4. Which of the following nervous systems directs the body's fight-or-flight response?

    A) Peripheral
    B) Central
    C) Parasympathetic
    D) Sympathetic

5. Which of the following is used in quantitative investigations?

    A) Sensory information
    B) Numerical information
    C) Phenomenological research
    D) Ethnographic research

6. Which of the following taxonomic ranks is the most general?

    A) Order
    B) Genus
    C) Phylum
    D) Family

7. Water undergoes relatively minor temperature and phase changes compared to other substances due to both its

    A) low specific heat and low heat of vaporization.
    B) low specific heat and high heat of vaporization.
    C) high specific heat and low heat of vaporization.
    D) high specific heat and high heat of vaporization.

8. A new species of bread mold that is genetically similar to the red bread mold *Neurospora crassa* is discovered; however, it is physically similar to the mold *Aspergillus nidulans*. Based on the current classification system, which of the following is the proper classification for this new species?

    A) *Neurospora crassa*
    B) *Neurospora novus*
    C) *Aspergillus nidulans*
    D) *Aspergillus novus*

9. Which of the following is an example of hydrocarbons containing double bonds?

    A) C_2H_6
    B) C_4H_8
    C) C_6H_{10}
    D) C_8H_{12}

10. Which of the following represents the correct order of the scientific process?

    A) Hypothesis, data, analysis
    B) Hypothesis, analysis, data
    C) Data, hypothesis, analysis
    D) Data, analysis, hypothesis

11. Which of the following organ systems supplies the body's cells with oxygen and nutrients?

    A) Cardiovascular
    B) Digestive
    C) Nervous
    D) Immune

12. Through which of the following does blood pass after leaving the right ventricle during contraction of the heart?

    A) Aorta
    B) Pulmonary artery
    C) Vena cava
    D) Mitral valve

13. Which of the following organ systems supplies the body with oxygen and removes carbon dioxide?

    A) Integumentary
    B) Endocrine
    C) Respiratory
    D) Renal

14. Which of the following is responsible for the peristalsis that occurs in the digestive tract?

    A) Smooth muscle
    B) Skeletal muscle
    C) Connective tissue
    D) Subcutaneous tissue

15. A proton should have which of the following two characteristics when compared to the charge and mass of an electron?

    A) The same charge and the same mass
    B) The same charge and a larger mass
    C) An opposite charge and the same mass
    D) An opposite charge and a larger mass

16. The spine is part of which of the following systems?

    A) Lymphatic
    B) Nervous
    C) Skeletal
    D) Endocrine

17. If two gases (A and B) that have detectable odors and the same temperature are released simultaneously on one side of a room, and the odor of Gas A is noticed 1 minute before that of Gas B, which of the following conclusions can be made?

    A) Gas A has a higher density than Gas B.
    B) Gas B has a higher density than Gas A.
    C) The opening in the container of Gas A is larger than that of Gas B.
    D) The opening in the container of Gas B is larger than that of Gas A.

18. Which of the following describes a substance that is completely ionized in its solution and has a pH of 2?

    A) Strong acid
    B) Strong base
    C) Weak acid
    D) Weak base

19. In which of the following organs are immune cells produced?

    A) Tonsils
    B) Spleen
    C) Lymph nodes
    D) Bone marrow

20. The heart is located _____ the sternum.

    Which of the following correctly completes the sentence above?

    A) to the right of
    B) to the left of
    C) behind
    D) in front of

21. A research student is determining the pollen count for a 24-hr period in a given location. The student's data would be most reliable if he decided to count pollen in

    A) a single decimeter square for one morning and one afternoon.
    B) multiple decimeter squares for one morning and one afternoon.
    C) a single decimeter square for one afternoon.
    D) multiple decimeter squares for one afternoon.

22. When two closely related species of flour beetles, *T. confusum* and *T. castaneum*, were placed in a culture in equal numbers, *T. castaneum* increased in numbers while *T. confusum* experienced population decline. The growth difference in the changes of population most likely indicate that the energy consumption efficiency of *T. castaneum* is _____ *T. confusum*.

    Which of the following correctly completes the sentence above?

    A) less than
    B) less variable than
    C) greater than
    D) more variable than

23. Exchange of oxygen occurs in which of the following structures of the respiratory system?

    A) Alveoli
    B) Bronchioles
    C) Trachea
    D) Pleura

24. Which of the following is true of fertility rates?

    A) They are lower in less-developed countries.
    B) They are higher in less-developed countries.
    C) They are higher in more-developed countries.
    D) They are the same in more-developed and less-developed countries.

25. Consider an atom that possesses 8 protons, 9 neutrons, and 7 electrons. This atom will have an overall charge of _____ and will have an overall mass of approximately _____ AMU.

    Which of the following correctly completes the sentence above?

    A) –1; 17
    B) –1; 15
    C) +1; 15
    D) +1; 17

26. Enzyme activity is driven by which of the following internal factors?

    A) pH
    B) Temperature
    C) Substrate concentration
    D) Amino-acid structure

27. A new organism has been recently discovered in the ocean. All that is known of the organism's cellular structure is that it lacks a membrane-bound nucleus. Which of the following indicates how this organism will be classified in terms of cell type?

    A) Plant
    B) Animal
    C) Prokaryote
    D) Fungus

28. In which of the following do mutations in human DNA originate?

    A) Protein
    B) Mitochondria
    C) Phenotype
    D) Genotype

29. Which of the following organelles found in heterotrophs is similar to the chloroplast?

    A) Vacuole
    B) Nucleus
    C) Lysosome
    D) Mitochondria

30.   UUA —   GCG   —   AUA   —   CGC   mRNA

       ? —   ? —   ? —   ?   Gene

Going from left to right on the diagram above, which of the following is the gene sequence that created the mRNA sequence?

A)   GGC-TAT-CGC-ATA
B)   AAU-CGC-UAU-GCC
C)   AAT-CGC-TAT-GCG
D)   CGC-TAT-CGC-AAT

31.   Which of the following organelles gives rough endoplasmic reticulum (ER) its signature rough characteristic?

A)   Ribosomes
B)   Mitochondria
C)   Centrosomes
D)   Vacuoles

32.   DNA is to genes as amino acids are to _____.

Which of the following correctly completes the sentence above?

A)   Cells
B)   Ribosomes
C)   RNA
D)   Protein

33.   Atoms having _____ bonds complete one another by the donation and acceptance of electrons to form stable outer electron shells.

Which of the following correctly completes the sentence above?

A)   Ionic
B)   Covalent
C)   Metallic
D)   Van der Waals

34.   Mutations in which of the following cells can be passed on to future generations?

A)   Brain cells
B)   Germ cells
C)   Skin cells
D)   Nerve cells

35.   ___ KOH + ___ $H_2SO_4 \rightarrow$ ___ H_2O + ___ K_2SO_4

Which of the following equations balances the acid/base reaction given above?

A) $KOH + H_2SO_4 \rightarrow H_2O + K_2SO_4$
B) $2\ KOH + H_2SO_4 \rightarrow 2\ H_2O + K_2SO_4$
C) $2\ KOH + H_2SO_4 \rightarrow H_2O + K_2SO_4$
D) $KOH + H_2SO_4 \rightarrow 2H_2O + K_2SO_4$

36. DNA codons encode which of the following?

    A) Blood
    B) Neurons
    C) Amino acids
    D) Cell walls

37. During cell replication, which of the following materials is duplicated by polymerase enzymes?

    A) Water
    B) Protein
    C) RNA
    D) DNA

38. Which of the following nitrogenous bases is unique to RNA?

    A) Uracil
    B) Guanine
    C) Thymine
    D) Adenine

39.   pH Scale

$[H^+]$	pH	$[OH^-]$
10^{-1}	1.0	10^{-13}
10^{-2}	2.0	10^{-12}
10^{-3}	3.0	10^{-11}
10^{-4}	4.0	10^{-10}
10^{-5}	5.0	10^{-9}
10^{-6}	6.0	10^{-8}
10^{-7}	7.0	10^{-7}
10^{-8}	8.0	10^{-6}
10^{-9}	9.0	10^{-5}
10^{-10}	10.0	10^{-4}
10^{-11}	11.0	10^{-3}
10^{-12}	12.0	10^{-2}
10^{-13}	13.0	10^{-1}
10^{-14}	14.0	10^{-0}

A difference of two units on the pH scale above represents a concentration difference of

    A) 2.
    B) 20.
    C) 100.
    D) 1,000.

40. A research student predicts that rats raised in a stimulating environment will learn faster than rats raised in an isolated environment. This prediction corresponds with which of the following steps in the scientific method?

    A) Formulating a hypothesis
    B) Conducting an experiment
    C) Analyzing the results
    D) Drawing a conclusion

41. The electron configuration for a certain neutral atom is $1s^22s^22p^63s^23p^64s^2$. This atom also has a mass number of 42. Which of the following indicates the number of protons and neutrons in this atom?

    A) 20 protons; 22 neutrons
    B) 20 protons; 42 neutrons
    C) 22 protons; 22 neutrons
    D) 22 protons; 42 neutrons

42. Consider 0.050 kilogram (kg) of water vapor at the boiling point. Which of the following is the amount of heat necessary to fully condense the gas? (Note: The heat of condensation is 540 calories/gram.)

    A) –27,000 kilocalories
    B) –27,000 calories
    C) 27,000 calories
    D) 27,000 kilocalories

43. A normal individual (*XX*) mates with an individual who is homozygous for a recessive trait (*xx*). Which of the following indicates the percent of offspring who will be carriers of the recessive trait?

    A) 0%
    B) 25%
    C) 50%
    D) 100%

44. Meiosis occurs in which of the following cells?

    A) Germ cells
    B) Skin cells
    C) Blood cells
    D) Brain cells

45. The liquid state of a substance is considered to have a _____ shape and a _____ volume.

    Which of the following correctly completes the sentence above?

    A) fixed; fixed
    B) fixed; changing
    C) changing; fixed
    D) changing; changing

46. Which of the following stars will provide the greatest energy for the Earth?

A) The Sun
B) A star with the same energy output as the Sun 4 light years away
C) A star with twice the energy output of the Sun 10 light years away
D) A star with 100 times the energy output of the Sun 100 light years away

47. A researcher conducts a study to examine the effects that time spent in extracurricular involvement has on college entrance exam scores. In this study, extracurricular involvement is which of the following types of variables?

A) Dependent
B) Independent
C) Extraneous
D) Qualitative

48. When an automobile traveling at 60 miles per hour is brought to a rapid stop, the two types of energy most involved are

A) potential and heat.
B) potential and kinetic.
C) kinetic and chemical.
D) kinetic and heat.

Section 4. ENGLISH AND LANGUAGE USAGE	Number of Scored Questions: 30
	Recommended Time Limit for Practice Test: 30 minutes*

*The proctored TEAS® has an additional four unscored questions for a total of 34 English and language usage questions. The time limit on the proctored English and language usage portion is 34 minutes.

1. Jane _____ broke the ceramic vase.

   Which of the following options correctly completes the sentence above?

   A) accidentilly
   B) acidentaly
   C) acidentily
   D) accidentally

2. If <u>Madelyn</u> doesn't arrive quickly, _____ will not be able to go to the concert with us.

   Which of the following options is the correct pronoun for the sentence above? The antecedent of the pronoun to be added is underlined.

   A) we
   B) she
   C) her
   D) they

3. Which of the following phrases follows the rules of capitalization?

   A) Professor Hopping
   B) Thanksgiving day
   C) uncle Larry
   D) Northern Canada

4. Which of the following is an example of correctly punctuated direct dialogue in a sentence?

   A) He told me, I plan on majoring in aeronautical engineering.
   B) He told me, "I plan on majoring in aeronautical engineering."
   C) Mark told me, "he plans on majoring in aeronautical engineering."
   D) Mark told me that "he plans on majoring in aeronautical engineering."

5. Which of the following sentences has correct subject-verb agreement?

   A) When the cafeteria serves lime gelatin for lunch, each of the children asks for more.
   B) As the car lurches forward, every one of the passengers brace for the impact.
   C) Because the bus broke down on the way, the group of swimmers are late to the meet.
   D) The family of four miss the flight because there was not enough parking at the airport.

6. The door swung open. We spun around. We saw Kyle Adams. He staggered into the room.

   To improve sentence fluency, which of the following best states the information above in a single sentence?

   A) When the door swung open and we saw Kyle Adams, he staggered into the room as we spun around.
   B) We saw Kyle Adams as the door swung open and he staggered into the room, as we spun around.
   C) When the door swung open, we spun around and saw Kyle Adams as he staggered into the room.
   D) As he staggered in the room, we saw Kyle Adams and the door swung open and we spun around.

7. Which of the following is a simple sentence?

   A) The woman who looked out of place.
   B) Looked out of place in the evening store.
   C) The woman in the convenience store looked out of place since she was dressed for an evening out.
   D) The woman in the elegant, gold evening gown and diamond-studded tiara looked out of place in the convenience store.

8. Which of the following underlined words is an example of correct spelling?

   A) My <u>deer</u> Aunt Jane was a wonderful cook.
   B) Her stomach is upset because she took <u>to</u> much medicine.
   C) They just left to go pick up <u>there</u> pizza at the restaurant.
   D) The dog got caught in the fence and broke <u>its</u> leg.

9. Which of the following is the best two-word definition of the word *multicellular?*

   A) Many units
   B) Few parts
   C) Hefty component
   D) Small entity

10. The girl wandered around the amusement park. She was astonished by the number of people in lines waiting for rides.

    Which of the following uses a conjunction to combine the sentences above so that the focus is more on the girl's astonishment and less on her wandering around?

    A) The girl wandered around the amusement park; she was astonished by the number of people in lines waiting for rides.
    B) The girl wandered around the amusement park and was astonished by the number of people in lines waiting for rides.
    C) As the girl wandered around the amusement park, she was astonished by the number of people in lines waiting for rides.
    D) The girl wandered around the amusement park, and she was astonished by the number of people in lines waiting for rides.

11. The owner of the <u>Labrador</u> puppy arrived <u>earlier</u> than expected, so I wasn't able to give it a bath.

    Which of the following correctly identifies the parts of speech in the underlined portions of the sentence above?

    A) Noun; adverb
    B) Noun; adjective
    C) Adjective; adverb
    D) Adjective; adjective

12. Which of the following sentences contains subject-verb agreement?

    A) Jerry and Karen, the new nurses on the floor, rushes to the nurse's station.
    B) Jerry and Karen, the new nurses on the floor, rush to the nurse's station.
    C) A group of nurses who are new to the floor rush to the nurse's station.
    D) All of the nurses who are new to the floor rushes to the nurse's station.

13. Which of the following book titles is correctly capitalized?

    A) *The Lion, The Witch, and The Wardrobe*
    B) *To Kill a Mockingbird*
    C) *A tale of two cities*
    D) *Computers for dummies*

14. The <u>ignoble</u> manner in which our stepmother treated us was unfair and made us feel like we were nothing to her.

    Which of the following is the meaning of the underlined word above?

    A) sarcastic
    B) impatient
    C) demeaning
    D) manipulative

15. Which of the following is an example of a simple sentence?

    A) The young boy in the white T-shirt had cried for 10 minutes but was silenced with a stale piece of gum from the bottom of my purse.
    B) The young boy in the white T-shirt had cried for 10 minutes, but he was silenced when I offered him a stale piece of gum from the bottom of my purse.
    C) The young boy in the white T-shirt had cried for 10 minutes until I offered him a stale piece of gum from the bottom of my purse.
    D) The young boy in the white T-shirt had cried for 10 minutes, although I offered him a stale piece of gum from the bottom of my purse.

16. Which of the following is an example of third-person point of view?

    A) The boy and the girl talked back and forth as they rode their bicycles.
    B) Due to the traffic noise, it was difficult to hear, and we frequently had to talk loudly to be heard.
    C) I took a deep breath and yelled, "Would you like to go out with me sometime?"
    D) You should never ask someone out in the middle of traffic.

17. Which of the following sentences correctly punctuates direct dialogue?

    A) The girl exclaimed, "My favorite new song is Elvis's 'Love Me Tender'!"
    B) The girl exclaimed, "My favorite new song is Elvis's "Love Me Tender!""
    C) The girl exclaimed, "My favorite new song is Elvis's "Love Me Tender"!
    D) The girl exclaimed, 'My favorite new song is Elvis's 'Love Me Tender!'

18. Which of the following sentences correctly applies the rules of punctuation?

    A) In the epic novel *Moby Dick*, Ahab utters, 'Towards thee I roll, thou all-destroying but unconquering whale; to the last I grapple with thee;' …
    B) In the epic novel *Moby Dick*, Ahab utters, 'Towards thee I roll, thou all-destroying but unconquering whale; to the last I grapple with thee; …'
    C) In the epic novel *Moby Dick*, Ahab utters, "Towards thee I roll, thou all-destroying but unconquering whale; to the last I grapple with thee;" …
    D) In the epic novel *Moby Dick*, Ahab utters, "Towards thee I roll, thou all-destroying but unconquering whale; to the last I grapple with thee; …"

19. _____ always complaining about the time of _____ curfew.

    Which of the following options correctly completes the sentence above?

    A) Their; they're
    B) They're; their
    C) There; they're
    D) They're; there

20. Each person should return to _____ own home.

    Which of the following is the correct pronoun to complete the sentence above?

    A) his
    B) its
    C) their
    D) him

21. The hot dog vendor on the corner of 8th and Mississippi Streets

    Which of the following completions for the above sentence results in a simple sentence structure?

    A) had to go out of business because customers began to prefer the vendor on the adjacent street corner
    B) lost many customers due to the opening of a competing vendor on another street.
    C) becomes overwhelmed on Thursdays, as the local school dismisses at lunchtime that day.
    D) sells a delicious hot dog, but it is much more expensive than most other vendors.

22. Her loss of focus was <u>notisable</u> to all around her.

    Which of the following words corrects the spelling of the underlined word in the sentence above?

    A) noticeible
    B) noticeable
    C) noticable
    D) noticible

23. Which of the following sentences uses capitalization rules correctly?

    A) My sister Abby traveled to the Red sea off the eastern coast of Egypt.
    B) My Sister Abby traveled to the Red Sea off the eastern coast of Egypt
    C) My sister Abby traveled to the Red Sea off the eastern coast of Egypt.
    D) My Sister Abby traveled to the Red sea off the eastern coast of Egypt.

24. Mr. Harris announced to the class, "Everyone is expected to do the following ____ sit quietly, raise your hand before speaking, and participate in discussion."

    Which of the following punctuation marks correctly completes the sentence above?

    A) ;
    B) ,
    C) -
    D) :

25. There is a girl _____ has talent.

    Which of the following correctly completes the sentence above?

    A) whom
    B) which
    C) that
    D) who

26. Which of the following sentences correctly applies the rules of punctuation?

    A) We did not make it in time for the 7:00 movie; however we were able to catch the 7:45 show time.
    B) We did not make it in time for the 7:00 movie, however, we were able to catch the 7:45 show time.
    C) We did not make it in time for the 7:00 movie, however; we were able to catch the 7:45 show time.
    D) We did not make it in time for the 7:00 movie; however, we were able to catch the 7:45 show time.

27. One day after school I strayed from my regular routine and decided to go home and fit in a workout. I loaded my gym bag onto the back of my bike and headed for my local fitness center. I'm so glad I chose that afternoon to work out, because I got the surprise of my life. Suddenly a bicycle whizzed past me, and I couldn't believe the rider was a girl I had a crush on in the sixth grade.

    From which of the following points of view is the above passage written?

    A) First person
    B) Second person
    C) Third person omniscient
    D) Third person limited

28. Which of the following is a simple sentence?

    A) Once I have finished, I will stop by.
    B) The blue and red cars collided, and I called the police.
    C) The dog and the young, active cat played together and chased each other.
    D) You may think I am getting very old, but I do not share your opinion.

29. The clerk absconded with the <u>company's</u> payroll.

    The underlined word in the sentence above is an example of which of the following parts of speech?

    A) Pronoun
    B) Noun
    C) Adverb
    D) Adjective

30. My aunt Jean asked the professor, "How will we get to Sunnyfield stadium given the construction road blocks on the west side of Cherry Street?"

Which of the following words in the sentence above should be capitalized?

A) aunt
B) west
C) stadium
D) professor

SOLUTIONS TO PRACTICE TEST 1

READING	MATHEMATICS	SCIENCE	ENGLISH AND LANGUAGE USAGE
1. A	1. C	1. B	1. D
2. D	2. C	2. C	2. B
3. D	3. C	3. D	3. A
4. B	4. C	4. D	4. B
5. C	5. B	5. B	5. A
6. A	6. A	6. C	6. C
7. A	7. C	7. D	7. D
8. B	8. A	8. B	8. D
9. B	9. C	9. B	9. A
10. A	10. B	10. A	10. C
11. D	11. B	11. A	11. C
12. C	12. C	12. B	12. B
13. C	13. B	13. C	13. B
14. D	14. A	14. A	14. C
15. B	15. C	15. D	15. A
16. A	16. B	16. C	16. A
17. D	17. C	17. B	17. A
18. C	18. A	18. A	18. D
19. C	19. A	19. D	19. B
20. A	20. D	20. C	20. A
21. C	21. B	21. B	21. B
22. B	22. C	22. C	22. B
23. C	23. A	23. A	23. C
24. A	24. A	24. B	24. D
25. B	25. D	25. D	25. D
26. D	26. D	26. D	26. D
27. C	27. D	27. C	27. A
28. B	28. D	28. D	28. C
29. D	29. A	29. D	29. D
30. B	30. B	30. C	30. C
31. B		31. A	
32. A		32. D	
33. C		33. A	
34. C		34. B	
35. A		35. B	
36. B		36. C	
37. A		37. D	
38. D		38. A	
39. A		39. C	
40. C		40. A	
41. D		41. A	
42. A		42. B	
		43. D	
		44. A	
		45. C	
		46. A	
		47. B	
		48. D	

READING
SOLUTIONS TO PRACTICE TEST 1

1.   A   This is a summary sentence that encapsulates the main idea of the article. Looking at the article, the reader can see that it covers three main subjects: the various problems faced by oaks, the chemical approach to solving those problems, and the nonchemical (or organic) approach to solving those problems. Along the way, it becomes clear that the article is strongly endorsing the chemical-free (organic) approach over the chemical approach. Therefore, this sentence illustrates the article's main idea.

2.   D   The author will most likely recommend that the homeowner let the tree die. The author has made his position on chemicals clear. He believes that their use should be avoided. Therefore, option A is unlikely, even though some tree specialists may be in favor of applying chemicals to help the tree live longer.

         The article suggests that chemical treatments are popular because they are inexpensive. The reader can infer that the alternative, nonchemical treatments the author recommends – like tree trimming and soil enrichment – are expensive. (Otherwise, they would be just as popular as chemicals.) Since this homeowner does not want to invest in expensive interventions, it seems unlikely that the author will recommend options B and C.

         Furthermore, the article clearly states that nothing can be done for a tree in some cases, and that one of those cases is when a tree has oak wilt. Since this tree has oak wilt, options B and C become even less likely. The only option left is to let the tree die a natural death.

3.   D   The author has selected this choice of words to convey meaning or feeling beyond what some may experience due to the death of an oak tree.

4.   B   The author is stating that a chemical-free approach is the best based on his experience; however, the experience of others may be different. Therefore, the author is offering only his opinion regarding the best approach.

5.   C   The author is using a comparison-contrast text structure to evaluate the two types of interventions before he concludes with his preference.

6.   A   This topic sentence appears at the very beginning of the text. It is clearly the topic sentence because it provides the theme that the remaining text will discuss. In this case, the theme is the American literary scene's lack of maturity. All the remaining text flows from this topic sentence, either elaborating upon this idea or explaining it.

7.   A   The topic of the article is literature, specifically American literature. The main idea is that American literature still has a way to go before it becomes truly relevant. In discussing the main idea, the article deals with the theme of isolation, suggesting that American poets' tendency toward isolation and solitary behavior is counterproductive. The supporting details are details of the passage that support the topic and main idea.

8.   B   This inference is based on a number of relatively subtle clues:
   - The article is slightly condescending towards American authors, minimizing their contributions and calling them antisocial loners.
   - The article presents British authors as a model for the Americans, which suggests that the author is exhibiting nationalistic pride.
   - The author paints American poets as unfamiliar, using terms like "bizarre" and "ghoulish"; meanwhile, British poets are described as "a social bunch," which is a much warmer, more familiar characterization.

9.   B   All four of the listed conclusions may be drawn from the article as a *whole*. However, paragraph three offers a specific explanation of how British poets enjoyed a vibrant literary and social environment, and how that environment gave them an advantage that the American poets lacked. Since social interaction is presented as a direct cause for British poets' superiority, the logical implication (or conclusion) is that social interaction must lead to better, more mature literature.

10.   A   The author's purpose is to compare the works of American and British poets with regard to maturity. Although the author does state options B, C, and D, those options are not the main purpose being conveyed in the writing.

11. D   The author's approach in the excerpt is to persuade the reader that American poetry is inferior to British poetry based on his personal opinions. Narrative, expository, and technical writing often employ the use of fact, rather than opinion.

12. C   This is a summary sentence. Option A is an example of a topic sentence. Options B and D are examples of supporting details.

13. C   While the paragraph never states that Marley is a thief, it strongly suggests that he is one. Marley blends into crowds, he is unusually interested in the location of people's items, he has money from an unknown source, and he appeared just before a series of neighborhood burglaries started. Option B offers the general conclusion that Marley prefers to be alone, but the paragraph is clearly trying to suggest something much more specific than that. In addition, there is no information presented in the paragraph that can allow the reader to conclude that Marley is a private investigator or to infer that the author does not care for Marley.

14. D   The paragraph is written in the typical style of a fiction novel; a narrator is telling the reader a story. It is not written in the typical style of a textbook or dissertation. In addition, given what is presented in the text, there is not enough information to conclude that the passage was taken from a science-fiction novel.

15. B   This paragraph was written to give the reader clues. The author is dropping strong hints that Marley is the burglar. This may turn out to be true, or it may later turn out that the author was leading the reader astray. Either way, these hints are the reason for the paragraph's existence.

16. A   Press releases are designed to release information about a company or government body. This press release provides succinct information about the new clinic in a format that is easy to read.

17. D   This document follows a structure that is very common for press releases. A typical press release states its topic and main idea right up front; in fact, the main idea is often the *title* of the press release. (The main idea is also echoed in the first sentence or two.) The remainder of the document provides supporting details that elaborate upon the main idea.

18. C   The author's primary intent is to recommend Alex Jones for the new job. While he does mention certain other facts – for example, that certain other departments need personnel more than the executive department and that Chinese food will be delivered later – these facts are mentioned casually, aside from the author's main purpose. The bulk of the letter is devoted to telling Debra about Alex Jones's suitability for the job.

19. C   The author has a bias toward Alex Jones and is open about that bias.

20. A   1. Jar contents: 1 red, 2 blue
         2. Jar contents: 1 red, 1 blue
         3. Jar contents: 1 red, 1 blue, 1 yellow
         4. Jar contents: 2 red, 1 blue, 1 yellow
         5. Jar contents: 2 red, 1 yellow
         6. Jar contents: 2 red, 2 yellow

21. C   According to the textbook's index, the first relevant entry regarding information about chromium alloys can be found on pages 221 and 222.

22. B   This scale measures up to 20 pounds; this is clear, because the maximum weight is identified on the scale face as 20 pounds. The current scale reading shows a measurement between 1 and 20 pounds.

23. C   An individual who is gregarious enjoys the companionship of others and can be viewed as sociable.

24. A   By comparing the height of the blue and red profit bars for a given month, the reader can tell whether the corporation did better (for that month) in 2007 or 2008. Looking at the chart, one can determine that in any given month, with the exception of May, the red (2008) bars are shorter than the blue (2007) bars, indicating less profitability overall for 2008.

25. B   This answer is obtained by looking for the month with the shortest profit bars for both years.

26. D   Following the route described, the family's car will pass through each of the two possible roadblocks twice, for a total of four times.

27. C   Southern Cleaning and Maintenance's free shipping rate for orders more than $100 makes it the least expensive shipping option. The other vendors would charge at least $20 for shipping this order.

28. B   In this context, the man in black is stealing from the older man's pocket. There is no information given in the context to support options A, C, or D.

29. D   This Web site is most likely to provide factual, unbiased information about a candidate's political position. The two Web sites devoted specifically to Bill Williamson are both likely to be filled with strongly biased opinions: one for the candidate and one against him. Finally, www.candidateblender.org seems to be devoted to political comedy, not necessarily the serious discussion of issues.

30. B   A road atlas will provide the information needed to map the shortest route to a destination. Options A, C, and D will not provide this specific information.

31. B   Undervale Car Audio is the only business of the four that is listed under Auto Radios & Stereo Systems; therefore, it is the appropriate choice for a customer wanting installation of a CD player.

32. A   Of the options listed, Comprehensive Auto Maintenance is the only car repair business that advertises that they offer free estimates.

33. C   Because the individual has been told to avoid blood thinners, aspirin and ibuprofen are not suitable choices. Because this person also has a history of addiction, morphine is not suitable. Therefore, the appropriate medication choice in this situation is acetaminophen.

34. C   The indented text is a quotation from another work. Specifically, the nonindented text above and below suggests that the indented text is an excerpt from William Altucher's journal.

35. A   *Diamagnetic* comes after *dextral* and before *diamond* in the dictionary.

36. B   The existing headings establish a definite pattern of continents. Of the available options, Europe is the only continent.

37. A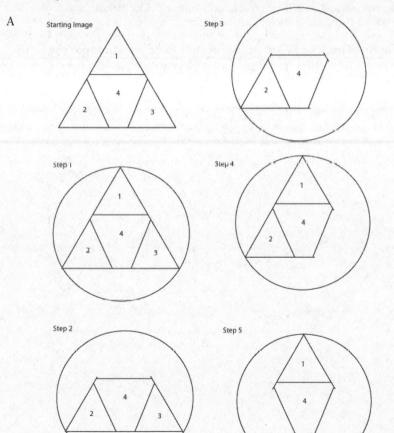

38. D   This article is current, unlike option B, and the title suggests that it covers Rotuma from an unbiased travel perspective, unlike option C. Because Rotuma is an island in the Pacific Ocean, and not a European country, option A is not a plausible choice.

39. A   Even if the meaning of diastolic blood pressure or how it is measured is unknown, clues are provided on the device. In this case, DIA represents the abbreviation for diastolic measurement, which is 72.

40. C   The first consideration is potential allergic reactions. Of the seven listed products, only two advertise that they will not cause allergic reactions. Therefore, the other five products can be immediately discounted. Of the two remaining products, the Champion Deluxe Flea Collar costs $15.00 and the Flea and Tick Control System costs $7.00. However, notice the descriptions: the Champion product lasts for 6 months, so the pet owner would need two of them to last 1 year. Meanwhile, the Flea and Tick product only lasts for 2 months, so the owner would need six of them to last 1 year. At this point it is a matter of basic math:

Champion: $15.00 × 2 = $30.00 for 1 year
Flea & Tick: $7.00 × 6 = $42.00 for 1 year

Therefore, the Champion product is the more economical of the two nonallergic options.

41. D   Only three of the seven listed products are collars: the Barton Flea Collar, the Champion Deluxe Flea Collar, and the Patton Flea Collar. All of the other products can be ignored. The pet owner wants to protect his cat for a year. Multiply each product's base cost by the number of products needed for a year's protection, to get the yearly price:

Barton: $5.00 × 4 = $20.00 for the year
Champion: $15.00 × 2 = $30.00 for the year
Patton: $12.00 × 3 = $36.00 for the year

The Patton collar may now be discarded since its yearly cost is more than $30.00. Finally, looking at the cat magazine's review ratings, the Barton is rated as a 5 and the Champion a 7. The Champion is the best-rated product that fits the buyer's criteria, so that is the correct answer.

42. A   A reader familiar with the convention of italicizing foreign words should understand that the words italicized here are not English – even if the actual meaning of those words is not understood.

MATHEMATICS
SOLUTIONS TO PRACTICE TEST 1

1. C The perimeter of the yard is found by adding up all four sides of the yard:
13.5 ft + 13.5 ft + 47.75 ft + 47.75 ft = 122.5 ft.
Note that:
  2 rolls × 50 ft per roll = 100 ft. This is not enough to fence the yard.
  3 rolls × 50 ft per roll = 150 ft. This is enough to fence the yard.
Therefore, the man should buy 3 rolls of fencing to fence his yard.

2. C $2\frac{1}{3} \times 4\frac{1}{2} = \frac{7}{3} \times \frac{9}{2} = \frac{63}{6} = 10\frac{3}{6}$ or $10\frac{1}{2}$

3. C $1,000 + (500 + 100 + 100 + 100) + 50 + (5 - 1) = 1,854$

4. C Gross pay − deductions = take-home pay
$1,278.00 − $422.25 = $855.75

5. B Add the three sides of the backyard 150 + 150 + 325 = 625 ft
Multiply the feet by the cost per foot: 625 × $13.00 = $8,125.00

6. A Total in symphony − women in symphony = men in symphony, so the ratio is
$\frac{\text{men in symphony}}{\text{total in symphony}} = \frac{125 - 75}{125} = \frac{50}{125} = \frac{2}{5}$.

7. C $6.95 + $2.45 + $1.49 + $1.19 = $12.08

8. A Previous balance + deposits − checks + interest − service charge.
$2,355.14 + $1,527.28 − $1,203.97 + $1.56 − $5.00 = $2,675.01

9. C $6 \times (5 + 7) \div 4 - 7 \times 2 + 3 \times 3 = 6 \times 12 \div 4 - 7 \times 2 + 3 \times 3$
$$= 72 \div 4 - 14 + 9$$
$$= 18 - 14 + 9$$
$$= 4 + 9$$
$$= 13$$

10. B To convert a decimal to a percent, move the decimal two places to the right and insert the % symbol. Moving the decimal in 0.003 to the right two places and inserting the % symbol gives 0.3%.

11. B 215.4% is 2.154 as a decimal. So, the equation looks like this:
2.154 × 55 = □. Then, 2.154 × 55 = 118.47

12. C (Number of nurses × cost per nurse) + (number of guests × cost per guest) = total cost
(315 × $18.00) + (53 × $25.00) = $6,995.00

13. B Round each number so there is only one nonzero digit. Then add the results.
$899.00 ≈ $900.00
$695.00 ≈ $700.00
$379.00 ≈ $400.00
$229.00 ≈ $200.00
$149.00 ≈ $100.00
$900.00 + $700.00 + $400.00 + $200.00 + $100.00 = $2,300.00

14. A The father's age (y) is equal to 3 times the daughter's age ($3x$) less 4 years, or $y = 3x - 4$.

15. C The chemist has the highest salary, $80,000.
The secretary has the lowest salary, $25,000.
The difference between the salaries is $80,000 − $25,000 = $55,000.

16. B $\frac{x}{2} + 5 = 9$

$\frac{x}{2} + \frac{10}{2} = \frac{18}{2}$

$\frac{x}{2} + 5 - 5 = 9 - 5$

$\frac{x}{2} = 4$

$x = 8$

17. C

$$\begin{array}{r} 7\ \ \cancel{8}^{7}\ \cancel{3}^{13} \\ -\ \ 4\ \ 5 \\ \hline 7\ \ 3\ \ 8 \end{array}$$

18. A To solve $|x + 2| = 5$, set up two equations and solve.
$x + 2 = 5$ or $x + 2 = -5$
       $x = 3$ $x = -7$

19. A The correct answer is a pie chart due to the fact that the data is categorical and totals 100%.

20. D Percent increase $= \frac{710 - 625}{625} = \frac{85}{625} = 0.136$ or 13.6%

21. B Pipettes are used to directly pour exact amounts of liquids. They are usually small and are not meant for large volumes. For the chemist, this is the best choice. Any of the other choices are not as good since there is always a chance of leaving a drop behind in the container after it is poured out. Pipettes eliminate this error to provide better accuracy and precision.

22. C Start with the measured distance on the map, then multiply by the ratio given on the map, making sure to leave the desired distance on top. In this case, miles should be on the top of the ratio.

$8 \text{ cm} \times \frac{10 \text{ mi}}{1 \text{ cm}} = 80 \text{ mi}$

23. A Since 1 teaspoon = 5 mL, mL would be a reasonable unit of measurement to choose to measure a liquid, oral medication. A liter is 1,000 times larger than a milliliter, so this would be too big. A liter, for example, is the size of a bulk IV bag. A kiloliter is 1,000 times larger than a liter, so it is also too large. Ten deciliters are the same size as 1 liter, so 1 deciliter could be a reasonable amount of liquid to drink, but this is still too large for oral medication. Therefore, milliliter seems like the most reasonable answer.

24. A The height of a person depends on his or her age, so height is the dependent variable. Therefore, age is the independent variable.

25. D 100 centimeters = 1 meter
400 centimeters = 4 meters

26. D $(x^2 + 3x - 2) - (x^2 - 2x - 5) = x^2 + 3x - 2 - x^2 + 2x + 5$
                                   $= 5x + 3$

27. D Since $\sqrt{25} = 5$ and $\sqrt{36} = 6$, then $\sqrt{27}$ must be between 5 and 6. Therefore, 5.2 is the only reasonable answer.

28. D $\frac{11}{3}$ is equal to 3.67; –3 is less than 3.67, which is less than 3.8, which is less than 4.

29. A Multiply 513 and 2 together. This equals 1,026. There are a total of four decimal places (two decimal places in 5.13 and two decimal places in 0.02). Counting back four decimal places from the end of 1,026 gives 0.1026.

30.   B   First, look at the denominators 8 and 12. The least common denominator (LCD) is 24. Therefore, each fraction needs to be changed to an equivalent fraction with a denominator of 24. This is what has been done in the first step.

$$\frac{7}{8} - \frac{5}{12} = \frac{7 \times 3}{8 \times 3} - \frac{5 \times 2}{12 \times 2} = \frac{21}{24} - \frac{10}{24}$$

In the second step, the fractions are subtracted since they have an LCD. Subtract the numerators, but keep the denominator unchanged.

$$\frac{21}{24} - \frac{10}{24} = \frac{11}{24}$$

Final Answer is $\frac{11}{24}$. This answer is simplified because the numerator and denominator do not share a common factor.

SCIENCE
SOLUTIONS TO PRACTICE TEST 1

1. B   Breakdown of fats begins in the small intestine. Breakdown of carbohydrates begins in the mouth, and breakdown of protein begins in the stomach. Fiber is not digestible.

2. C   A paradigm shift is considered to be a radical change from previous thinking.

3. D   Adaptation is the increase of alleles of certain genes from generation to generation that allows a species to survive and reproduce better. Natural selection is the means by which adaptation occurs.

4. D   The sympathetic nervous system activates the body's fight-or-flight response. In the presence of stress, the heart beats faster and stronger, more blood is carried to the vital organs, and the pupils dilate to prepare the body to defend itself.

5. B   Quantitative data deal with numbers that can be measured.

6. C   The biological classification system starts broad at domain and becomes more specific as it descends to species. Phylum is the most general level of those options listed.

7. D   Water's high specific heat and high heat of vaporization mean that a great deal of energy is required to cause increases in temperature, as well as large-scale phase changes. These two large, energy-related values are responsible for the moderation of Earth's climate and contribute greatly to sustaining life.

8. B   Because this mold is a new species, a different species classification, rather than an established one, is required. The new classification system relies more heavily on DNA sequence similarities to name and classify organisms than on physical characteristics. The mold would not be named with the same name as another known organism, *Neurospora crassa* or *Aspergillus nidulans*. Since it is genetically similar to the *Neurospora* species, it would be named *Neurospora novus*, not *Aspergillus novus*.

9. B   Hydrocarbons with double bonds obey the general formula C_nH_{2n}, and are referred to as alkenes. Notice that the number of hydrogen atoms is always double the number of carbon atoms.

10. A   Scientific arguments are communicated according to the scientific method. A hypothesis (or claim) must be supported by analyzed data. After this point, a potential conclusion may be reached.

11. A   The role of the cardiovascular system is to provide the body's cells with oxygen and nutrients via a system of arteries and arterioles. Although the digestive system breaks down food into nutrients that can then be transported via the cardiovascular system, it is not primarily responsible for that transport. Options C and D are not responsible for providing the body's cells with oxygen and nutrients.

12. B   After passing through the right ventricle of the heart during contraction, blood then travels through the tricuspid valve into the pulmonary artery.

13. C   The respiratory system is responsible for supplying the body with oxygen and removing carbon dioxide. Options A, B, and D are not responsible for this vital function.

14. A   The lining of the hollow organs of the digestive system, such as the esophagus, stomach, and intestines, is comprised of smooth muscle tissue, which creates the peristalsis needed to push undigested food through the body. Options B, C, and D are not examples of tissues that involuntarily contract.

15. D   Protons have a charge of +1, and electrons have a charge of –1. However, in regard to mass, protons are about 2,000 times more massive than electrons.

16. C   The spine, which is part of the skeletal system, provides protection for the spinal cord.

17. B   Since B has a higher density than A, it travels more slowly. Consequently, the molecules of A will reach the other side of the room sooner than the molecules of B.

18. A   Since acidic solutions have pH values that range from 1 to 7 (where 7 indicates neutrality), a substance with a pH value of 2 that is completely ionized in its solution indicates a strong acidic solution.

19. D   Immune cells are produced in the body's bone marrow.

20. C The heart is located behind the sternum. Although the apex of the heart is located to the left of the sternum, the majority of the heart is covered and protected by the sternum.

21. B Counts in several squares provide a sufficient sample size, and counts from morning and afternoon indicate the pollen distribution throughout the day.

22. C Energy consumption is necessary for growth in all animals. Therefore, population growth is positively correlated with the consumption of food (i.e., energy).

23. A The alveoli are the structures in the respiratory system in which the exchange of gases occurs. Although options B, C, and D are components of the respiratory system, they are not directly responsible for the exchange of oxygen.

24. B Fertility rates are higher in less-developed countries than they are in more-developed countries.

25. D Since protons are positive, electrons are negative, and neutrons are neutral, the overall charge is imbalanced in favor of the protons by +1 (since the neutrons do not contribute to the charge). Since the mass of a proton and a neutron is nearly the same (and the mass of an electron is negligible compared to both), the overall mass is largely determined by the number of protons and neutrons.

26. D The amino-acid structure found within protein molecules is considered an internal factor, and the other choices are important external influences.

27. C A prokaryotic cell lacks a membrane-bound nucleus, and all other options contain a membrane-bound nucleus.

28. D The genotype of an individual is comprised of its various genes, which are made up of DNA. The changes at the genotypic level are seen at the phenotypic level, such as hair or eye color.

29. D In heterotrophs, mitochondria are the powerhouses of cells. They produce ATP for the cell to use. They are physically similar to chloroplasts.

30. C The base pairings on the mRNA must be compatibly matched with those of the DNA as follows:

UUA GCG AUA CGC
AAT CGC TAT GCG

31. A Ribosomes on the surface of the ER give it a rough characteristic, as opposed to smooth ER, which lacks ribosomes.

32. D Genes are composed of DNA, and protein is composed of amino acids.

33. A While covalent bonds require the sharing of electrons, ionic bonds are viewed as having electrons donated and accepted by atoms to complete the valence structure.

34. B Germ cells are the only type of cell capable of passing along mutations to offspring.

35. B There are 2 moles of potassium (K), 6 moles of oxygen (O), 4 moles of hydrogen (H), and 1 mole of sulfur (S) on both sides of the reaction equation.

36. C DNA codons found in genes encode amino acids that comprise proteins.

37. D During a cell replication cycle, the DNA of the cell should be fully and correctly duplicated.

38. A Uracil is found only in RNA, thymine only in DNA, and guanine and adenine are found in both RNA and DNA.

39. C A difference of two units on the pH scale represents a difference of 100 in strength of concentration, based on $\log_{10}[H^+]$.

40. A Formulating a hypothesis involves predicting what may happen in a study.

41. A The sum of all the raised numbers equals the number of electrons found within the neutral atom for that element. For a neutral atom, the number of protons equals the number of electrons. Also, the mass number equals the number of protons and neutrons.

42.   B   The appropriate expression to calculate heat removal is H = – M L. The given mass must first be converted to grams. Then, H = – (0.050 kg)(540 cal/g) = – (50 g)(540 cal/g) = –27,000 cal.

43.   D   All of the offspring will be carriers of the recessive trait (Xx).

44.   A   Meiosis only occurs in germ cells. Mitosis occurs in all other cells.

45.   C   Although a liquid has a distinctly measurable volume, it will conform to the shape of the container in which it resides.

46.   A   Even though the Sun only provides an average energy output for stars, it is so close to Earth that any other star's energy output is too far away to contribute significantly to Earth.

47.   B   In this study, the exam scores depend on the extracurricular involvement. Stated another way, the extracurricular involvement influences the exam scores; therefore, it is the independent variable.

48.   D   The automobile has energy of motion (kinetic energy) until it stops. To stop, it relies on friction. The friction generates heat during the course of braking.

ENGLISH AND LANGUAGE USAGE
SOLUTIONS TO PRACTICE TEST 1

1. D *Accidentally* is a commonly misspelled word. The word has two c's and two l's

2. B The antecedent, Madelyn, is singular and feminine, which means that *she* is the only correct answer. The other options are incorrect either in number, gender, or case.

3. A A person's title is capitalized when it appears before the name. Both words in option B require capitalization, as this is the full title of the holiday. In option D, it is not necessary to capitalize the word *northern*. This word is used only as an adjective in this case rather than as part of the place's name.

4. B Option B contains direct dialogue and is punctuated properly with quotation marks. Option A incorrectly omits the quotation marks. Both options C and D confuse direct and indirect dialogue.

5. A Option A contains correct subject-verb agreement: "each . . . asks." Options B, C, and D contain incorrect subject-verb conjugation with regard to number. When a prepositional phrase modifies the subject of a sentence, it is important to remember to conjugate back to the original subject rather than to the object of the prepositional phrase.

6. C Option C effectively uses transitional words to combine the sentences into a single sentence that still reflects the original meaning of the group of sentences.

7. D Option D is constructed as a simple sentence containing one subject and one verb. Although the description of the woman is detailed, there are no clauses adding to the complexity of the sentence structure, as is the case in option C. Options A and B are not complete sentences.

8. D It is a common mistake to place an apostrophe in the word *its* to indicate possession. However, for this sentence, an apostrophe indicates a contraction for *it is*. Options A, B, and C are all examples of incorrect usage of the underlined words.

9. A The word, *multicellular* is made up of the prefix *multi-*, which means "many," and the root word *cell*, which is defined as a "unit."

10. C Only option C makes one clause subordinate to the other by the addition of a subordinating conjunction. All other options contain two clauses of equal weight.

11. C Only option C correctly identifies *Labrador* as an adjective and *earlier* as an adverb.

12. B Option B is an example of a sentence containing subject-verb agreement: "Jerry and Karen...rush." Options A, C, and D contain verbs with regard to number.

13. B Capitalize the first word and all subsequent important words in titles of books, periodicals, poems, stories, articles, documents, movies, paintings, and other works of art.

14. C Within this context, the word *ignoble* is used to describe a manner of treatment that is demeaning, that is employed to make one feel less worthy. This is strengthened by the contextual clue "made us feel like we were nothing to her."

15. A Option A is constructed as a simple sentence containing one subject and a compound verb. Although the sentence is detailed, there are no clauses adding to the complexity of the sentence structure, as is the case in the other options.

16. A This option is an example of third-person point of view. Options B and C are examples of first-person point of view. Option D is an example of second-person point of view.

17. A Option A correctly contains double quotation marks around the whole quote, with single quotation marks around the song title. The exclamation point appears outside of the single quotes, as it is not a part of the song's title but the ending punctuation for the entire quote.

18. D Option D is the only example that contains correct punctuation. This option correctly punctuates Ahab's quotation with double quotation marks and includes the ellipsis within the quotation marks.

19. B Option B correctly completes the sentence. In the first part of the sentence, the contraction for *there are* is appropriate. In the second part of the sentence, *their* is the correct pronoun to use.

20. A   The antecedent *person* is singular; therefore, option A is the only correct option. The other options are incorrect in number or person.

21. B   Option B is constructed as a simple sentence containing one subject and one verb. There are no clauses adding to the complexity of the sentence structure, as is the case in options A, C, and D.

22. B   Noticeable is a commonly misspelled word. Since notice ends in *-ce* and the added suffix is *-able*, keep the letter *e*.

23. C   The word *sister* should not be capitalized in this context. The words *Red* and *Sea* should both be capitalized, because together they make up the name of a proper noun.

24. D   To correctly punctuate the sentence, a colon is required after the word *following*. A colon is used following an independent clause that precedes a list.

25. D   The word *who* or *whom* should be used in reference to people, while the words *which* and *that* should be used to refer to things. The word *whom* should be used to reference a direct or indirect object, and the word *who* should be used in reference to the subject of a sentence (in this case, *the girl*).

26. D   Option D is correctly punctuated with the conjunctive adverb preceded by a semicolon and followed by a comma.

27. A   The passage is written from the first-person point of view, which is signified by the use of the words *I*, *my*, and *me*.

28. C   Although this sentence contains a compound subject and a compound verb, it is a simple sentence because it has only one clause.

29. D   The word *company's* is used as an adjective in the above context, modifying the word *payroll*.

30. C   The word *stadium* should be capitalized, as it is used as a proper noun in this context. There is no need to capitalize the words in options A, B, or D.

PRACTICE TEST 2

READING	MATHEMATICS	SCIENCE	ENGLISH AND LANGUAGE USAGE
1.____	1.____	1.____	1.____
2.____	2.____	2.____	2.____
3.____	3.____	3.____	3.____
4.____	4.____	4.____	4.____
5.____	5.____	5.____	5.____
6.____	6.____	6.____	6.____
7.____	7.____	7.____	7.____
8.____	8.____	8.____	8.____
9.____	9.____	9.____	9.____
10.____	10.____	10.____	10.____
11.____	11.____	11.____	11.____
12.____	12.____	12.____	12.____
13.____	13.____	13.____	13.____
14.____	14.____	14.____	14.____
15.____	15.____	15.____	15.____
16.____	16.____	16.____	16.____
17.____	17.____	17.____	17.____
18.____	18.____	18.____	18.____
19.____	19.____	19.____	19.____
20.____	20.____	20.____	20.____
21.____	21.____	21.____	21.____
22.____	22.____	22.____	22.____
23.____	23.____	23.____	23.____
24.____	24.____	24.____	24.____
25.____	25.____	25.____	25.____
26.____	26.____	26.____	26.____
27.____	27.____	27.____	27.____
28.____	28.____	28.____	28.____
29.____	29.____	29.____	29.____
30.____	30.____	30.____	30.____
31.____		31.____	
32.____		32.____	
33.____		33.____	
34.____		34.____	
35.____		35.____	
36.____		36.____	
37.____		37.____	
38.____		38.____	
39.____		39.____	
40.____		40.____	
41.____		41.____	
42.____		42.____	
		43.____	
		44.____	
		45.____	
		46.____	
		47.____	
		48.____	

Section 1. READING	Number of Scored Questions: 42
	Recommended Time Limit for Practice Test: 51 minutes*

*The proctored TEAS® has an additional six unscored questions for a total of 48 reading questions. The time limit on the proctored reading portion is 58 minutes.

UFO Watcher

On a late December afternoon last year, Pam Markesan looked into the New Mexico sky and saw three pulsing blue lights. The lights crossed the sky overhead, and as they did, Ms. Markesan saw that they belonged to a spinning, disc-shaped craft unlike any plane she had ever seen. Inquiries with the Federal Aviation Administration showed no records of any planes or other aircraft within hundreds of miles of the Markesan property that evening.

Later that same evening, on the other side of town, Alvin Mendez, 92, disappeared in his own backyard. A neighbor reported that he saw pulsing blue lights from the vicinity of Mr. Mendez's property; as he walked out to look, he saw Mr. Mendez walking up the ramp to a giant, disc-like craft, where he was awaited by an indistinct, glowing being that, in the neighbor's words, "could not have come from this world." The ramp then retracted and the disc flew into the sky, blue lights still pulsing. Mr. Mendez is still reported missing.

UFO Watcher Today contacted the local army base by phone for comment on this story, but the army spokesman refused to talk. The reporter then drove out to the base for a personal interview, but was again denied. He then took up a position on a hillside overlooking the base, and waited for nightfall. Shortly after dusk a large hangar on the far side of the army base opened up. Inside, the reporter saw the remains of a large, saucer-shaped craft. The damage to the craft seemed consistent with what one might expect from a missile attack.

Baffled but excited, scientists in white laboratory coats were inspecting the debris and pointing to the sky. Later, a pilot who was still wearing his flight suit came and spoke to one of the scientists. He gestured as he spoke. He seemed to be describing a midair battle, indicating that he had fired a missile at an enemy. Then he pointed to the damaged portion of the saucer-like craft inside the hangar.

When *UFO Watcher Today* contacted the army base again, this time relaying startling new information about the damaged vessel in the hangar, the reporter was told to "mind his own business."

The next seven questions are based on this passage.

1. Which of the following is a logical conclusion that may be drawn based on the first two paragraphs of the passage?

   A) Aliens appeared in New Mexico last December and abducted an older adult man.
   B) A series of strange, unexplained events happened in New Mexico last December.
   C) A woman in New Mexico saw something bizarre in the sky last December, and on that same night, an older adult man disappeared.
   D) *UFO Watcher Today* suggested that aliens abducted a man in New Mexico last December. However, since UFOs have never been proven to exist, there is likely a nonparanormal explanation for these events.

2. Which of the following is a logical conclusion based on the last three paragraphs of the passage?

   A) Some sort of wreckage is being kept at a local army base. The army refused to comment about it. It is unclear what the wreckage is or what its significance may be.
   B) The army is secretly building UFO-like aircraft. One of these aircraft was damaged and is now being held at a local army base.
   C) A fighter pilot shot down a UFO that is now being kept in a hangar at a local army base. The army is trying to cover up the story.
   D) Some aircraft wreckage at a local army base may or may not be a UFO. The army has decided not to disclose information about this wreckage, maintaining that it has the right to keep some programs secret.

3. Which of the following excerpts from the passage contains an opinion?

   A) Shortly after dusk, a large hangar on the far side of the army base opened up.
   B) He seemed to be describing a midair battle, indicating that he had fired a missile at an enemy.
   C) Mr. Mendez is still reported as missing.
   D) *UFO Watcher Today* contacted the local army base by phone for comment on this story, but the army spokesman refused to talk.

4. "When *UFO Watcher Today* contacted the army base again, this time relaying startling new information about the damaged vessel in the hangar, the reporter was told to 'mind his own business.'"

   Which of the following is a characteristic of the above passage type?

   A) Narrative
   B) Expository
   C) Technical
   D) Persuasive

5. Based on prior knowledge and personal experience, which of the following statements is likely to be true?

   A) The magazine that published this story does not have high standards of fact-checking.
   B) The magazine that published this story is very highly regarded.
   C) The magazine that published this story has high standards of fact-checking.
   D) The magazine that published this story is now out of print.

6. Three eyewitnesses are cited in the article: Pam Markesan, Mr. Mendez's neighbor, and the reporter sent out to the military bases. Which of the following statements best describes these eyewitness accounts?

   A) None of them are primary sources.
   B) All of them are primary sources.
   C) Pam Markesan and the neighbor are primary sources; the reporter is not.
   D) The reporter is a primary source; Pam Markesan and the neighbor are not.

7. Is the following a topic, main idea, supporting detail, or theme of the UFO article?

   Conspiracy and cover-up

   A) Topic
   B) Main idea
   C) Supporting detail
   D) Theme

Grading Scheme

The teacher of a college class has several assistants. These assistants are given the task of calculating grades for all the students in the class. The following document, written by the teacher, explains how to calculate the grades. Read the document carefully, and then answer the following questions.

To all assistants:

I am aware that my grading technique is unusual. However, I have my reasons for it, and I assure you that it is here to stay – so please, no more discussion. It is time to assign grades.

Below, please find a summary of the technique. Use these rules when calculating grades for my students.

There have been four exams this semester: three section exams and one final exam. These exams are the main basis for class grades, though participation in discussion sections can be a factor.

If a student achieved the same grade on all four of the exams, then the student receives that grade for the class.

If a student received the same grade on three out of four exams, but a different grade on the fourth, you must look at the circumstances:

* If the fourth grade is only one step above or below that of the identical three (e.g., if the student received three B's and an A), the student's class grade is the grade scored on the three exams (in this case, the B), and the fourth exam is discarded.

* If the student's single different grade is more than one step different from the identical three (e.g., the student earned three C's and an A), you must look at which exam yielded the different grade. If it was the final exam, the student's grade should be pushed one step toward the final exam grade. So, in the case of the student with three C's and an A, if the A came on the final, the student's grade for the class is B.

* If the lone grade was more than one step different from the other three, but was *not* on the final exam, simply ignore it and use the grade the student earned on the other three exams.

In all cases other than those described above (in other words, when the student has not scored the same grade on at least three exams), take the final exam grade and adjust it up or down according to discussion participation: up one step for a *plus*, down one step for a *minus*, and no adjustment for a *satisfactory*. So, a student with a final exam grade of B and a *plus* discussion group rating will get a final class grade of an A.

I hope things are now clear.

Professor H.

The next five questions are based on this passage.

8.

Exam	Grade
First	D
Second	B
Third	A
Final	C
Discussion-group participation:	Minus

Using the instructions given in the letter, which of the following class grades should a student receive if she earned the grades displayed in the table above?

A)　A
B)　B
C)　C
D)　D

9. Which of the following is the intention of the professor's letter to his assistants?

   A) To inform
   B) To persuade
   C) To entertain
   D) To express feeling

10. Which of the following sentences is the topic sentence for the professor's letter?

    A) "I am aware that my grading technique is unusual."
    B) "It is time to assign grades."
    C) "The teacher of a college class has several assistants."
    D) "I hope things are now clear."

11. Which of the following inferences may logically be drawn from the letter?

    A) Most students like the professor's unusual grading style.
    B) Some assistants have complained about the unusual grading style.
    C) This grading style results in more passing grades than a typical grading style.
    D) This grading style results in more failing grades than a typical grading style.

12. Refer to the first bullet point (*) in the letter. Is this part of the letter best described as narrative, expository, technical, or persuasive writing?

    A) Narrative
    B) Expository
    C) Technical
    D) Persuasive

Cora must have been 90 years old, or possibly more – nobody knew for certain. She lived alone in a creaky, old house on a hilltop just outside of town. Her husband had been dead for 40 years, and her only son had disappeared a decade ago. No one visited her, at least not that I could ever recall.

One afternoon, my mother, feeling sorry for the old lady, told me to go check on her. I said I would, but I was afraid of the old house and the old lady, and had other things I would much rather do. I went fishing instead, and lied to my mother that Cora was fine.

A month later, a traveling salesman found Cora dead in her house. She had been gravely ill for some time, it seemed, but nobody had known. Possibly I could have helped her, if only I had listened to my mother that afternoon. Not a day goes by that don't I wish I had.

The next two questions are based on this passage.

13. Which of the following is the author's intent in the passage?

    A) To inform
    B) To entertain
    C) To persuade
    D) To express feelings

14. Which of the following are likely motives for the author?

    A) He wants the reader to despise him.
    B) He wants the reader to sympathize with him.
    C) He wants the reader to believe he should be punished.
    D) He wants the reader to believe his actions were justified.

Three candidates showed up for an interview. Of all the candidates, only one was appropriate for the job. The first candidate arrived promptly and was dressed professionally. She spoke articulately and seemed a good fit for the organization. The next candidate was also on time, but his dress shirt was stained, his tie was crooked, and he seemed to struggle with the standard interview questions. His performance during the interview was not as impressive as the first candidate's performance. The final candidate, dressed in a T-shirt and ripped jeans, arrived a full hour past the scheduled interview time. Because of her tardiness, we did not interview her.

The next two questions are based on this passage.

15. Which of the following text structures is used to organize the above passage?

    A) Cause-Effect
    B) Comparison-Contrast
    C) Problem-Solution
    D) Sequence

16. Which of the following sentences is most representative of a summary sentence for this passage?

    A) "Three candidates showed up for an interview."
    B) "Of all the candidates, only one was appropriate for the job."
    C) "His performance during the interview was not as impressive as the first candidate's performance."
    D) "Because of her tardiness, we did not interview her."

It is human nature to glorify past leaders, raising them to the level of heroes or demigods. However, closer inspection typically reveals these historical figures to be merely men – very often, flawed and unremarkable men, undeserving of their legends. That is not the case with George Washington.

While Washington was indeed a man, and not without flaws, close scrutiny validates his legend. He was not merely a man in the right place at the right time, swept along by the tide of current events. Rather, he was a man of extraordinary conviction and ability, someone who changed the fortunes of battle – and, by extension, the fortunes of a nation. It is not exaggeration to suggest that, had a different man stood in Washington's shoes, America as we know it might never have existed.

The next three questions are based on this passage.

17. Which of the following describes this type of writing?

    A) Persuasive
    B) Narrative
    C) Technical
    D) Expository

18. Which of the following statements accurately represents the historical context of this text?

    A) It was written during Washington's presidency. Because the author was writing about current events, he needed to sift through popular opinions about Washington to get to the truth.
    B) It was written right after Washington's presidency. Because not much time had passed, the author had a difficult time deciding how historically significant Washington's deeds were.
    C) It was written by a personal friend of Washington. Because of this, the author had a hard time being objective.
    D) It was written well after Washington's lifetime. Because of this, the author's main difficulty was deciding whether or not the legend of Washington's deeds had been inflated by the passage of time.

19. Which of the following indicates how the author would likely state his position on history?

A) History is most accurate when it comes from first-person accounts. Once those accounts are written down, they should not be re-evaluated.
B) It's important to periodically re-evaluate our impressions of history.
C) It's impossible to go back and see what really happened, so our understanding of history is quite limited.
D) Historical figures cannot be judged according to our modern values. They can only be judged according to the opinions of their peers.

20. Follow the numbered instructions to transform the starting word into a different word.

1. Start with the word "STARTING."
2. Remove both T's from the word.
3. Remove the letter G from the word.
4. Remove the letter R from the word.
5. Add the letter D to the end of the word.
6. Remove the letter I from the word.

What new word has been spelled?

A) SAND
B) SEND
C) STAR
D) SEAR

21. The Wall Street trader hated to hold his stocks overnight. Instead, his preferred technique was to <u>scalp</u>. Sometimes he held a stock for only a matter of minutes.

Based on context, which of the following is a definition for the underlined word in the sentences above?

A) A token of victory
B) To resell items at other-than-legal rates
C) To collect small profits from quick buying and selling
D) The skin and subcutaneous structure of the upper head

22. Chapter 11 Analyzing Nursery Rhymes
   - *Jack and Jill*
   - *Three Blind Mice*
   - *Macbeth*
   - *Three Men in a Tub*

Analyze the headings above. Which of the following is out of place?

A) *Jack and Jill*
B) *Three Blind Mice*
C) *Macbeth*
D) *Three Men in a Tub*

Map of Blackstone Recreational Area

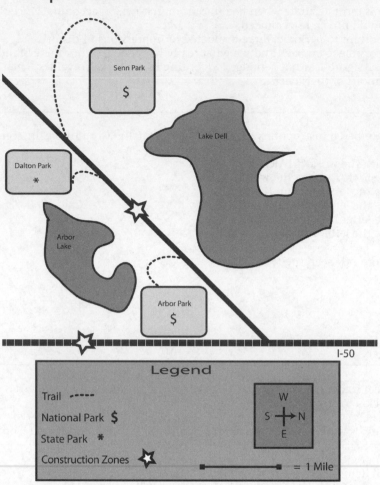

The next two questions are based on this map.

23. On any given day, the roadblocks in Blackstone Recreational Area may be open (allowing traffic through), or closed (blocking traffic). Today, both roadblocks are closed. If a driver arrives from the southwest on County Highway CV, which of the following can he visit?

A) Arbor Park
B) Dalton and Senn Parks
C) All three parks
D) None of the parks

24. On any given day, the roadblocks in Blackstone Recreational Area may be open (allowing traffic through), or closed (blocking traffic). Today, both roadblocks are closed. A driver appears on Interstate 50 traveling from north to south. This driver has not paid for a national parks license; therefore, she is only permitted to visit state parks. Which of the following describes the driver's situation?

A) She can visit a park today because no roadblocks will interfere with her route.
B) She can visit only one of the two state parks today because a roadblock blocks the other.
C) She cannot visit a park today because roadblocks prevent her from reaching any of the parks in the area.
D) She cannot visit a park today because the only park accessible from her starting point is a national park.

Pricing Chart: Cases of Cleaning Fluid

Store	Unit price (1 to 3 cases)	Unit price (4 to 10 cases)	Unit price (11+ cases)	Shipping and handling
Janitor Depot	$10.00	$9.00	$8.00	$30.00 total for any order
Hyperion Cleaning Supplies	$11.00	$10.00	$7.00	$40.00 total for any order
Southern Cleaning & Maintenance	$9.00	$8.00	$8.00	$30.00 for orders under $100.00; free for orders $100.00 or more
Maid Central	$10.00	$9.00	$8.00	$2.00 per case

The next two questions are based on this pricing chart.

25. A company in Oregon needs to purchase 15 cases of cleaning fluid. Which of the following stores will provide the best total order price?

   A) Southern Cleaning & Maintenance
   B) Hyperion Cleaning Supplies
   C) Janitor Depot
   D) Maid Central

26. As a back-to-school special, Janitor Depot is currently waiving shipping charges. Considering this information, which of the following stores will provide the best total price on 50 cases of cleaning fluid?

   A) Maid Central
   B) Janitor Depot
   C) Hyperion Cleaning Supplies
   D) Southern Cleaning & Maintenance

27.

> Maria –
>
> When feeding the cats, remember to use the **Kitten Formula XL**, not the Mr. Meow Factory Plus. Feed the cats small portions **twice a day**, as they will overeat if you try to feed them all at once. **Never** let Paws outside, as he likes to run away. And thank you for looking after them while I am on vacation.
>
> – Yolanda

The bold text in the above note indicates which of the following?

   A) Brand names
   B) Emphasis
   C) Commands
   D) Proper nouns

28. An individual is interested in placing an advertisement in a newspaper to sell his car. To which of the following departments of the newspaper should this person e-mail the information?

   A) Editorial
   B) Business
   C) Local news
   D) Classified

29.

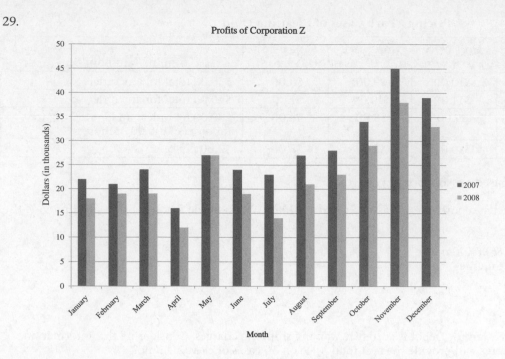

Profits of Corporation Z

Based on the chart above, which of the following is the approximate amount of money Corporation Z made in November of 2007?

A) $38.00
B) $45.00
C) $38,000.00
D) $45,000.00

30.

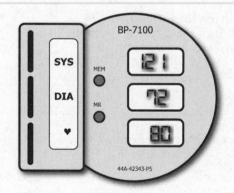

Based on the blood pressure monitor above, which of the following is the patient's pulse rate?

A)   44
B)   72
C)   80
D)   121

31.

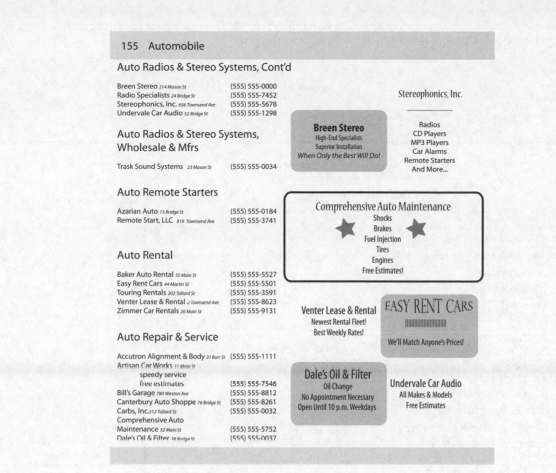

An individual wants to buy a remote starter for her car so she can let the car warm up while she's still inside her house. Which of the following is the number of businesses listed above that can sell her a remote starter?

A) 1
B) 2
C) 3
D) 4

32. Luu appeared <u>rapturous</u> when he received a C in chemistry; his mother, on the contrary, looked displeased.

Which of the following is the definition of the underlined word in the sentence above?

A) Rattled
B) Ecstatic
C) Dismayed
D) Ravenous

33. An aspiring author wants to be sure that her novel is properly formatted and wants to avoid making errors of which her English teacher would disapprove. Which of the following resources is most appropriate in this case?

A) *The Philadelphia Manual of Grammar Style*
B) "How to Plot a Breakthrough Novel"
C) *New Literary Horizons: A Journal of Contemporary Fiction*
D) *The Personal Web Site of Author Kevin Handel*

34. A student needs to review the description of flower parts for a test. To find out where this information is located in her biology textbook, which of the following will be most helpful?

A) Preface
B) Index
C) Appendix
D) Glossary

Abacus Accounting Software

Table of Contents

The next two questions are based on this table of contents.

35. A reader has just used the Abacus Accounting Software package to submit his taxes. Now he wants to verify that the IRS received his tax information. Based on the table of contents, in which of the following sections and subsections in Chapter 3 can he find this information?

A) Section A, subsection 2
B) Section A, subsection 3
C) Section B, subsection 1
D) Section B, subsection 5

36. A reader is having problems with the Abacus Accounting Software. Whenever he looks through his accounting tables, he sees a lot of empty spaces. In which of the following sections and subsections in Chapter 4 may he find an answer?

A) Section C, subsection 3
B) Section C, subsection 4
C) Section D, subsection 2
D) Section D, subsection 3

---

37.   Chapter 4: Valuable Gemstones

A. How to Identify Gold
B. How to Identify Emeralds
C. How to Identify Rubies
D. How to Identify Diamonds

Analyze the headings above. Which of the following headings is out of place?

A) How to Identify Gold
B) How to Identify Emeralds
C) How to Identify Rubies
D) How to Identify Diamonds

---

38. The palace guard was an impressive man. He held a ceremonial spear in one hand, a shield in the other. His uniform consisted of a silver helmet, dark pants, and an elaborate jacket that was held together with golden-threaded _frogs_ instead of buttons.

Based on the context of the passage above, which of the following is the definition of the underlined word?

A) A tailless amphibian
B) A hoarseness in the throat
C) An ornamental coat fastening
D) A device used to hold flower stems in position in a vase

---

39.   Flea Control Products for Cats

Product name	Manufacturer	Cost	Rating from a cat magazine's product review (out of 10)	Description
Barton Flea Collar	Barton	$5.00	5	Standard 2-ounce flea collar lasts a typical cat 3 months.
Champion Deluxe Flea Collar	Champion	$15.00	7	Heavy-duty 3-ounce flea collar lasts a typical cat 6 months. Guaranteed to not cause allergic reaction for pets or owners.
Super Flea Prevention Bath	Granville	$6.00	8	Bathe cat in this solution to prevent fleas for 4 months at a time.
Nordson Flea Inhibitor Spray	Nordson	$10.00	6	Spray on the back of the cat's neck to deter flea infestation. Enough sprays to last a typical cat 4 months.
Patton Flea Collar	Patton	$12.00	8	Standard 2-ounce flea collar lasts a typical cat 4 months.
Flea and Tick Control System	Redding	$7.00	7	Bathe cat in this solution to prevent fleas for 2 months at a time. Guaranteed to not cause allergic reaction for pets or owners.
ZenPet Flea Spray	ZenPet	$11.00	9	Spray on the back of the cat's neck to deter flea infestation. Enough sprays to last a typical cat 6 months.

A man has a cat that has developed a flea problem. He prefers a collarless solution that is inexpensive. Based on the chart above, which of the following companies manufactures the best option for this cat owner?

A)   Barton
B)   Granville
C)   Redding
D)   ZenPet

40.   A young boy has an allergy to all types of nuts. Which of the following candy bars is safe for him?

A)   Indulge Bar – Ingredients: dark chocolate, cocoa butter, skim milk, corn syrup, sugar, soy protein, peanut butter, artificial flavor
B)   Chocolate Extreme – Ingredients: milk chocolate, cocoa butter, raisins, skim milk, corn syrup, chopped pecans, sugar, soy protein, artificial flavor
C)   Vanilla Blast – Ingredients: white chocolate, whey protein, skim milk, vanilla flavor, almond extract, corn syrup, sugar, soy protein
D)   Chocolate Crunch – Ingredients: milk chocolate, rice puffs, skim milk, corn syrup, sugar, soy protein, malt powder, soybean oil, artificial flavor

41. A customer at an electronics store is describing to a salesperson the ideal computer for her. The following is a list of the customer's criteria:

- Dual-core processor
- Dedicated graphics system
- Minimum 400 gigabyte hard drive
- G speed wireless connectivity

Which of the following is an appropriate choice for this customer?

A)

Processor:	2.5 ghz dual core
Graphics Subsystem:	Dedicated
Front-Side Bus:	800 ghz
Hard drive:	800 gigabytes
Memory:	6 gigabytes
Connectivity:	Wireless G, optional cellular modem

B)

Processor:	3 ghz dual core
Graphics Subsystem:	Dedicated
Front-Side Bus:	800 ghz
Hard drive:	750 gigabytes
Memory:	4 gigabytes
Connectivity:	Wireless B, optional cellular modem

C)

Processor:	2.5 ghz dual core
Graphics Subsystem:	Dedicated
Front-Side Bus:	600 ghz
Hard drive:	350 gigabytes
Memory:	4 gigabytes
Connectivity:	Wireless G, optional cellular modem

D)

Processor:	3 ghz single core
Graphics Subsystem:	Dedicated
Front-Side Bus:	600 ghz
Hard drive:	750 gigabytes
Memory:	6 gigabytes
Connectivity:	Wireless G, optional cellular modem

42. As an incentive to purchase a computer from his store, the salesperson offered additional software to the customer at no additional cost. Which of the following is an appropriate resource for the customer to obtain detailed information about this software and instructions for its use?

A) An online encyclopedia
B) Computer owner's manual
C) Software developer's Web site
D) Computer manufacturer's technical support line

Section 2. MATHEMATICS	Number of Scored Questions: 30
	Recommended Time Limit for Practice Test: 45 minutes*

*The proctored TEAS® has an additional four unscored questions for a total of 34 mathematics questions. The time limit on the proctored mathematics portion is 51 minutes.

1. $\frac{4}{5} \div \frac{8}{15}$

    Simplify the expression above. Which of the following is correct?

    A) $\frac{2}{3}$
    B) 1
    C) $1\frac{1}{2}$
    D) $1\frac{2}{3}$

2. A model car is scaled to a 1:25 scale. If the model car measures 7 inches (in) from bumper to bumper, which of the following is the length of the actual version of the vehicle?

    A) 100 in
    B) 118 in
    C) 132 in
    D) 175 in

3. A population decreases from 404 million to 288 million. Which of the following is the percent decrease of the population? (Round the solution to the nearest tenth of a percent.)

    A) 2.9%
    B) 3.5%
    C) 28.7%
    D) 71.3%

4. Which of the following is the number of inches in $2\frac{1}{2}$ yards? (Note: 1 yard = 3 feet; 1 foot = 12 inches.)

    A) 7
    B) 14
    C) 30
    D) 90

5. A penny must be measured to the nearest $\frac{1}{32}$ of an inch. Which of the following is the most appropriate measurement tool for this task?

    A) Caliper
    B) Ruler
    C) Scale
    D) Pipette

6. If a person weighs about 220 pounds, which of the following is the person's approximate weight in metric measurement? (Note: 1 kilogram ≈ 2.2 pounds.)

   A) 2.2 grams
   B) 100 grams
   C) 100 kilograms
   D) 440 kilograms

7. During an 8-hour shift, a quality inspector finds three defective CD players in the 135 players that are inspected. Based on this rate, if a shipment of 900 CD players will be sent to retailers at the end of the week, which of the following is the number of them that may be defective?

   A) 13
   B) 18
   C) 20
   D) 45

8. A coat was marked down to 15% of its original price, which made the new price $18.00. Which of the following was the original price of the coat?

   A) $27.00
   B) $83.00
   C) $120.00
   D) $270.00

9. A nursing student is purchasing books and supplies for the semester. A set of scrubs for clinicals is $27.95, a math textbook is $150.25, a beginning nursing textbook is $215.16, and an anatomy textbook is $195.15. Which of the following is an accurate estimate of the cost for the semester?

   A) $580.00
   B) $700.00
   C) $830.00
   D) $900.00

10. 7,535 – 72

    Simplify the expression above. Which of the following is correct?

    A) 7,443
    B) 7,463
    C) 7,543
    D) 7,563

11. Which of the following is the decimal equivalent of 3.2%?

    A) 0.032
    B) 3.2
    C) 32.0
    D) 320.0

12. In a baseball tournament, a boy hit the ball 11 out of 15 times he was at bat. Which of the following is the decimal equivalent for the boy's average?

    A) 0.733
    B) 1.36
    C) 4.0
    D) 26.0

13. Write the number 1910 in Roman numerals.

    A) MCMX
    B) IXXX
    C) MMCX
    D) MDCCCCX

14. $(x - 7)(2x + 1)$

    Simplify the expression above. Which of the following is correct?

    A) $2x^2 - 7$
    B) $3x - 7$
    C) $2x^2 - 13x - 7$
    D) $2x^2 + 15x - 7$

15. As the seasons change, the temperature outside changes.

    Which of the following is the dependent variable in the event described above?

    A) Temperature
    B) Season of the year
    C) Winter
    D) Summer

16.

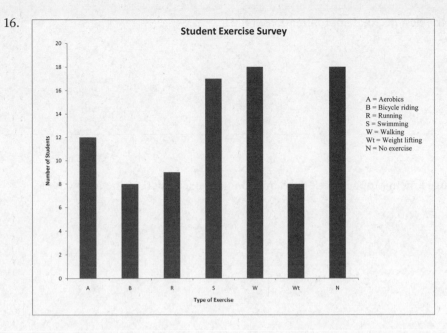

Student Exercise Survey

A = Aerobics
B = Bicycle riding
R = Running
S = Swimming
W = Walking
Wt = Weight lifting
N = No exercise

The graph above represents the results of a survey of 90 students regarding the types of exercise in which they regularly participate.

Which of the following is the percent of the surveyed students that reported that they walk regularly?

A) 0.18%
B) 0.20%
C) 18%
D) 20%

17. A certified medical assistant receives $1,460.16 each pay period. The deductions per pay period are: federal tax $136.21, federal insurance $76.68, state tax $106.24, retirement plan $50.00, and health insurance $89.51. Which of the following is the take-home pay per pay period?

A) $271.44
B) $839.28
C) $996.60
D) $1,001.52

18. Reconcile this checking account for the month of May 2009. The previous balance was $853.91. Deposits were made for $1,910.15. Checks were written for $1,339.11. There is a returned check charge of $35.00. Which of the following is the balance after reconciling this account?

A) $1,354.95
B) $1,389.95
C) $1,424.95
D) $1,459.95

19. Which of the following numbers is the best decimal approximation of 8.2?

    A) $\sqrt{10}$
    B) $\sqrt{17}$
    C) $\sqrt{67}$
    D) $\sqrt{79}$

20. $3\frac{3}{4} + 2\frac{5}{6}$

    Simplify the expression above. Change any improper fractions to mixed numbers. Which of the following is correct?

    A) $2\frac{1}{5}$

    B) $4\frac{3}{5}$

    C) $5\frac{1}{2}$

    D) $6\frac{7}{12}$

21. $|x-8| < 7$

    Solve the inequality above. Which of the following is correct?

    A) $x < 1$ or $x > 15$
    B) $1 < x < 15$
    C) $x < 1$
    D) $x < 15$

22. $-\frac{28}{3}, -9.1, -\frac{15}{2}, -9$

    Arrange the numbers above from greatest to least. Which of the following is correct?

    A) $-\frac{15}{2}, -9, -9.1, -\frac{28}{3}$

    B) $-\frac{28}{3}, -9.1, -9, -\frac{15}{2}$

    C) $-9.1, -9, -\frac{28}{3}, -\frac{15}{2}$

    D) $-9, -9.1, \frac{15}{2}, -\frac{28}{3}$

23. $10 \div 2 \cdot 5 + (3 - 8 + 2) + 2^3$

    Simply the expression above. Which of the following is correct?

    A) 6
    B) 26
    C) 28
    D) 30

24. The local shoe store is having a buy one pair of shoes get the second pair, of equal or lesser value, for half off sale. A customer wants to purchase a pair of shoes for $79.95 and a second pair that is priced at $54.95. Which of the following is the cost of both pairs?

    A) $67.45
    B) $94.93
    C) $107.43
    D) $134.90

25. $2(x + 1) = 3x - 1$

    Solve the equation above. Which of the following is correct?

    A) $x = \dfrac{3}{5}$
    B) $x = 2$
    C) $x = 3$
    D) $x = 8$

26. A fisherman wants to present his yearly catch totals in terms of the number and types of fish he caught. Which of the following graphs is most appropriate for the fisherman to use?

    A) Line graph
    B) Pie chart
    C) Scatterplot
    D) Bar graph

27. 0.013×0.04

    Simplify the expression above. Which of the following is correct?

    A) 0.00052
    B) 0.0052
    C) 0.052
    D) 52

28. One number, y, is 3 more than $\dfrac{1}{2}$ of another number, x.

    Which of the following algebraic equations correctly represents the sentence above?

    A) $y = \dfrac{1}{2}(x + 3)$

    B) $y = \dfrac{1}{2}x + 3$

    C) $x = \dfrac{1}{2}y + 3$

    D) $y + 3 = \dfrac{1}{2}x$

29. A graduating class of nurses is planning a 1-day workshop, and 125 nurses have registered so far. Each nurse will receive a notebook, pen, logo bag, and flash drive. The supply company charges $1.75 for notebooks, $1.25 for pens, $3.25 for bags, and $5.85 for flash drives. Which of the following will be the cost of supplies for this workshop?

    A) $1,501.40
    B) $1,512.50
    C) $1,523.75
    D) $1,546.25

30. A young couple is buying their first home for $183,500. A contractor gave them a $12,335 bid for needed renovations. Which of the following will be the actual cost of their home if they make the renovations?

    A) $171,165
    B) $171,265
    C) $195,835
    D) $196,835

<table>
<tr><td rowspan="2">Section 3. SCIENCE</td><td>Number of Scored Questions: 48</td></tr>
<tr><td>Recommended Time Limit for Practice Test: 59 minutes*</td></tr>
</table>

*The proctored TEAS® has an additional six unscored questions for a total of 54 science questions. The time limit on the proctored science portion is 66 minutes.

Periodic Table of the Elements

1																	18
IA	2											13	14	15	16	17	0
1 H	IIA												IIIA	IVA	VA	VIA	VIIA	2 He
3 Li	4 Be	3	4	5	6	7	8	9	10	11	12		5 B	6 C	7 N	8 O	9 F	10 Ne
11 Na	12 Mg	IIIB	IVB	VB	VIB	VIIB	[	- VIIIB -	]	IB	IIB	13 Al	14 Si	15 P	16 S	17 Cl	18 Ar
19 K	20 Ca	21 Sc	22 Ti	23 V	24 Cr	25 Mn	26 Fe	27 Co	28 Ni	29 Cu	30 Zn	31 Ga	32 Ge	33 As	34 Se	35 Br	36 Kr
37 Rb	38 Sr	39 Y	40 Zr	41 Nb	42 Mo	43 Tc	44 Ru	45 Rh	46 Pd	47 Ag	48 Cd	49 In	50 Sn	51 Sb	52 Te	53 I	54 Xe
55 Cs	56 Ba	71 Lu	72 Hf	73 Ta	74 W	75 Re	76 Os	77 Ir	78 Pt	79 Au	80 Hg	81 Tl	82 Pb	83 Bi	84 Po	85 At	86 Rn
87 Fr	88 Ra	103 Lr	104 Unq	105 Unp	106 Unh	107 Uns	108 Uno	109 Une									

Lanthanide Series	57 La	58 Ce	59 Pr	60 Nd	61 Pm	62 Sm	63 Eu	64 Gd	65 Tb	66 Dy	67 Ho	68 Er	69 Tm	70 Yb
Actinide Series	89 Ac	90 Th	91 Pa	92 U	93 Np	94 Pu	95 Am	96 Cm	97 Bk	98 Cf	99 Es	100 Fm	101 Md	102 No

1. Which of the following indicates the number of neutrons and electrons for a neutral isotope of iridium (Ir) that has a mass number of 191?

A) 77 neutrons and 114 electrons
B) 114 neutrons and 77 electrons
C) 191 neutrons and 114 electrons
D) 191 neutrons and 77 electrons

2. When examining electronegativity values, which of the following atoms will form the least polar bond with hydrogen (H)?

A) Hydrogen (H)
B) Fluorine (Fl)
C) Chlorine (Cl)
D) Bromine (Br)

3. Which of the following elements is the best electrical conductor?

A) Bromine (Br)
B) Arsenic (As)
C) Carbon (C)
D) Potassium (K)

4. A large saturated hydrocarbon will contain

   A) the same number of hydrogen atoms as carbon atoms.
   B) exactly twice as many hydrogen atoms as carbon atoms.
   C) less than twice as many hydrogen atoms as carbon atoms.
   D) more than twice as many hydrogen atoms as carbon atoms.

5.

Soil sample		
Nutrient	Sample 1	Sample 2
Nitrates	Yes	Yes
Phosphates	Yes	No

A student is testing the materials in two different soil samples. Which of the following assumptions can be inferred from the data presented in the table above?

   A) Different soils contain different nutrients.
   B) Sample 1 is the best soil.
   C) Nitrates are more frequently found in soil than are phosphates.
   D) Most plants thrive in nitrate-rich soil.

6. _____ are at a higher taxonomic level of organization than _____.

   Which of the following completes the sentence above?

   A) Organs; organ systems
   B) Cells; molecules
   C) Atoms; molecules
   D) Tissues; organs

7. Which of the following is considered least useful in conducting quantitative scientific research?

   A) Modeling data
   B) Applying empirical formulas
   C) Using highly precise measurement tools
   D) Recording qualitative observations

8. Which of the following is needed for cellular waste recycling?

   A) Centrosome
   B) Lysosome
   C) Chromosome
   D) Golgi apparatus

9. A researcher wishes to test the hypothesis that soy is a superior diet compared to whole wheat for the reproductive purposes of a certain type of beetle. Which of the following describes how the researcher should best test this hypothesis?

   A)   Record the number of eggs recovered from a single culture reared on soy versus a single culture reared on whole wheat.
   B)   Count the eggs recovered from 10 separate cultures reared on soy versus a single culture on whole wheat.
   C)   Compare the eggs from 10 soy cultures versus 10 whole-wheat cultures.
   D)   Record the eggs from one soy culture versus 10 whole-wheat cultures.

10. Which of the following systems includes organs between the mouth and anus?

   A)   Respiratory
   B)   Digestive
   C)   Endocrine
   D)   Skeletal

11. Which of the following describes how a Punnett square can help predict the genotype of the offspring if the alleles of both parents are known?

   A)   Provides information on dominant traits in the parents
   B)   Shows what genotypes are possible in the offspring
   C)   Provides probabilities of getting an incomplete dominance
   D)   Shows exactly what genotypes will occur in the offspring

12. A substance with a pH of 7.0 when dissolved in water is

   A)   a strong acid.
   B)   a weak base.
   C)   a weak acid.
   D)   a neutral substance.

13. Which of the following by-products of cellular respiration is used by autotrophs in the production of glucose?

   A)   ATP
   B)   Carbon dioxide
   C)   Chlorophyll
   D)   Oxygen

14. A certain disease is carried on the allele (a) which is recessive the normal condition (A). If a normal (AA) male mates with a female who has the disease (aa), which of the following is the percentage of offspring that are carriers of the disease?

   A)   0%
   B)   25%
   C)   75%
   D)   100%

15.

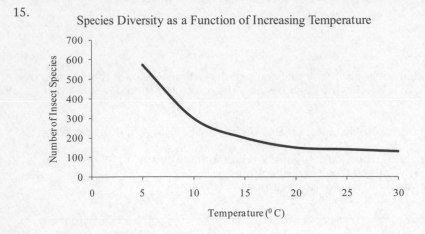

Species Diversity as a Function of Increasing Temperature

Based on the diagram above, which of the following describes the correlation between the diversity of insect species and temperature?

A) Direct
B) Scattered
C) Inverse
D) Linear

16. The pancreas is a component of which of the following systems?

A) Lymphatic
B) Nervous
C) Endocrine
D) Muscular

17. Which of the following types of bonds is primarily responsible for base pairing in complementary strands of DNA?

A) Ionic
B) Covalent
C) Dative
D) Hydrogen

18. A cell uses which of the following as the first-line defense against mutations during DNA replication?

A) Cell death
B) Excision repair
C) Mismatch repair
D) DNA polymerase proofreading

19. After passing through the stomach, food continues into which of the following structures?

A) Duodenum
B) Jejunum
C) Ileum
D) Cecum

20. Suppose a 2-kilogram mass is traveling at 3 meters/second. Which of the following is the object's kinetic energy (KE)?

    A)   3 Joules
    B)   6 Joules
    C)   9 Joules
    D)   18 Joules

21. Three different liquids with different densities were placed together in a container as shown. The liquids, when stirred and allowed to resettle, returned to the same arrangement.

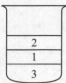

    Which of the following statements is true about these liquids?

    A)   Liquid 1 has a lower density than Liquid 2.
    B)   Liquid 1 has a higher density than Liquid 2.
    C)   Liquid 3 has a lower density than Liquid 1.
    D)   Liquid 2 has a higher density than Liquid 3.

22. Which of the following is the term given to multiple forms of a gene that are produced by mutation?

    A)   Adaptation
    B)   DNA
    C)   Allele
    D)   Natural selection

23. During mitosis and cell division, spindle fibers are associated with which of the following organelles?

    A)   Centrosomes
    B)   Lysosomes
    C)   Mitochondria
    D)   Vacuoles

24. In which of the following parts of the gastrointestinal tract does the absorption of water primarily occur?

    A)   Stomach
    B)   Small intestine
    C)   Cecum
    D)   Colon

25. During which of the following stages of development do individual tissue layers begin to form?

    A)   Embryo formation
    B)   Zygote development
    C)   Gastrulation
    D)   Differentiation

26. Which of the following represents the number of different cells formed upon completion of meiosis II?

    A)   1
    B)   2
    C)   3
    D)   4

27. Which of the following is a property of bases?

    A)   Tastes sour
    B)   Dissolves metal
    C)   Turns blue litmus paper red
    D)   Liberates OH^- in solution

28. During which of the following stages of interphase is mRNA synthesized?

    A) G^1
    B)   Prophase
    C)   S
    D)   M

29. A harmful example of a catalytic reaction involves the breakdown of ozone by the use of _____ .

    Which of the following correctly completes the sentence above?

    A)   chlorine ions
    B)   fluorine ions
    C)   manganese dioxide
    D)   rhodium

30. Phenotypes are seen due to the production of _____ from the genotypic code found in the cell nucleus.

    Which of the following correctly completes the statement above?

    A)   Cell membranes
    B)   Golgi bodies
    C)   Lysosomes
    D)   Proteins

31. Receiving a vaccination against a particular disease results in which of the following types of immunity?

    A)   Passive
    B)   Active
    C)   Humoral
    D)   Cell-mediated

32. The veins of the upper part of the body are responsible for transporting blood to which of the following areas of the heart?

    A) Superior vena cava
    B) Inferior vena cava
    C) Ascending aorta
    D) Descending aorta

33. The spleen and thoracic duct are parts of which of the following systems?

    A) Endocrine
    B) Reproductive
    C) Lymphatic
    D) Urinary

34. Nucleotides are to DNA as amino acids are to _____ .

    Which of the following correctly completes the sentence above?

    A) proteins
    B) ribosomes
    C) RNA
    D) cells

35. Which of the following taxonomic ranks is the most specific?

    A) Class
    B) Domain
    C) Kingdom
    D) Species

36. For a given substance, the gas phase (compared to the liquid phase) is considered to have _____ intermolecular attractions and to exist at _____ temperatures.

    Which of the following correctly completes the sentence above?

    A) weaker; higher
    B) weaker; lower
    C) stronger; higher
    D) stronger, lower

37. Which of the following pulls air into the body during inspiration?

    A) Diaphragm
    B) Trachea
    C) Bronchioles
    D) Pleura

38. Which of the following is the chemical formula for octyne?

    A) C_8H_{12}
    B) C_8H_{14}
    C) C_8H_{16}
    D) C_8H_{18}

39. A culture for the flour beetle *Tribolium confusum* was started with 10 males and 10 females in a 20-milliliter flask. Over a period of time, the beetle population increased to 940 insects, after which, the number remained constant for several days, followed by an increase in the death rate.

    Which of the following is a reasonable hypothesis related to this experiment?

    A) The population is controlled by density-dependent factors.
    B) The population is controlled by density-independent factors.
    C) The male beetles have a shorter life span than the female beetles.
    D) The female beetles have a shorter life span than the male beetles.

40. Which of the following describes how inhibitors affect the reaction rate of enzymes?

    A) They cause violent collisions, which in turn, cause the substrate molecule to break.
    B) They have little to no affect on reaction rates.
    C) They block the active sites of the substrate, causing greatly reduced activity.
    D) They cause reverse reactions to act similarly to forward reactions so that equilibrium is maintained.

41. _____ CH_4 + _____ O_2 → _____ CO_2 + _____ H_2O

    Which of the following correctly balances the combustion reaction above?

    A) $CH_4 + O_2 \rightarrow CO_2 + H_2O$
    B) $CH_4 + 3O \rightarrow CO + 2H_2O$
    C) $CH_4 + O_2 \rightarrow CO_2 + 2H_2O$
    D) $CH_4 + 2O_2 \rightarrow CO_2 + 2H_2O$

42. Water's _____ bonding results in a _____ ratio of hydrogen to oxygen.

    Which of the following correctly completes the sentence above?

    A) ionic; 1:2
    B) ionic; 2:1
    C) covalent; 1:2
    D) covalent; 2:1

43. During which of the following processes does RNA relay information to the ribosomes?

    A) Translation
    B) Transcription
    C) Mitosis
    D) Double-helix formation

44. In which of the following is urine stored?

    A) Ureter
    B) Prostate
    C) Bladder
    D) Kidneys

45. In a medication study, population A is given the medication, and population B is given a placebo. Which of the following describes population B?

    A) Control group
    B) Treatment group
    C) Dependent variable
    D) Independent variable

46. A boy is throwing a baseball at a target. The baseball travels at 15 miles per hour (mph) during his first throw and 30 mph during his second throw. Which of the following statements correctly compares the energy of the baseball in these two situations?

    A) The kinetic energy of the second throw is twice that of the first throw.
    B) The kinetic energy of the second throw is four times that of the first throw.
    C) The potential energy of the second throw is twice that of the first throw.
    D) The potential energy of the second throw is four times that of the first throw.

47. A researcher predicts that nursing students who have taken extensive science courses will score significantly higher on their national licensing exams, when compared to nursing students who have only taken required science courses. This prediction corresponds with which of the following steps in the scientific method?

    A) Formulating a hypothesis
    B) Conducting an experiment
    C) Analyzing the results
    D) Drawing a conclusion

48. Which of the following organs produces bile that begins the breakdown of fats?

    A) Gallbladder
    B) Liver
    C) Pancreas
    D) Kidneys

Section 4. ENGLISH AND LANGUAGE USAGE	Number of Scored Questions: 30
	Recommended Time Limit for Practice Test: 30 minutes*

*The proctored TEAS® has an additional four unscored questions for a total of 34 English and language usage questions. The time limit on the proctored English and language usage portion is 34 minutes.

1. Which of the following is an example of a correctly punctuated sentence?

   A) I asked her "Since when are you an Elvis fan?"
   B) I asked her "since when are you an Elvis fan"?
   C) I asked her, "Since when are you an Elvis fan?"
   D) I asked her, "Since when are you an Elvis fan"?

2. Which of the following is an example of a simple sentence?

   A) The man wandering into the store.
   B) The man in the green overalls with the steel-toed boots wandered into the upscale department store.
   C) The man in the green overalls with the steel-toed boots wandering into the upscale department store.
   D) The man in the green overalls with the steel-toed boots had wandered into the upscale department stores as if he felt perfectly at home there.

3. The PTA held _____ annual fundraiser.

   Which of the following correctly completes the sentence above?

   A) its
   B) there
   C) their
   D) it's

4. It was hoped that the lines for the roller coaster would be shorter in the afternoon.

   Which of the following changes the sentence above so that it is written in the active rather than in the passive voice?

   A) In the afternoon, it was hoped that the lines would be shorter.
   B) She hoped that the lines for the roller coaster would be shorter in the afternoon.
   C) It was expected that the lines for the roller coaster would be shorter in the afternoon.
   D) It was hoped by her that the lines for the roller coaster would be shorter in the afternoon.

5. Which of the following is correctly punctuated?

   A) Due to the time-sensitive nature of the request the lawyer faxed the document to the judge.
   B) Due to the time-sensitive nature of the request. The lawyer had faxed the document to the judge.
   C) Due to the time-sensitive nature of the request, the lawyer faxed the document to the judge.
   D) Due to the time-sensitive nature of the request; the lawyer had faxed the document to the judge.

6. Which of the following phrases follows the rules of capitalization?

   A) English language
   B) professor Henry
   C) History class
   D) Christmas day

7. Because of his credulous nature, they took advantage of him and tricked him time and time again.

   Which of the following is the meaning of the word *credulous* as used in the sentence above?

   A) Dependable and responsible
   B) Easily cheated or fooled
   C) Believable and trustworthy
   D) Socially popular and outgoing

8. In the eastern part of Kansas, after the tornado last summer, governor Stevens declared a state of emergency.

   Which of the following words in the sentence above should be capitalized?

   A) state
   B) eastern
   C) summer
   D) governor

9. Which of the following sentences provides an example of correct subject-verb agreement?

   A) The group of children are ecstatic that Santa is coming to visit.
   B) The family, after hearing the weather report, agree to postpone the trip.
   C) The committee, upon reviewing the budget, votes to increase sales tax.
   D) The couple decide to leave the restaurant after waiting more than an hour to be seated.

10. The puppy has lost ____ way home, and ____ getting dark.

    Which of the following sets of words should be used to fill in the blanks in the sentence above?

    A) its; its
    B) it's; it's
    C) it's; its
    D) its; it's

11. I hope that the <u>choir</u> in the front row sits down soon; I cannot see the concert because _____ blocking my view.

    Which of the following is the correct pronoun and verb for the sentence above? The antecedent of the pronoun to be added is underlined.

    A) it is
    B) they are
    C) their
    D) its

12. Which of the following is an example of a correctly punctuated sentence?

    A) I was planning to stop by the grocery store, however, I realized that my tire had gone flat.
    B) I was planning to stop by the grocery store, however; I realized that my tire had gone flat.
    C) I was planning to stop by the grocery store however, I realized that my tire had gone flat.
    D) I was planning to stop by the grocery store; however, I realized that my tire had gone flat.

13. Which of the following sentences contains the appropriate use of an apostrophe?

    A)   The Malone's are coming over for dinner this evening.
    B)   The storm was beginning to rear it's ugly head.
    C)   The players on the soccer team left they're sports equipment all over the gym.
    D)   The group of employees arranged to have flowers delivered on Boss's Day.

14. The client made an appointment with a cosmetic surgeon to discuss possible rhinoplasty.

    In the sentence above, the prefix *rhino-* in the word *rhinoplasty* indicates that this client is interested in cosmetic surgery related to which of the following?

    A)   Eyes
    B)   Chin
    C)   Forehead
    D)   Nose

15. Which of the following sentences in the set of instructions below is an example of third-person voice?

    A)   To begin with, one should have a loaf of very fresh bread.
    B)   Remove the twist-tie, take out two pieces of bread, and set them aside.
    C)   Then, you should use a knife to spread one tablespoon of peanut butter on one side of the pieces of bread.
    D)   Finally, I place the unbuttered slice of bread on top of the buttered slice.

16. Which of the following words is written correctly?

    A)   pro-active
    B)   antiinflammatory
    C)   un-American
    D)   re-active

17. Which of the following nouns is written in the correct plural form?

    A)   data
    B)   crisises
    C)   diagnosises
    D)   mooses

18. I lost my book bag. My book bag contained my lunch money. I was very hungry. I had a difficult time staying awake in class that afternoon.

    Which of the following options best uses grammar for style and clarity to combine the sentences above?

    A)   I was very hungry because I lost my book bag. It contained my lunch money, and it was difficult to stay awake in class that afternoon.
    B)   Because I lost my book bag that contained my lunch money, I was very hungry in the afternoon and had a difficult time staying awake in class.
    C)   It was difficult to stay awake in class that afternoon, because I lost my lunch money. It was in my book bag, and I was very hungry.
    D)   My book bag contained my lunch money, and I lost it. I was so hungry that afternoon that I had a difficult time staying awake in class.

19. Because the thief broke his ankle during the robbery, he was unable to abscond with the cash.

Which of the following is the meaning *of abscond* as it is used in the sentence above?

A)   remain
B)   return
C)   confess
D)   escape

20. Which of the following is an example of a grammatically correct sentence?

A)   I cannot remember who I lent the book to.
B)   I cannot remember to who I lent the book.
C)   I cannot remember to whom I lent the book.
D)   I cannot remember whom lent me the book.

21. Which of the following phrases follows the rules of capitalization?

A)   uncle Elson
B)   your Mother
C)   my cousin Michelle
D)   his Aunt

22. The woman's arm ached badly after playing tennis for 3 hours.

The word *badly* serves as which of the following types of speech in the sentence above?

A)   Adjective
B)   Adverb
C)   Verb
D)   Possessive

23. She interviewed for two jobs; however, she accepted the second job, as it offered a higher _____.

Which of the following is the correct completion of the sentence above?

A)   sallary
B)   salery
C)   salary
D)   sallery

24. Which of the following is an example of a complex sentence?

A)   I so enjoy riding my bike.
B)   When I ride my bike along a country lane, I feel a harmony with the world around me.
C)   That harmony does not reveal itself to me in the same way at other times or during other tasks.
D)   The simplicity of the movement and the peacefulness of the countryside offers serenity.

25. Which of the following sentences contains a correct example of subject-verb agreement?

    A) One of the children are hungry.
    B) The coach, as well as her team, are nervous about the game.
    C) Either of the options are correct.
    D) The lady with her dogs walks every morning.

26. The woman who lives in the last house on our street is _____

    Which of the following allows the above sentence to be completed as a simple sentence?

    A) reclusive and is rarely seen outside of her home.
    B) reclusive, and we have actually never seen her.
    C) very cheerful, despite the fact that neighbors say she is strange.
    D) very cheerful because her son is coming home from college today.

27. Although I have not had much practice, I feel _____ in my ability to train the puppy.

    Which of the following is the correctly spelled word to complete the sentence?

    A) confidante
    B) confidents
    C) confident
    D) confidense

28. Which of the following sentences is most clear and correct?

    A) The kittens were found when they were 6 weeks old by the couple.
    B) The couple found the kittens when they were 6 weeks old.
    C) The couple found the kittens at the age of 6 weeks.
    D) Six weeks old, the couple found the kittens.

29. Which of the following sentences contains an example of correct subject-verb agreement?

    A) My sister or my brother is picking me up from school today.
    B) Neither my mom nor I are attending the concert.
    C) Mary and Tom is arriving around 5 o'clock this evening.
    D) Each of the girls play the piano well.

30. The child enjoyed watching the _____ dogs at the petting zoo.

    Which of the following words correctly completes the sentence above?

    A) prarie
    B) prairie
    C) prayer
    D) prairy

SOLUTIONS TO PRACTICE TEST 2

READING	MATHEMATICS	SCIENCE	ENGLISH AND LANGUAGE USAGE
1. A	1. C	1. B	1. C
2. C	2. D	2. A	2. B
3. B	3. C	3. D	3. A
4. D	4. D	4. D	4. B
5. A	5. A	5. A	5. C
6. B	6. C	6. B	6. A
7. D	7. C	7. D	7. B
8. D	8. C	8. B	8. D
9. A	9. A	9. C	9. C
10. A	10. B	10. B	10. D
11. B	11. A	11. B	11. A
12. C	12. A	12. D	12. D
13. D	13. A	13. B	13. D
14. B	14. C	14. D	14. D
15. B	15. A	15. C	15. A
16. A	16. D	16. C	16. C
17. A	17. D	17. D	17. A
18. D	18. B	18. D	18. B
19. B	19. C	19. A	19. D
20. A	20. D	20. C	20. C
21. C	21. B	21. B	21. C
22. C	22. A	22. C	22. B
23. B	23. D	23. A	23. C
24. D	24. C	24. D	24. B
25. A	25. C	25. C	25. D
26. C	26. D	26. D	26. A
27. B	27. A	27. D	27. C
28. D	28. B	28. A	28. B
29. D	29. B	29. A	29. A
30. C	30. C	30. D	30. B
31. C		31. B	
32. B		32. A	
33. A		33. C	
34. B		34. A	
35. D		35. D	
36. C		36. A	
37. A		37. A	
38. C		38. B	
39. B		39. A	
40. D		40. C	
41. A		41. D	
42. C		42. D	
		43. A	
		44. C	
		45. A	
		46. B	
		47. A	
		48. B	

READING
SOLUTIONS TO PRACTICE TEST 2

1. A   Remember that the reader does not need to agree with the logical conclusion; the logical conclusion only needs to be logical in the context of the ideas in the text.

    Options B and C are not conclusions, even though the writer is clearly implying the existence of an alien encounter. Both options B and C summarize a few ideas from the text, but neither tries to wrap up the ideas in a conclusive statement. Option D is a conclusion, but it is not the logical conclusion of the text. It is an example of using personal knowledge or opinions to draw the conclusion, rather than drawing the conclusion solely from what is written in the text.

    A logical conclusion follows directly from the text. To deduce that option A is the author's main point in this passage, the reader must decide what is being implied, but not specifically stated, by the author. After identifying the logical conclusion, the reader can make a decision about whether or not that conclusion is worthwhile.

2. C   Based on the information presented in the article, the craft in the army hangar is a UFO. The pilot mentioned in the article shot the UFO down, and the army is trying to cover up the story.

    The writer never explicitly refers to the wrecked craft as a UFO, never states that the pilot shot the UFO down, and never states that the army is attempting to cover things up; however, all of these conclusions are strongly implied by the writer though the details of the text.

    Option A summarizes a few items from the text, but it is not a conclusion. Option B concludes that the army is building UFO-type aircraft itself. While this is an interesting idea, none of the article's details point directly to that conclusion.

    Option D concludes that, whatever the wreckage is, the army has the right to keep it secret. This may be a valid point, but it is not the logical conclusion of the article. The article is trying to convince the reader that a UFO is being held at an army base.

3. B   When determining opinion versus fact, words such as *seemed* can be used as clues for the reader. The author is intending for the reader to understand that this statement is a personal conclusion based on the actions of the pilot. Options A, C, and D are facts, as they can be confirmed by an independent source.

4. D   It is the author's intent to persuade with this last paragraph of the passage. The reader can infer from the use of the quote "mind his own business" that the army base has something to hide, even though the author does not state this specifically. This passage is not an example of narrative, expository, or technical writing.

5. A   The article's claims are farfetched, and much of the information comes from potentially unreliable sources: residents with wild stories, a not-very-official-sounding statement from an unnamed military official, and a reporter (again unnamed) who describes something straight out of a science fiction novel. Based on the strangeness of the story, and also the lack of concrete, well-respected sources, the reader may safely assume that this magazine doesn't place a high priority on checking its facts.

6. B   All three sources claim to have personally seen or experienced events that are related to the article. Eyewitness accounts are considered primary sources.

7. D   The topic of the article is UFOs. The main idea is that a UFO (or UFOs) recently visited a New Mexico town, and that the government knows something about it. Most of the article consists of (admittedly implausible) supporting details that elaborate upon this main idea.

    There are several themes of the passage: paranormal events, aliens, conspiracies, and cover-ups. Themes are topics that, while not the central focus of the article, are raised along the way.

8. D   Since the student did not get at least three identical test grades, she must be graded according to the rules in the second-to-last paragraph of the professor's letter. That paragraph explains that students like the one mentioned should receive a class grade equal to their final exam grade, modified according to their mark from discussion group. This student received a C on her final exam, so that is the starting point for her class grade. Since she scored a minus for discussion group, that grade is adjusted down one step – so her final class grade is a D.

9. A   It is the intention of the professor to inform his assistants about the process used to calculate grades for

students in his class. Although the professor's tone in specific parts of the document may be entertaining to read, it is not the professor's purpose to entertain, persuade, or express feeling with his letter.

10. A   This is the topic sentence because it provides the theme that the remaining text will discuss and clarify. In this case, the remainder of the professor's letter details his unusual process of assigning grades. Although the sentence presented in option C is the first sentence of the overall passage, it is not the topic sentence of the professor's letter.

11. B   Options A, C, and D are incorrect because there's no reason to draw these inferences. The actual statements in these options may be true, or they might be false – but their truth is irrelevant, because there's nothing in the letter to suggest them.

Option B suggests the following: "I am aware that my grading technique is unusual. However, I have my reasons for it, and I assure you that it is here to stay – so please, no more discussion." This passage suggests that someone has complained about the grading style – possibly because it is unusual or complex – and this letter has been written to address those complaints.

12. C   The bulleted text tells the reader exactly how to accomplish a task. Specifically, it gives detailed, step-by-step instructions on how to determine a student's grade. This type of detailed, step-by-step instruction is the hallmark of technical writing.

13. D   The reader is intended to feel sorry for Cora's lonely situation – and more importantly, to feel the narrator's shame about his failure to visit (and possibly save) the old lady. Most fiction is written to entertain.

14. B   In telling his side of the story, the author explains how his failure to visit Cora came from a combination of fear and youthful thoughtlessness. He doesn't say his actions were justified, but he also doesn't say they were inexcusable. Rather, he explains his motives, inviting the reader to consider why an otherwise decent child might fail to visit an older adult lady. He also expresses his deep regrets for what happened as a result of his actions.

By presenting both his motivations and his regrets, the author invites the reader to stand in his shoes. The reader is meant to sympathize with the author, not condemn him.

15. B   Each of the three candidates' clothing and behavior is listed one after the other so that the reader can compare and contrast the impression that each candidate made on the interviewer. This is a particularly effective use of the comparison-contrast structure, because the candidates are very different. The first candidate's appropriate dress and skillful conversation stand out because of the inappropriate dress and unprofessional behavior demonstrated by the other two candidates.

Although cause and effect can be inferred by the reader, the main focus of the passage is to describe the narrator's use of comparison and contrast to describe each of the three candidates.

16. A   Option A is the summary sentence because the paragraph discusses each of the three candidates that showed up for the interview, giving them each equal weight. Options C and D are not summary sentences because they do not include information that is relevant to the paragraph as a whole. Option B may appear to be a summary sentence, because it tells the outcome of the interview. However, the paragraph does not focus on the one candidate who got the job. She is not given more attention than the candidates that did not get the job.

17. A   The author is trying to persuade the reader that George Washington was a great man who was fully deserving of his place in history. When a writer offers conclusions or summaries that are not based entirely on fact, the text is likely to be an example of persuasive writing. Even though the author's conclusion may be sound, it is still a subjective judgment. Someone else could reach a different conclusion based on different facts or by interpreting the same facts that the author used, but in a different way.

18. D   The author refers to "past leaders," "historical figures," and "legends." Therefore, it is clear that the text was written long after Washington's death. Generally, these terms are not used about one's contemporaries. Because of this, options A and B can be eliminated. So can option C, since a personal friend of Washington's could not have lived long enough to look back this far.

Also, the author makes it clear that the question of hero worship – the tendency to glorify past leaders and think of them as something more than ordinary men – is something he has wrestled with, which is another clue that the author is looking back across a span of many years.

19. B   Options A, C, and D are directly contradicted by the text.

Option B is correct because the text is concerned with the reevaluation of modern perceptions of history – in this case, the history of George Washington.

20. A   1. STARTING
         2. SARING
         3. SARIN
         4. SAIN
         5. SAIND
         6. SAND

21. C   Context shows that "quick buying and selling," in this case, of stocks, is the definition of scalp in this scenario. One could try to make a case for "to resell items at other-than-legal rates," but there is no contextual suggestion that the trader is doing anything illegal. Furthermore, context states that the trader sometimes holds stocks for "only a matter of minutes," lending further backing to the definition that includes "quick buying and selling."

22. C   Chapter 11 is about nursery rhymes. *Macbeth* is out of place because it is a Shakespearian play, not a nursery rhyme.

23. B   The following chain of logic leads to the correct answer:
         • The compass rose shows that the upper left corner of the map corresponds to the southwest.
         • The driver will appear on the Highway CV line at the spot nearest the upper left corner of the map.
         • Tracing the driver's possible routes from this spot and following the roads and trails, it is clear that the driver may visit both Dalton and Senn Parks (via the unlabeled trails) without encountering a star that indicates a roadblock. However, Arbor park is behind one of the stars.

24. D   Referring to the map legend, the reader can work out the following details:
         • The driver starts out near the bottom-right corner of the map.
         • From there, the driver can only get to one park – Arbor Park – without hitting a roadblock.
         • Arbor Park is depicted with the $ symbol, which according to the legend, indicates that it is a national park.
         • The driver does not have the necessary license to visit a national park; therefore, she cannot visit a park today, because the only park accessible from her starting point is a national park.

25. A   Southern Cleaning and Maintenance's free shipping rate on any order of $100.00 or more makes this the appropriate choice. The other vendors would charge a shipping rate of at least $30.00, which would make the total order price higher than that of Southern Cleaning and Maintenance.

26. C   The following table shows the math for each vendor.

	Number of cases × base price	Shipping and handling	Total
Janitor Depot	50 × $8.00	Free	$400.00
Hyperion Cleaning Supplies	50 × $7.00	$40.00	$390.00
Southern Cleaning and Maintenance	50 × $8.00	Free	$400.00
Maid Central	50 × $8.00	$100.00	$500.00

Hyperion Cleaning Supplies is the price leader for this order.

27. B   The writer is trying to make sure the reader understands which pieces of information are important. Options C and D are incorrect, as not all of the bolded words are nouns, and the first bolded words name a brand of cat food, which is not a command. It may be tempting to think the answer is Option A, since the first instance of bold text is the brand name of a cat food. However, later bolded text does not contain a brand name. Also, there is a different brand of cat food mentioned in the note, which is not in bold.

28. D   The section of a newspaper that contains advertisements to buy and sell is called the classified section; therefore, to place an advertisement in the newspaper to sell a car, one would need to notify that newspaper's classified section or this section.

29. D   Looking at the chart, find November. Then look at the blue bar, which represents 2007 profits for that month. Notice that this bar tops out near a horizontal line. Follow that line to the left to see the number *45*. Since the chart label explains that all numbers represent millions of dollars, 45 = $45,000,000. So, Corporation Z made about $45,000,000 in November of 2007.

30. C There are three labels on the left that correspond to the three boxes on the right that contain numbers. The abbreviations SYS and DIA are not likely to correspond to pulse rate. However, the heart symbol of the bottom label does make sense for a pulse rate label. The number to the right of that label is 80; therefore, 80 is the correct answer.

31. C Two businesses are listed under "Auto Remote Starters." These are Azarian Auto and Remote Start, LLC. Both will be able to do the job. A third business, Stereophonics, is not listed under Auto Remote Starters, but it does list Remote Starters in its display advertisement. It is important to remember that category titles are not always representative of all services a business may provide.

32. B *Rapturous* means "ecstatic" or "delighted." *On the contrary* is a clue that indicates that *rapturous* is an antonym of *displeased*. Ecstatic is also an antonym of the word *displeased*, which is used to describe the mother's response.

33. A The author's goals are to format the novel correctly and to avoid basic English errors. A manual of grammar and style is an appropriate choice, as it likely covers these topics. None of the other choices is likely to provide assistance with grammar or formatting.

34. B An index is a list of specific topics and the corresponding page numbers on which those topics can be found; therefore, to guide her toward information regarding the parts of flowers, the student should consult the textbook's index for page numbers containing that information.

35. D Chapter 3, Section B, Subsection 5, is entitled, "Checking Tax Submission Status," and will likely contain the information needed. Tables of contents rarely contain the exact words the reader expects. In this case, for example, the phrase "verify that the IRS got my taxes" does not appear in the table of contents. That is why it is important to read each section title carefully, looking for descriptions that approximately match what is sought.

36. C Chapter 4, Section D, Subsection 2 is entitled, "Empty Columns in Data Tables." Since the reader's problem is empty spaces that appear in his accounting tables, this subsection appears to be a direct match.

37. A Three of the four headings discuss how to identify specific gemstone. Based on these three examples, the reader should expect the other heading to follow this pattern. But "How to Identify Gold" fails to follow the pattern.

38. C All of the options are correct definitions of frogs, but in this case the word means "an ornamental coat fastening." The surrounding sentences tell the reader that these frogs are part of a coat and that they are used in place of buttons, which indicates that they are coat fastenings. The reader can use logic to determine that the other options are inappropriate given the context of the passage.

39. B Following is a chain of logic that leads to the answer:
- The cat owner prefers a collarless solution; therefore, several products can be eliminated. The remaining products are manufactured by Granville, Nordson, Redding, and ZenPet.
- In addition, the cat owner prefers an inexpensive solution; therefore, it is a matter of comparing the prices on the remaining products. The Granville product is the least expensive collarless solution.

40. D Chocolate Crunch is the only candy bar that doesn't list any nut products. It contains a variety of soy and dairy products, but no nuts. Chocolate Extreme contains chopped pecans. Also, cocoa butter can be problematic for people with nut allergies. Vanilla Blast contains almond extract, and cocoa butter. The Indulge Bar contains peanut butter, and cocoa butter.

41. A Option A is the only computer that meets all of the customer's criteria. Option B does not have wireless G connectivity. Option C has only a 350 gigabyte hard drive. Option D has a single-core, not a dual-core, processor. These computer terms and numbers may mean nothing to some readers, but the answer may be discovered even without any knowledge of computers. The correct answer is revealed through a process of elimination.

42. C The software developer's Web site will likely include the most comprehensive information regarding the additional software. Options A and B may provide general information about the type of software; however, the customer is seeking more detailed information. Option D is an inappropriate source, as a computer manufacturer will likely not have information regarding specific software.

MATHEMATICS
SOLUTIONS TO PRACTICE TEST 2

1. C   Multiply by the reciprocal: $\frac{4}{5} \div \frac{8}{15} = \frac{4}{5} \times \frac{15}{8} = \frac{4 \times 15}{5 \times 8} = \frac{1 \times 3}{1 \times 2} = \frac{3}{2}$.

    Written as a mixed number, the solution is $1\frac{1}{2}$.

2. D   Start with the measured length of the model car, then multiply by the ratio of 1 to 25 inches. Twenty-five inches is the numerator of the ratio, since it reflects the actual vehicle.

    $7 \text{ in} \times \frac{25 \text{ in}}{1 \text{ in}} = 175 \text{ in}$

3. C   Percent decrease = $\frac{404{,}000{,}000 - 288{,}000{,}000}{404{,}000{,}000} = \frac{116{,}000{,}000}{404{,}000{,}000} = \frac{116}{404} = 0.2871$ or about 28.7%.

4. D $\frac{1 \text{ yard}}{36 \text{ inches}} = \frac{2.5 \text{ yards}}{x}$

    $x = 36 \times 2.5$
    $x = 90 \text{ inches}$

5. A   Calipers are used to measure smaller lengths with greater precision than a ruler. At $\frac{1}{32}$ of an inch, this is more precise than a ruler with standard $\frac{1}{16}$ markings.

6. C $\frac{1 \text{ kilogram}}{2.2 \text{ pounds}} = \frac{x}{220 \text{ pounds}}$

    $x = 220 \div 2.2$
    $x = 100 \text{ kilograms}$

7. C $\frac{\text{known defective}}{\text{known inspected}} = \frac{\text{unknown defective}}{\text{total to be sent}}$

    $\frac{3}{135} = \frac{x}{900}$

    $135x = 2{,}700$

    $x = 20$

8. C   15% can be rewritten as 0.15, then $0.15 \times \square = \$18.00$. Solving for the unknown amount, $\square = \frac{\$18}{0.15} = \$120.00$.

9. A $27.95 = \$30.00$
         $150.25 = \$150.00$
         $215.16 = \$200.00$
         $195.15 = \$200.00$
         $\$30.00 + \$150.00 + \$200.00 + \$200.00 = \$580.00$

10. B
         $$\begin{array}{r} 7\ \overset{4}{\cancel{8}}\ \overset{13}{\cancel{3}}\ 5 \\ -\quad\ 7\ \ 2 \\ \hline 7{,}4\ 6\ 3 \end{array}$$

11. A   To convert a percent to a decimal, move the decimal two places to the left and remove the % symbol. Moving the decimal in 3.2% two places left and remove the % symbol gives 0.032.

12. A $\frac{11}{15} = 0.733$

13. A $1910 = 1000 + (1000 - 100) + 10$
         $1910 = \text{MCMX}$

14.   C $(x - 7)(2x + 1) = (x)(2x) + (x)(1) + (-7)(2x) + (-7)(1)$
$$= 2x^2 + x - 14x - 7$$
$$= 2x^2 - 13x - 7$$

15.   A   Since the temperature depends on the season, the temperature is the dependent variable.

16.   D   18 of the 90 students who were surveyed reported that they walk regularly.
18 out of 90 = 0.20 = 20%

17.   D   Gross pay – deductions = take-home pay
$1,460.16 – $458.64 = $1,001.52

18.   B   Previous balance + deposits – checks – returned check charge.
$853.91 + $1,910.15 – $1,339.11 – $35 = $1,389.95

19.   C   Since $\sqrt{64} = 8$ and $\sqrt{81} = 9$, $\sqrt{67}$ and $\sqrt{79}$ are both possible answers. However, 8.2 would make the answer closer to 64 than 81. Therefore, $\sqrt{67}$ is the best answer.

20.   D   First change the mixed numbers into improper fractions.

$$3\frac{3}{4} + 2\frac{5}{6} = \frac{15}{4} + \frac{17}{6}$$

Next, find the least common denominator (LCD) for 6 and 4. The LCD is 12. Therefore, each fraction needs to be changed to an equivalent fraction with a denominator of 12.

$$\frac{15}{4} + \frac{17}{6} = \frac{15 \cdot 3}{4 \cdot 3} + \frac{17 \cdot 2}{6 \cdot 2} = \frac{45}{12} + \frac{34}{12}$$

Then add the fractions together. Add the numerators, but keep the denominator unchanged.

$$\frac{45}{12} + \frac{34}{12} = \frac{79}{12} = 6\frac{7}{12}$$

Final Answer is $6\frac{7}{12}$. This answer is simplified since the numerator and denominator do not share a common factor.

21.   B $|x - 8| < 7$
$7 < x \quad 8 < 7$
$1 < x < 15$

22.   A $-\frac{15}{2}$ is equal to –7.5; –7.5 is larger than –9, which is larger than –9.1, which is larger than $-\frac{28}{3}$, which is equal to –9.3.

23.   D $10 \div 2 \cdot 5 + (3 - 8 + 2) + 2^3$ Simplify inside parenthesis from left to right.

$10 \div 2 \cdot 5 + (-5 + 2) + 2^3$

$10 \div 2 \cdot 5 + (-3) + 2^3$ Simplify exponents.

$10 \div 2 \cdot 5 + (-3) + 8$ Multiply and divide from left to right.

$5 \cdot 5 + (-3) + 8$

$25 + (-3) + 8$ Add and subtract left to right.

$22 + 8$

30 is the answer.

24.   C $79.95 + \frac{1}{2} \times $54.95 = $107.43

25.   C $2(x + 1) = 3x - 1$

$2x + 2 = 3x - 1$

$2x + 2 - 2x = 3x - 1 - 2x$

$2 = x - 1$

$3 = x$

26. D A bar graph is the most appropriate because he is graphing the frequency of the type of fish he caught (i.e., he is graphing the frequency of qualitative data).

27. A Multiply 13 and 4. This gives 52. There are three decimal places in 0.013 and there are two decimal places in 0.04. This gives a total of 5 decimal places. Count back from the end of 52 by five decimal places. This gives 0.00052.

28. B $\frac{1}{2}$ of a number is $\frac{1}{2}x$. Three more than $\frac{1}{2}x$ is $\frac{1}{2}x + 3$. This quantity equals y

29. B (Cost for notebooks + cost for pens + cost for bags + cost for flash drives) × number of nurses = total cost ($1.75 + $1.25 + $3.25 + $5.85) × 125 = $1,512.50

30. C Add listed cost of home and cost of renovations: $183,500 + $12,335 = $195,835.

SCIENCE
SOLUTIONS TO PRACTICE TEST 2

1. **B** Since the mass number represents the total number of protons and neutrons, subtract the number of protons to find the number of neutrons. The number of protons is known from the atomic number for Iridium (77) on the periodic table. So, the number of neutrons = 191 – 77 = 114. Also, a neutral atom will have the same number of electrons as protons in this case, 77.

2. **A** By looking at the difference between electronegativity values, the combination with the smallest difference is considered the least polar. While it is true that chlorine and bromine both form covalent bonds with H, H bonds with itself in the most covalent, or least polar, sense (no difference in electronegativity).

3. **D** Metals are good conductors, but nonmetals are not. Potassium is the only metal of the options listed.

4. **D** Since the general formula for saturated hydrocarbons is $C_nH_{2n}+2$, the number of hydrogen atoms must be more than twice the number of carbon atoms. The number $2n$ would be exactly twice, but single-bonded hydrocarbons, called alkanes, will always possess two more than twice the number (2n+2).

5. **A** The other options do not reflect the basic information presented in the table.

6. **B** Cells are at a higher level of organization than molecules.

7. **D** Scientific research relies on modern methods of data collection, display, and analysis. Collection often involves precise measuring tools. Display may involve three-dimensional modeling with computer software. Analysis may make use of high-powered mathematics, such as calculus. Qualitative descriptions can serve a useful function in scientific investigation, but often in a secondary fashion.

8. **B** A lysosome is required for waste processing because it contains the enzymes needed for that process.

9. **C** The protocol in option C gives enough replications on each diet to determine the accuracy and precision of the experiment and increase the statistical significance of the data.

10. **B** The digestive system consists of all the organs between the mouth and anus.

11. **B** A Punnett square is useful for predicting what offspring are possible and what proportion of the offspring will have each genotype if there is a very large number of offspring.

12. **D** A substance with a pH of 7.0 is a neutral substance $[H^+] = 10^{-7}$, $[OH^-] = 10^{-7}$.

13. **B** Heterotrophs release carbon dioxide, which is used to produce glucose in autotrophs during cellular respiration. Oxygen is a by-product of glucose production in autotrophs that is used by heterotrophs for ATP production in cellular respiration.

14. **D** The disease is carried on the gene (*a*), which occurs in all offspring in a heterozygous (*Aa*) state.

15. **C** The curve indicates that as temperature increases, the number of species decreases.

16. **C** The pancreas is a component of the endocrine system.

17. **D** Hydrogen bonds between bases allow two complementary strands of DNA to form a double helix. The other bonds do not form between the bases to form the double helix.

18. **D** The proofreading abilities of DNA polymerase are the first mechanism used by cells to prevent mutations during DNA replication. If this fails, mismatch repair can be used. Excision repair is used after exposure to mutagens.

19. **A** After passing through the stomach, food continues into the duodenum.

20. **C** Since kinetic energy is calculated by the expression $KE = \frac{1}{2}mv^2$, we can determine from the given information that $KE = \frac{1}{2}(2\text{ kg})(3\text{ m/s})^2 = 9$ Joules. The appropriate units are Joules, which match units of kg and m/s.

21.   B   A liquid with less density than that of another liquid will float on the latter liquid if these two are placed together. Liquid 3 is the densest of the three liquids shown.

22.   C   Alleles of genes form from genetic changes (mutations), which can occur in genes. These mutations modify the gene and produce a different allele.

23.   A   Spindle fibers grow from the centrosomes during mitosis to aid in chromosome separation.

24.   D   Absorption of water occurs primarily in the colon.

25.   C   Gastrulation is the stage at which individual tissue layers begin to form.

26.   D   After meiosis II, 4 haploid cells are produced. After meiosis I, diploid cells are produced.

27.   D   The liberation of OH^- ions in aqueous solutions is a property of bases. Tasting sour, dissolving in metal, and turning blue litmus paper red are properties of acids.

28.   A   During the G_1 portion of interphase, protein is produced via RNA being decoded by ribosomes.

29.   A   Since the ozone layer acts as a protective lay of the atmosphere, shielding off ultraviolet radiation from space, the breakdown of ozone is considered harmful. The chlorine ions from chlorofluorocarbons contribute to this breakdown.

30.   D   Proteins are the workhorses of organisms. When a change in a gene is able to be seen as a phenotype, it is probably due to actions of protein.

31.   B   Receiving a vaccination against a particular disease involves a process whereby a person is injected with a pathogen that causes the body to produce antibodies to protect against future infections of that same pathogen.

32.   A   The superior vena cava receives blood from the veins of the upper body. The inferior vena cava receives blood from the lower veins of the body. Options C and D receive blood from the heart itself.

33.   C   The lymphatic system consists of lymphatic nodes and vessels, the spleen, and the thoracic duct.

34.   A   DNA is formed from nucleotides, and proteins are formed from amino acids.

35.   D   The biological classification system starts broad at domain and becomes more specific as it descends to species. Because it is the most specific level, species contains the highest number of entries.

36.   A   The random movement of gases is related to the weak nature of the intermolecular forces. The greater atomic separation within gases is related to the higher temperatures required for their existence.

37.   A   The diaphragm is the muscle that pulls air into the body during inspiration.

38.   B   Hydrocarbons containing triple bonds obey the general formula C_nH_{2n-2}. Since n = 8, the number of hydrogen atoms would be 14, called octyne. Note that the prefix *oct-* found in *octyne* refers to the number 8, and *–yne* refers to triple bonds.

39.   A   The size of the flask limited the population increase to 940 insects. Growth would have continued exponentially, independent of population density, had the size of the environment not been a factor.

40.   C   Inhibitors, such as alcohol and poisons, have structures that allow for matching with certain molecular substrates, reducing any potential activity.

41.   D   Since the combustion of propane is given as an example of an oxidation-reduction reaction within the explanation, writing the reaction for methane follows suit. Then, balancing the atoms is a matter of inspection.

42.   D   Water's dominant bonding type (covalent) involves the sharing of valence electrons between hydrogen and oxygen atoms. The H_2O molecule's structure is seen to have a 2:1 ratio between the hydrogen and oxygen.

43. A Translation is the process by which the message is relayed from RNA to ribosomes to create proteins. Transcription is the process where the message from DNA is transferred to RNA. Mitosis involves the splitting of nuclei into two daughter nuclei. A double helix forms due to the complementary bases of DNA forming hydrogen bonds.

44. C Urine is stored in the bladder. Although urine is produced in the kidneys and passes through the ureter, it is stored in the bladder for release during urination. It is not stored in the prostate.

45. A Bias in an experiment can be minimized by the use of a control. Control groups allow unexpected influences to be removed from the scientific argument.

46. B Applying the equation, kinetic energy = $\frac{1}{2}$ mv^2 (m = mass; v = velocity); doubling the velocity of an object increases the kinetic energy of the object by a factor of four.

47. A Formulating a hypothesis involves predicting what may happen in the study.

48. B The liver produces bile necessary for the breakdown of fat. Options A, C, and D are not responsible for this function.

COMPREHENSIVE PRACTICE TESTS

ENGLISH AND LANGUAGE USAGE
SOLUTIONS TO PRACTICE TEST 2

1. **C**   Option C is an example of correctly punctuated direct dialogue. A quote is preceded by a comma after an introductory clause. Also, in this case, the word *since* should be capitalized. And the question mark should be contained within the quotation marks.

2. **B**   Option B is a simple sentence containing one subject, one conjugated verb, and no clauses. Options A and C are sentence fragments. Option D is not a simple sentence, as it contains a dependent clause.

3. **A**   The pronoun *its* correctly refers back to its antecedent *PTA*. Although consisting of several members, the PTA is one group; therefore, it is a singular antecedent. Options B and C are incorrect pronouns with regard to number, and option D is only used as the contraction for *it is*.

4. **B**   Option B is an example of active voice, which can enhance clarity in writing. The passive voice construction exists in all other options.

5. **C**   Option C is an example of a correctly punctuated sentence in which the dependent clause is offset from the main clause by a comma. Option A is considered a run-on sentence. Option B contains a sentence fragment. A semicolon is not necessary in option D, as the two clauses are not both independent.

6. **A**   Names of languages, professional titles of people, and full names of holidays are always capitalized. Because option C is not an example of the exact name of a class, there is no need to capitalize the word *history*.

7. **B**   Using the context of the sentence, one can draw the conclusion that the word *credulous* is an adjective that means "easily cheated or fooled." There are not contextual cues in the sentence to support options A, C, or D.

8. **D**   The word *governor* should be capitalized, as it refers to the title of a specific person. It is not necessary to capitalize the words *state*, *eastern*, or *summer* given the context of the sentence.

9. **C**   Option C correctly conjugates the subject *committee* with the verb *votes*. Options A, B, and D are examples of incorrect subject-verb agreement in which singular subjects are conjugated with plural verbs.

10. **D**   The first blank in the sentence requires the possessive pronoun *its*, which should not be used with an apostrophe. When used with an apostrophe, the word *it's* is always the contraction for *it is*. Therefore, *it's* is the word required for the second blank in the sentence.

11. **A**   Option A agrees in number with its antecedent, *choir*. Option B is a plural pronoun that cannot be used with the singular antecedent. Options C and D are examples of possessive pronouns that are incorrect given the context of the sentence.

12. **D**   Option D is properly punctuated with a semicolon between two independent clauses. The conjunction *however* is also correctly followed by a comma. Options A, B, and C are examples of incorrectly punctuated sentences.

13. **D**   Option D contains an example of the correct use of an apostrophe: Boss's Day. The apostrophe in option A is unnecessary because in this case, the *s* is being used only to indicate that the subject is plural. Option B contains the contraction for *it is*, as opposed to the corrective possessive *its*. Option C contains the contraction for *they are*, as opposed to the correct possessive *their*.

14. **D**   The prefix *rhino-* originates from the Greek language. It means "of or pertaining to the nose." Therefore, it can be concluded that this client is interested in surgery of his nose.

15. **A**   Option A is an example of third-person voice. Options B and C are examples of second-person voice, option B being implied. Option D is an example of first-person voice.

16. **C**   Prefixes should always be hyphenated when they appear before proper nouns. It is inappropriate to hyphenate between the two vowels in option A, as the vowels are different; however, a hyphen is required between the vowels in option B, as they are the same. A hyphen should always be used after the prefix *ex-*.

336   **TEAS® STUDY MANUAL**

17. A   The plural form of *datum* is *data*. The plural form of *crisis* is *crises*. The plural form of *moose* is *moose*. And the plural form of *diagnosis* is *diagnoses*.

18. B   Option B is an example of the use of grammar to enhance clarity and readability. The four sentences are combined into one clear, succinct sentence that is easy to read and understand. Options A, C, and D, while employing correct grammar to condense the four sentences, do not do so in a manner that clearly expresses the writer's intent.

19. D   Given the context of the sentence, the conclusion can be drawn that the definition of the word *abscond* is "depart unnoticed" or "escape." There is not context to support options A, B, or C.

20. C   Option C is an example of a grammatically correct sentence in which the objective pronoun *whom* is appropriately used. Options A, B, and D are examples of incorrect usages of this same pronoun.

21. C   A word showing family relationship should be capitalized when used with the person's name; however, not when preceded by a possessive adjective. Options A, B, and D are examples of incorrect capitalization with regard to this same rule.

22. B   The word *badly* serves as an adverb in the sentence, because it modifies the word *ached*. It is not used as an adjective, verb, or pronoun.

23. C   *Salary* is the correct spelling of the word that completes the sentence.

24. B   Option B is an example of a complex sentence that contains one dependent and one independent clause. Options A, C, and D are examples of simple sentences.

25. D   The singular verb *walks* is correctly paired with its singular subject, *lady*. Options A, B, and C are examples of incorrect subject-verb agreement with regard to number.

26. A   Option A completes the above sentence as a simple sentence. Option B is an example of a compound sentence. Options C and D are examples of complex sentences.

27. C   *Confident* is the correct spelling of the word that completes the sentence.

28. B   Option B clearly and succinctly conveys the writer's intent to describe that the couple found the kittens when the kittens were 6 weeks old. The plural pronoun *they* refers back to the plural antecedent *kittens*. Options A, C, and D are written in ways in which the writer's intent might be confused.

29. A   Two singular subjects connected by the word *or* require a singular verb. Options B, C, and D are all examples of incorrect subject-verb agreement.

30. B   Option B is the correctly spelled completion of the sentence above. Options A, C, and D are misspelled.

absolute value	distance between a number and zero on the number line
acid	any compound with a hydrogen ion activity greater than water (pH < 7)
acidic solutions	solutions that have a pH scale value less than 7
activation energy	energy necessary for a chemical reaction to occur
active verb	verb that shows an action performed by the subject of the sentence
active voice	state of a sentence that contains an active verb
adaptation	increase from generation to generation of alleles of genes that allows a species to survive in their environment
addition principle	rule that makes it possible to move terms from one side of an equation to the other by adding opposites to each expression
adenosine triphosphate (ATP)	cellular fuel; produced in the mitochondria
adjective	descriptive word that modifies nouns or pronouns
adverb	word modifying a verb, adjective, or other adverb indicating when, how, where, why, or how much
alkane	hydrocarbon with only single bonds (C_nH_{2n+2})
alkene	hydrocarbon with one double bond (C_nH_{2n})
alkyne	hydrocarbon with one triple bond (C_nH_{2n-2})
alleles	two or more different forms of a certain gene
alveoli	structure in the lungs that permits the exchange of oxygen and carbon dioxide to occur
amino acid	building blocks of proteins
anatomical position	a standard position in which the body is facing forward, the feet are parallel to each other, and the arms are at the sides with the palms facing forward
anatomy	study of the structure of various organs and body systems
anion	atom or molecule with a negative charge
antecedent	noun that a pronoun refers back to (replaces)
anterior	toward the front of the body or body structure (opposite of posterior)
antibody	protein produced by a B cell in response to an antigen
antigen	a foreign protein, such as a pathogen, that stimulates antibody production.
apostrophe	punctuation mark (') used to indicate possessiveness or the omission of letters or numbers
Arabic numerals	written numbers that use a combination of the whole numbers 0, 1, 2, 3, 4, 5, 6, 7, 8, and 9
arteries	blood vessels that transport blood away from the heart to the capillaries
article	word that is used to limit a noun, either indefinite – *a, an* – or definite – *the*
atom	smallest part of an element that still retains all the original properties of the element
atomic mass	number of protons and neutrons within the nucleus of an atom; the average mass of all of the known isotopes of an element
atomic number	number of protons in the nucleus of the chemical element; the number of protons that defines a specific atom
attributive tag	part of a sentence that indicates who said a direct quote
audience	person or persons who will be reading a piece of writing
author's intent	underlying reason why the author wrote the text

autonomic nervous system	branch of the peripheral nervous system that controls automatic body functions like heartbeat and digestion
autotroph	organism that is able to produce its own food
axon	part of the nerve cell that carries impulses away from the cell body and connects one neuron with another neuron over a synapse
B cell	type of lymphocyte that produces antibodies in response to antigens; responsible for humoral immunity
bar graph	graph used to compare the frequency of an event; frequencies are displayed as vertical or horizontal, nontouching bars; data is usually noncontinuous
base	any compound with a hydrogen ion activity less than water (pH > 7)
basic solutions	solutions that have a pH scale value greater than 7
biases	opinions or beliefs that affect a person's ability to make fair, unclouded judgments or decisions
binomial	polynomial that has two terms
binomial nomenclature	two-word naming system that includes the universally accepted genus and species of each organism; developed by Carolus Linnaeus
bronchial tubes	small respiratory passages that connect the trachea to the lungs
calories	*see* Joules
capillaries	tiny blood vessels that transport blood between arteries and veins within the body
catalyst	substance that controls the rate of a chemical reaction
cation	atom or molecule with a positive charge
cause-effect text structure	first presents an action, and then describes the effects that result (or may result) from that action
cell	basic unit of all life
cell wall	outside, rigid layer that helps separate the inside and outside of both prokaryotic and plant cells
cellular respiration	process in which glucose is used to produce adenosine triphosphate
Celsius	metric temperature scale defined (at standard pressure) by the melting point of ice (0° C) and the boiling point (100° C) of liquid water
central nervous system	branch of the nervous system that includes the brain and spinal cord
centrosome	microtubule organizing center that helps to form and organize the mitotic spindle during mitosis
charge	positive or negative distribution within an object
Charles Darwin	evolutionary biologist who studied wild life on the Galapagos Islands in the 1800s and wrote *On the Origin of Species*, in which he explained adaptation and natural selection
chemical bonding	chemical attraction of atoms due to their electron arrangement
chemical reaction	dynamic event that alters the chemical makeup of a molecule; a process that chemically transforms a set of substances into another set
chemotaxis	release of chemicals by damaged cells that attract white blood cells
chlorophyll	green pigment in plants
chloroplast	organelle that contains chlorophyll and is found in plants; used to carry out photosynthesis
chromatid	one of a pair of newly duplicated chromosomes that are still attached to one another; a pair of matching "sister" chromatids make up the duplicated chromosome
chromosomes	condensed, single, very long strands of DNA double helix located in the nucleus of a cell and containing hundreds of genes
chyme	mixture of food, chemicals, and enzymes in the stomach

cilia	tiny hairs in the bronchial tubes that keep the airway clear by removing unwanted matter from the lungs
circle graph	divided into sectors representing the frequency of an event; sectors total 100%
circulatory system	transportation highway for the entire body (also known as the cardiovascular system)
clause	group of words that are related and contain both a subject and a properly conjugated verb
codon	group of three nucleotides on RNA or DNA that encodes for a single, specific amino acid
coefficient	numerical part of a term
colon	punctuation mark (:) used to indicate that there is information to follow
comma	punctuation mark (,) used to indicate a break or pause within a sentence
comparison-contrast text structure	presents two different cases, usually with the intent of making the reader consider the differences (or similarities) between the two cases
compass-rose	symbol that indicates the cardinal directions (north, south, east, and west) as they relate to the map
complex sentence	sentence that contains an independent clause and a dependent clause
compound sentence	two (or more) independent clauses joined together with a coordinating conjunction
connective tissue	connects different structures of the body; includes bones, cartilage, adipose tissues (fats), and blood vessels
constant	quantity that does not change; it's what students refer to as "numbers" such as 8, –3, ½, ¼, 0.45, etc.
context	text surrounding a word, phrase, or passage
context clues	words surrounding an unfamiliar word that can help a reader discern the meaning of the unfamiliar word
coordinating conjunctions	words that join two or more words, phrases, or clauses so that each conjoined element is equal; in English, there are only seven, and they may be remembered using the acronym FANBOYS (*for, and, nor, but, or, yet,* and *so*)
covalent	sharing of electrons between atoms
cristae	series of folds formed by the inner membrane of a mitochondrion
critical reading	reading style where the reader carefully analyzes the text, judging its credibility and the author's intentions, rather than simply accepting the material as fact
crude birth rate	number of childbirths per 1,000 people per year
crude death rate	number of deaths per 1,000 people per year
crystalline order	atoms arranged in a highly ordered state
cumulative sentence	contains an independent clause followed by a parallel string of modifiers; modifiers may be adjectives, prepositional phrases, or dependent clauses
cytokines	chemical messengers that are released by damaged tissues
cytokinesis	division and separation of the cytoplasm from one cell into two new cells; is accomplished by pinching off of the cell membrane to form two cells while simultaneously synthesizing an additional membrane to help in the process; begins in late anaphase and completes in telophase
cytoplasm	rich protein fluid with gel-like consistency that houses organelles
deductions	items that are subtracted from a beginning salary (i.e., state taxes, federal taxes, health insurance, and retirement contributions).
deductive reasoning	method whereby conclusions follow from a general principle
deep	away from or below the body surface (opposite of superficial)
degree	exponent or sum of exponents of the variable(s) of a term
dendrites	branched extensions of the neuron that receive impulses (electric messages) from other neurons and stimuli

denominator	b in the fraction $\frac{a}{b}$
density	ratio of mass per volume for a substance
dependent clause	group of words containing a subject with a properly conjugated verb that is made dependent or incomplete because of the addition of a subordinating conjunction
dependent variable	depends on another variable
description	passage of text that describes or characterizes a person, thing, or idea
diapedesis	process of white blood cells squeezing through the capillary slits in response to cytokines
diaphragm	dome-shaped muscle located immediately below the lungs that stimulates inhalation and exhalation by contracting and relaxing
diatomic molecule	molecule consisting of two atoms
digestion	mechanical and chemical breakdown of foods
digestive system	manufactures enzymes that break down food so that nutrients can be easily passed into the blood for use through the body; consists of all the organs from the mouth to the anus involved in the ingestion, breakdown, and processing of food
diploid cell	containing two sets of chromosomes
direct dialogue (or direct discourse)	writing that reflects someone's exact words, often with an attributive tag, using quotation marks
direct object	noun or pronoun that receives the action of the verb and answers the question *whom* or *what*
distal	away from the origin of the body part or point of attachment (opposite of proximal)
distance scale	information in the legend that tells the reader how to interpret distances on the map
distributive property	property that removes parentheses in an expression, such as $a(x + y) = ax + ay$
dividend	quantity to be divided
divisor	quantity by which another quantity is divided
DNA (deoxyribonucleic acid)	a molecule that exists as a double-stranded helix made from sugars, phosphates, and nitrogenous bases
dorsal body cavity	contains the cranial cavity and spinal column
duodenum	first section of the small intestine
effectors	glands and muscles that are innervated and extend away from the spinal cord
electrolysis	use of electric current to drive the breakdown of a molecule
electromagnetic waves	waves of radiation that are characterized by electric and magnetic fields; waves are members of a spectrum, a continuum of wavelengths ranging from very short (trillionth of a meter) to very long (kilometers) that are divided into bands of wavelengths, ordered from short to long in the order of gamma rays, x-rays, ultraviolet, visible, infrared, microwave, and radio waves; visible part of the spectrum can be further subdivided by color bands from short to long in the order of violet, indigo, blue, green, yellow, orange, and red
electronegativity	ability of an atom to attract electrons to itself
electrons	negatively charged subatomic particles found in various orbits around the nucleus
element	substance that cannot be decomposed by ordinary chemical means; each chemical element is characterized by the number of protons in the nucleus (e.g., all atoms of hydrogen have 1 proton, and atoms of oxygen have 8 protons)
ellipsis	punctuation mark (…) used to indicate a pause or omission of material
embryo	early development of an animal or a plant after fertilization
emigration	act of an individual moving out of one region or country to live in another
endocrine system	controls body functions; glands in this system secrete hormones that travel through the blood to organs throughout the body to regulate processes such as growth and metabolism

endoplasmic reticulum (ER)	tubular transport network with the cell that appears as a stack of flattened membranous sacs
enzyme	protein catalyst; chemical that changes the rate of a chemical reaction in living tissue without itself being chemically altered; a chemical that breaks down proteins, carbohydrates, and fats into nutrients that can be absorbed through the wall of the intestine into the bloodstream
epithelial tissue	provides covering (such as skin tissue) or produces secretions (such as glandular tissue); commonly exists in sheets and does not have its own blood supply
equation	mathematical sentence in which two expressions are set equal to each other
estimate	approximate value
etymology	history of a given word; a word's origin
eukarya	organism that contains cellular organelles; organism that has cells that contain nuclei (protists, plants, fungi and animals)
excision repair	mechanism that inspects the DNA for damage and attempts to repair it
expiration	act of exhaling carbon dioxide from the body
exponent	number written as a superscript that is used to denote the number of times a number should be multiplied by itself
expository writing	introduces a topic or provides background information for later remarks
expression	one or more terms consisting of any combination of constants and/or variables
fact	information based on real, provable events or situations
fertility rate	average number of children a woman will have during her childbearing years (from the ages of 15 to 44)
first-person point of view	perspective in which the narrator is the one speaking, evidenced by the use of the first-person pronoun *I* or *we*
flagella	long, whip-like structure used for cellular movement in certain prokaryotic cells
FOIL	acronym that represents the order in which two binomials can be multiplied; stands for *first, outer, inner, last*
frontal section	cut made along a longitudinal plane that divides the body into front and back regions; coronal section
gametes	cells of reproduction
ganglia	collection of nerve cell bodies
gendered language	specifies male or female gender using words such as *he* or *she*; neuter gender words like *it* do not specify male or female gender, but are rare in English
gene	portion of DNA on a chromosome that provides information for an organism's characteristics; genetic blueprint for the formation of proteins that make up the machinery of the cell
genome	complete set of DNA for an individual; contains all genes
genotype	organism's underlying genetic makeup or code
germ cells	reproductive cells that give rise to sperm and ovum
globular protein	protein that is roughly spherical in shape
Golgi apparatus	structure involved in packaging and transporting proteins in the cell
greatest common factor	greatest number that will divide evenly into two or more numbers
haploid cell	one set of chromosomes
headings	titles that preface a section of text; advertise the subject of the text below, making it easier to skim or search for a particular topic; give the text structure
heart	organ that rhythmically contracts and pumps blood throughout the body
heat	flow of energy due to a difference in temperature

heat of vaporization	amount of heat necessary to cause a phase transition between a liquid and a gas
heterotroph	organism that cannot produce its own food
heterozygous	having received different alleles for a particular trait from each parent
histogram	graph used to compare the frequency of an event; frequencies are displayed as vertical, touching bars, and data is usually continuous
historical context	time and place in which a text was written; style and content of a text are part of its historical context
homeostasis	a stable state in which all the needs of a body are met and all of the organ systems are working properly together
homologous	similar in size and function
homozygous	having received the same allele for a particular trait from both parents
hydrocarbon	compound whose structure is entirely composed of hydrogen and carbon atoms
hyphen	punctuation mark (–) used to connect parts of a word or to join separate words together
hypothesis	possible explanation formulated to answer questions that are being investigated; involves making predictions that follow from the initial statement of a problem.
immigration	act of an individual moving into a region or country to live
immune system	tissues, cells, and organs that work together to fight off illness and disease
improper fraction	fraction whose numerator is greater than its denominator
incomplete dominance	dominant and recessive genotypes interact to produce an intermediate phenotype
independent clause	clause that has a complete meaning
independent variable	does not depend on another variable; affects the dependent variable
index	listing of important names, ideas, and topics from the publication, along with page numbers (or links to those items); traditionally appears at the end of the publication
indirect dialogue (or indirect discourse)	writing that reflects the idea of someone else's words but does not quote them directly
inductive reasoning	arriving at general principles from specific facts
inequality	mathematical sentence in which one expression may not be equal to another expression
inference	logical conclusion or next step; inferred conclusion not actually written in the text, but deduced by the reader, based on information that is in the text
inferior	toward the lower end of the body or body structure (opposite of superior)
inspiration	act of breathing in oxygenated air
integumentary system	protects internal tissues from injury, waterproofs the body, and helps regulate body temperature; serves as a barrier to pathogens; consists of the skin, mucous membranes, hair, and nails
interferon	protein that inhibits the reproduction of a virus
intermediate	between the medial and lateral aspects of the body or body structure
interphase	process that occurs prior to mitosis; occurs when the cell must duplicate its DNA, increase the amount of organelles and cytoplasm, and synthesize protein in preparation for cell division; three stages of interphase are Gap 1 (G1), Synthesis (S), and Gap 2 (G2)
ion	positively or negatively charged atom
ionic	electrical attraction between ions of opposite charges
irrational number	any real number that cannot be written as a fraction
isotope	atoms with the same number of protons but differing numbers of neutrons
Joule	a common metric unit of energy (1 calorie = 4.2 Joules)
Kelvin	metric temperature scale defined by an absolute zero reference point (0 Kelvin = – 273° C, the temperature at which molecular motion ceases)

kinetic energy	the energy of motion
latent heat	heat per mass needed for a phase change at a constant temperature
lateral	toward the outer sides of the body or body structure (opposite of medial)
Law of Conservation of Energy	if a system is closed, the total amount of energy in the system does not change; however, energy can be changed from one form to another
least common denominator (LCD)	smallest common multiple of the denominators; the LCD of two fractions is the least number that both denominators divide into evenly
legend	small portion of a map devoted to explaining the symbols and notations used in the main portion of the map
leukocytes	white blood cells
Lewis structure	symbolic representation of covalent bonding between atoms
light-year	distance that light will travel within 1 year
like terms	terms that have the same variable and the same exponent associated with that variable
line graph	shows change over time; compares the relationship between two or more quantities
logical conclusion	well-reasoned idea that stems from the information in the text, not from the reader's personal ideas or biases
loose sentence	*see* cumulative sentence
lungs	paired organs that take in oxygen and exhale carbon dioxide
lymphatic system	supports the immune system by housing and transporting white blood cells to and from lymph nodes; returns fluid that has leaked from the cardiovascular system back into the blood vessels; consists of the lymph nodes, the lymph vessels that carry lymph, the spleen, the thymus, and the tonsils
lyse	Latin word for *break*; used in biology and chemistry to mean rupture or destruction of the cell membrane, a cell structure, or a molecule
lysosome	organelle containing digestive enzymes capable of disposing of cellular debris and worn cellular parts
main idea	specific message of a writing
mass	quantity of matter within an object
mass number	total number of protons and neutrons found within the nucleus of an atom matter anything that takes up space and has mass
medial	toward the middle of the body or body structure (opposite of lateral)
meiosis	process by which gametes reduce their DNA content
metabolic pathways	chemical reactions within a cell
metabolism	chemical reactions in living organisms used to maintain life
metalloids	elements that may accept or donate electrons readily; possess a mixture of metallic and nonmetallic properties
metals	elements that readily donate electrons and are good conductors of electricity; donate highly conductive electrons to their environment
metaphase plate	disc extending across the nuclear area on which the chromosomes are found at metaphase just prior to separation of the chromosomes during mitosis
microtubules	cellular tracks that form the mitotic spindle during mitosis
microvilli	microscopic projections of tissues that make up the villi
midsagittal section	sagittal section made down the median of the body
mismatch repair	mechanism that scans over the DNA to find any mismatches of nitrogenous bases
mitochondrion	powerhouse of the cell
mitosis	process of cell duplication in which two daughter cells receive exactly the same nuclear material as the original cell

mixed number	number that represents the sum of a whole number and a proper fraction
molecule	group of chemically bonded atoms that possesses characteristics independent of the atoms themselves
monomial	polynomial that has only one term
multiplication principle	rule that states that the equality of an equation does not change if both sides of an equation are multiplied by the same nonzero number
muscle tissue	dedicated to producing movement; three types include skeletal, cardiac, and smooth
muscular system	consists of skeletal muscles, tendons that connect muscles to bones, and ligaments that attach bones together to form joints
mutagen	substance that induces mutations
mutation	permanent change in DNA sequence
narrative writing	relates a chain of events or tells a story
natural selection	process in which individuals of a species carrying certain mutations are better able to survive and reproduce in their natural environment than others members of the species (survival of the fittest)
nervous system	serves as the body's control system; consists of the brain, spinal cord, and nerves
nervous tissue	structure for the brain, spinal cord, and nerves; made up of neurons that send electrical impulses throughout the body
neurons	specialized cells that make up the nervous system and transmit electrical impulses
neutron	neutral subatomic particle found in the nucleus of an atom
nitrogenous base	molecule found in DNA and RNA that encodes the genetic information in cells
nominalization	changing a verb, adverb, or adjective to a noun
nonrestrictive clause	group of words that contains a subject and a properly conjugated verb but does not contain information that is necessary to interpreting the meaning of the sentence
nonrestrictive phrase	group of words that does not contain both a subject and a verb and does not contain information that is necessary to interpreting the meaning of the sentence
noun	a word for a person, place, or thing
nucleic acid	chain of nucleotides
nucleoid	condensed DNA of a cell
nucleolus	small body within the nucleus that functions to produce ribosomes that are then moved to the cytoplasm to make cell proteins
nucleotide	molecule that consists of a pentose, a phosphate group, and a nitrogenous base
nucleus	central region of an atom; large organelle that is the control center of the entire cell
numerator	a in the fraction
object of the preposition	noun, pronoun, phrase, or clause to which the preposition refers
opinion	belief based on personal judgment, rather than on indisputable facts
orbital shell	arrangement of electrons within a specific region around the nucleus
ordered pair	denotes the x-coordinate (position of a point along the horizontal axis) and y-coordinate (position of the point along the vertical axis) on a graph, written (x, y)
organ	two or more tissue types that work together to perform a specific function
organ system	group of organs in an organism working together to perform a specific function
organelle	tiny organ
organic chemistry	study of the structure and properties of carbon compounds
organism	living body made up of several organ systems
oxidation	electron donation by a chemical group that leaves that group with one less electron and a more positive charge

paragraph	group of sentences that forms a cohesive whole due to a similar topic or theme
parasympathetic nerve	branch of the autonomic nervous system that is active when a person is eating or at rest
parentheses	punctuation marks ( ) used to indicate interjectory, explanatory, or qualifying material; parentheses always come in pairs
passive verb	comprised of *be* plus a past participle that shifts the action of a sentence from the subject to the object
passive voice	state of a sentence that contains a passive verb
pathogen	any disease-causing agent
pentose	type of sugar
percent	ratio whose denominator is 100; per 100
perforin	pore-forming protein
periodic sentence	independent clause is delayed until the end of the sentence and is often preceded by parallel strings of modifiers
peripheral nervous system	branch of the nervous system that extends outside of the central nervous system and consists of the cranial and spinal nerves
peristalsis	rhythmic contractions of the stomach and intestines that propel food toward the colon and anus
peroxisome	organelle used to rid the body of toxic components
persuasive writing	writing intended to change the reader's mind or form the reader's opinions on a particular topic
pH	measure of hydrogen ion concentration within a solution; the scale used to measure the strength of acidic solutions; pH = –log (hydrogen ion concentration)
pH indicator	chemical detector of hydrogen ions to visually determine acidity (color change)
phagocytosis	engulfing of pathogens by white blood cells
phase transition	alteration of the physical state of a substance between a solid, liquid, and gas
phenotype	physical expression of genetic traits
phosphate group	molecule in the backbone of DNA and RNA that links adjoining bases together
photosynthesis	process carried out by green plants, green algae, and certain bacteria, in which the energy from sunlight is trapped by chlorophyll and used for synthesis of glucose
phrase	group of words that are related but do not contain a verb and a subject together
physical bonding	physical connection between atoms (or molecules) that does not alter the chemical nature of the atoms (or molecules)
physiology	study of the function of the various organs and body systems
pie chart	*see* circle graph
plasmids	small circular portions of DNA not associated with the nucleoid
point of view	perspective from which an author writes
polar molecule	possesses both positive and negative regions
polynomial	term or combination of terms
possessive pronoun	used to indicate ownership
posterior	toward the back of the body or body structure (opposite of anterior)
potential energy	stored energy
prefix	group of letters added to the beginning of a word that modifies or extends the word's meaning

preposition	words such as *by, at, to,* and *from* that give additional information, usually in relationship to something else
primary source	firsthand record of events, theories, opinions, or actions; either published or unpublished documents, recordings, or artifacts that are contemporary to the events, people, or information that is at issue
problem-solution text structure	presents a problem or question, and then responds with a solution or answer
products	substances formed as the result of chemical reactions
prokaryote	single-celled organism lacking defined cellular organelles or a nucleus
pronoun	word that replaces a noun
proper fraction	fraction whose numerator is less than its denominator
proportion	two ratios that are set equal to each other
protein	compound composed of a large number of amino acids joined in a particular type of chemical bond called a peptide bond
proton	positively charged subatomic particle found in the nucleus of an atom
proximal	close to the origin of the body part or point of attachment (opposite of distal)
Punnett square	graphical way to show all possible combinations of alleles given the two parents' genotypes
purine	nitrogenous base with two rings (adenine and guanine)
purpose of a passage	main reason or intent for writing a particular piece
pyloric sphincter	muscle that separates the stomach from the duodenum and slowly releases chyme from the stomach into the small intestine (duodenum)
pyrimidine	nitrogenous base with one ring (thymine, cytosine, uracil)
quantitative	relating to numbers
quotation marks	punctuation marks (" ") used to indicate the exact phrasing of material or to show dialogue; always come in pairs
quotient	c in the equation $= c$
rate of change	speed at which something changes
ratio	relationship between two quantities
rational number	any real number that can be written as a fraction
reactants	substances consumed or altered in a chemical reaction
real number	any number on the number line
reciprocal	the multiplicative inverse of a number; the reciprocal of $^a/_b$ is $^b/_a$
reduction	electron acceptance by a chemical that produces a more negative charge on the group
reflex	automatic response to a stimulus that occurs when neurons transmit a message to the spinal cord, which in turn sends a message back to the muscles to react before the message is transmitted to the brain
reproductive system	main purpose is to produce offspring; houses hormones that encourage or suppress activities within the body (e.g., libido and aggression) and influences the development of masculine or feminine body characteristics; consists of the testes and penis or the ovaries, vagina, and breasts
respiratory system	organ system that provides for air exchange by supplying tissues with oxygenated blood and removing carbon dioxide
ribosome	organelle responsible for synthesizing protein within the cell from amino acids
RNA (ribonucleic acid)	single-stranded molecule made from sugars, phosphates, and nitrogenous bases; required for the transfer and translation of the DNA code within a cell
Roman numerals	written numbers that use a combination of M, D, C, L, X, V, and I
root word	a word in its simplest form before any affixes are attached

sagittal section	cut made along a longitudinal plane that divides the body into right and left parts
salt	neutral product of an anion and a cation
saturated hydrocarbon	chemical structure composed entirely of single bonds
scale	any standard instrument of measurement that has marking at established intervals
second-person point of view	perspective in which the writer directly addresses the reader using the pronoun *you*
secretion	process of moving proteins outside of the cell
semicolon	punctuation mark (;) used to indicate division between equal elements in a sentence
sensory neurons	neurons that carry messages from sense organs to the brain and spinal cord
sensory-somatic nervous system	part of the peripheral nervous system that consists of 12 pairs of cranial nerves, 31 pairs of spinal nerves, and associated ganglia; controls voluntary actions of the body
sequence	ordered list of thoughts or ideas
simple sentence	contains only one independent clause and no dependent clauses
simplified fraction	has no common factors between the numerator and the denominator except for the number 1 (a reduced fraction)
skeletal system	supports and protects the body and its organs; supplies a framework that, when used in conjunction with the muscles, creates movement; serves as storage for minerals, such as calcium and phosphorus; consists of bones, cartilage, ligaments, and joints
specific heat	energy required to raise one unit of mass in a substance by $1°$ C
stem cells	can divide and remain undifferentiated; gives rise to a variety of more-specialized cells
stereotypes	oversimplified opinions about an entire group of people or things that do not account for individual differences
stimulus	change in the environment that triggers a physical response
subheadings	headings that appear below other headings; appear in a smaller typeface than headings, so that they may easily be distinguished; single heading may have many subheadings, and these subheadings may have their own subheadings
subject	noun or pronoun that performs the action of the verb in a sentence; if a sentence contains a verb of being or a linking verb such as *be, feel, become,* or *look,* the subject of the sentence is the noun or pronoun being described
subordinating conjunction	word that joins two or more clauses and makes the clause that contains it dependent on another clause, and therefore of slightly less importance; there are many subordinating conjunctions, but some common ones are *because, though, although, while, if,* and *as if*
substrate	molecule acted upon by an enzyme
suffix	group of letters added to the end of a word that modifies or extends the word's meaning
summary sentence	recaps the essential point(s) of a paragraph, or of a larger work, such as an essay; gives the reader the take-away message for the paragraph, or for the larger work
superficial	toward or at the body surface (opposite of deep)
superior	toward the upper end of the body or body structure (opposite of inferior)
support	examples and details that explain the topic of a paragraph; follows the topic sentence
supporting details	details that explain the main idea
sympathetic nerve	branch of the autonomic nervous system that is activated when a person is excited or scared
synapse	fluid-filled gap that connects the axon of one nerve cell with the cell body of another
T cell	lymphocyte that is responsible for cellular immunity
table of contents	listing of a publication's chapters, sections, or other organizational units; includes page numbers (Web documents may have links to the various sections)
take-home pay	money received after deductions are subtracted from the beginning salary

taxonomy	classification of organisms into universally accepted taxons; names reflect the organism's evolutionary heritage
technical writing	writing that passes along specific information or knowledge in a formal or standardized way
term	constant, variable, or product of a constant and variable
text features	formatting that serves a consistent purpose in a document; add meaning to the text that they modify, change the text's meaning, or add structure and clarity to the document
text structure	way of organizing text to better present thoughts or ideas; includes sequence, problem-solution, comparison-contrast, description, and cause-effect
themes	subjects that a written work frequently touches upon
third-person point of view	perspective in which the narrator is distanced from the story and tells it as an outsider; third-person pronouns such as *he, she,* or *they*
tissue	collection of cells in an organism that have a similar function and structure
topic	general subject matter covered by a writing
topic sentence	generally at or near the beginning of a paragraph; gives the topic or point of the paragraph and often explains that topic in relation to the overall theme of the writing
trachea	airway that connects the larynx to the bronchial tubes; also known as the windpipe
transcription	process of cells copying the instruction from the DNA into the RNA
transition	smooth movement from one idea to the next, from one sentence to the next, or from one paragraph to the next; transition words may include *additionally, finally, similarly, next, however,* and *furthermore*
translation	process of protein reduction from messenger RNA
transverse section	cut made along a horizontal plane that divides the body into upper and lower regions; cross section
triple-point	temperature and pressure at which a substance will coexist as a solid, liquid, and gas
unsaturated hydrocarbons	a chemical molecule containing at least one double or triple bond
urinary system	helps maintain the water and electrolyte balance within the body; regulates the acid-base balance of the blood; removes all nitrogen-containing wastes from the body
vaccine	inactivated form of a pathogen that stimulates the body to produce antibodies for future protection
vacuole	basic storage unit of a cell that can hold various compounds
valence electrons	electrons in the outermost shell of an atom
variable	unknown quantity in an expression or equation
veins	blood vessels that transport unoxygenated blood from the capillaries back to the heart
ventral body cavity	contains all the structures within the chest and abdomen; the diaphragm divides the ventral cavity into the thoracic cavity (superior to the diaphragm); below the diaphragm are the abdominal and pelvic cavities
verb	word that shows an action or state of being
verbal	word that is sometimes used as a verb but is currently being used as another part of speech
vesicles	small membrane-bound sacs within the cytoplasm used to transport proteins or other substances in and out of a cell
villi	finger-like projections in the mucosa of the small intestine lining; produce a pleated appearance; each villus is supplied with blood and has lymphatic vessels for absorption
whole numbers	nonzero, positive integer (0, 1, 2, 3, 4, 5, 6, etc.)
word structure	way in which the parts of a word are arranged together
work	result of any change in energy
zygote	mass of cells formed after an egg is fertilized and begins dividing